Craniofacial identification in forensic medicine

Edited by

JOHN G CLEMENT BDS PhD (Lond) LDS RCS (Eng) DipForOdont (LHMC)

Associate Professor in Oral Anatomy and Forensic Odontology,
University of Melbourne; Consultant in Charge of Forensic Odontology,
Victorian Institute of Forensic Medicine; Honorary Associate Professor (Clinical),
Department of Forensic Medicine, Monash University;
President of the Australian Society of Forensic Dentistry;
past President of the British Association for Forensic Odontology

DAVID L RANSON BMedSci BM BS (Notts) LLB FRCPath FRCPA DMJ

Deputy Director, Victorian Institute of Forensic Medicine (VIFM);
Head of Forensic Pathology Division, VIFM; Honorary Associate Professor (Clinical),
Department of Forensic Medicine, Monash University; Senior Associate,
School of Dental Science, University of Melbourne; Associate,
Department of Pathology, University of Melbourne; Associate, Faculty of Law,
Monash University, Australia

ARNOLD

A member of the Hodder Headline Group
LONDON • SYDNEY • AUCKLAND
Co-published in the USA by Oxford University Press, Inc., New York

First published in Great Britain 1998 by
Arnold, a member of the Hodder Headline Group,
338 Euston Road, London NW1 3BH

Co-published in the United States of America by
Oxford University Press, Inc.,
198 Madison Avenue, New York, NY 10016
Oxford is a registered trademark of Oxford University Press

Whilst the advice and information in this book is believed to be true and
accurate at the date of going to press, neither the author[s] nor the publisher
can accept any legal responsibility or liability for any errors or omissions
that may be made. In particular (but without limiting the generality of the
preceding disclaimer) every effort has been made to check drug dosages;
however it is still possible that errors have been missed. Furthermore,
dosage schedules are constantly being revised and new side-effects
recognized. For these reasons the reader is strongly urged to consult the
drug companies' printed instructions before administering any of the drugs
recommended in the book

British Library Cataloguing in Publication Data
A catalogue record for this book is available from the British Library

Library of Congress Cataloging-in-Publication Data
A catalog record for this book is available from the Library of Congress

ISBN 0 340 60759 9

Publisher: Georgina Bentliff
Project Editor: Catherine Barnes
Production Editor: Julie Delf
Production Controller: Sarah Kett

Typeset in Times and Optima by J&L Composition Ltd, Filey, North Yorkshire
Printed and bound in Italy by G. Canale & Co, Turin

Contents

Contributors   v
Foreword   vii
Preface   ix
Acknowledgements   xi

PART 1   Principles

1. **Craniofacial identification**   *JG Clement, DL Ranson*   3
2. **Management of the scene and forensic evidence**   *MA Raymond, WJ Ashley*   9
3. **The autopsy in human identification**   *DL Ranson*   25
4. **Craniofacial anatomy**   *CA Briggs, M Martakis*   37
5. **Anthropological assessment**   *CA Briggs*   49
6. **Dental identification**   *JG Clement*   63

PART 2   Techniques

7. **Preservation, restoration and duplication of remains** *PJG Craig, JL Leditschke, RG Taylor*   85
8. **Craniofacial dissection** *DL Ranson*   95
9. **Scene photography** *K Byrne*   105
10. **Photography of remains** *A Henham*   123
11. **Craniofacial photography in the living** *T Dobrostanski, CD Owen*   137
12. **Superimposition techniques** *JA Taylor, KA Brown*   151
13. **Quantification of facial shape and form** *CDL Thomas*   165
14. **Facial reconstruction and approximation** *RG Taylor, C Angel*   177
15. **Computer modelling of facial form** *A Linney, AM Coombes*   187

PART 3   The changing face

16. **Growth of children's faces** *SA Feik, JE Glover*   203
17. **Age changes to the face in adulthood** *R Neave*   225

PART 4   Medico-legal issues

18. Forensic 'art' in human identification *W Haglund*   235
19. Reporting and presentation of evidence *DL Ranson*   245
20. Identification and the law *I Freckelton*   257

Appendixes

Appendix I   **Recovery of remains** *CA Briggs, WB Wood*   267
Appendix II   **Packaging of evidence** *MA Raymond, WJ Ashley*   273
Appendix III **Commonly used dental charts** *DH Clark, E Dykes*   275
Appendix IV   **Chronology of dental development** *E Dykes, DH Clark*   279
Appendix V   **Laboratory materials** *JL Leditschke, RG Taylor, CJ Scane*   283
Appendix VI   **Guides for post mortem cranial radiography** *JG Clement*   287
Appendix VII **Guides and checklists for medico-legal reports** *DL Ranson*   291

Glossary   297

Index   299

Contributors

Christopher Angel MB BS BDSc MDSc (Melb) FRACDS FFOP (RCPA)

Sessional Oral Pathologist, School of Dental Science, University of Melbourne; Assistant Forensic Odontologist to the Victorian Institute of Forensic Medicine, Australia

Wayne J Ashley BA MAComm

Senior Sergeant, Crime Scene Investigation, Victoria Police; Victorian Forensic Science Centre, Melbourne, Australia

Christopher A Briggs MS PhD (Oregon) DipPhysEd (Exe)

Associate Professor in Anatomy, University of Melbourne; Honorary Senior Lecturer, Department of Forensic Medicine, Monash University; Forensic Osteologist to the Victorian Institute of Forensic Medicine, Australia

Kenneth A Brown BDS (Adel) FICD

Director of Forensic Odontology Unit, University of Adelaide; Formerly Senior Lecturer in Forensic Odontology, University of Adelaide; Founding President, Australian Society of Forensic Dentistry; Past President of the International Organisation for Forensic Odontostomatology, Australia

Karen Byrne BAppSci (Photog) (Hons) (RMIT) RN

Forensic Photographer to the Victorian Institute of Forensic Medicine, Australia

Derek H Clark CStJ BDS PhD (Lond) LDS RCS DFO SRN

Scientific Director, Kenyon International Emergency Services, London, UK; Visiting Lecturer in Disaster Victim Identification, Universities of Hertfordshire and Coventry, UK; WHO Adviser to the Commission on Identification in former Yugoslavia; Past President, British Association of Forensic Odontology; Formerly Course Organiser of Diploma in Forensic Odontology, London Hospital Medical College, UK

John G Clement BDS PhD (Lond) LDS RCS (Eng) DipForOdont (LHMC)

Associate Professor in Oral Anatomy and Forensic Odontology, University of Melbourne; Consultant in Charge of Forensic Odontology, Victorian Institute of Forensic Medicine; Honorary Associate Professor (Clinical), Department of Forensic Medicine, Monash University; President of the Australian Society of Forensic Dentistry; Past President of the British Association for Forensic Odontology

Anne M Coombes BSc PhD CPhys MInstP

Linney & Coombes, Forensic Consultants

Pamela Craig BDSc MDSc DipFOd (Melb)

Lecturer in Radiology, School of Dental Science, University of Melbourne; Consultant to the Transport Accident Commission, Victoria, Melbourne; Assistant Forensic Odontologist to the Victorian Institute of Forensic Medicine, Australia

Tadeusz Dobrostanski

Photographer in Charge, Clinical Photography and Audio-Visual Section, School of Dental Science, University of Melbourne, Australia

Eric Dykes BSc PhD DipFOd MIEM

Director, Civil Emergency Management Centre and President, Institute of Emergency Management, University of Hertfordshire, UK

Sophie A Feik MDS
Senior Lecturer in Growth Studies, School of Dental Science, University of Melbourne, Australia

Ian Freckelton BA (Hons) LLB (Syd)
Barrister at Law; President, Australian and New Zealand Association of Psychiatry, Psychology and Law; Honorary Associate Professor, Department of Forensic Medicine, Monash University; Fellow, Criminology Department, University of Melbourne; Honorary Senior Lecturer, Faculty of Law, Monash University; Owen Dixon Chambers, Melbourne, Australia

John E Glover RFD BEd ARMIT GradDipEd SCVH FIR MRSH MNZIMRT MACE
Radiographer, Senior Lecturer in Medical Radiation Science, Royal Melbourne Institute of Technology, Australia

William Haglund PhD
Senior Forensic Consultant, United Nations International Crimes Tribunal, Rwanda; 20410 25th Avenue, NW Shoreline, Washington 98177, USA

Amanda Henham BAppSc (Photog) RN
Formerly Forensic Photographer to the Victorian Institute of Forensic Medicine, Australia

Jodie L Leditschke PhD (Monash)
Chief Scientist and Manager of Mortuary Services, Victorian Institute of Forensic Medicine; Honorary Lecturer, Department of Forensic Medicine, Monash University, Australia

Alfred D Linney BSc PhD ARCS DIC MIPEMB
Head of Medical Graphic and Imaging, Department of Medical Physics and Bioengineering, University College, London, UK

Mark Martakis MB BS
Medical Practitioner; Lecturer in Department of Anatomy, University of Melbourne, Australia

Richard Neave FMAA AIMI
Artist in Medicine and Life Sciences, Faculty of Medicine, Dentistry and Nursing, University of Manchester, UK

Christopher D Owen BAppSci (Photog) (RMIT)
Clinical Photographer, School of Dental Science, University of Melbourne; Professional Member of AIMBI, Australia

David Ranson BMedSci BM BS (Notts) LLB FRCPath FRCPA DMJ
Deputy Director, Victorian Institute of Forensic Medicine (VIFM); Head of Forensic Pathology Division, VIFM; Honorary Associate Professor (Clinical), Department of Forensic Medicine, Monash University; Senior Associate, School of Dental Science, University of Melbourne; Associate, Department of Pathology, University of Melbourne; Associate, Faculty of Law, Monash University, Australia

MA Raymond BSc(Hons) MSc PhD
Director, Forensic Services Group, Sydney, NSW, Australia

Christopher J Scane BAppSc(MLS) (RMIT)
Resources Manager, School of Dental Science, University of Melbourne, Australia

Jane A Taylor BDS (Adel) BScDent (Hons) (Adel) MScDent (Adel)
Lecturer in Forensic Odontology, University of Adelaide, Australia

Ronn Taylor FAISDT
Advanced Dental Technician; Tutor Technician, School of Dental Science, University of Melbourne; Forensic Sculptor to the Victorian Institute of Forensic Medicine, Australia

C David L Thomas HNC (AppPhys) GradDipDigCompEng (RMIT) MEng (IT) MIEEE
Professional Officer, School of Dental Science, University of Melbourne, Australia

Walter B Wood MB BS BSc
Forensic Anthropologist; Senior Lecturer, Department of Anatomical Sciences, University of Queensland, Australia

Foreword

The lot of the forensic pathologist is sometimes a difficult one, but it is always fascinating. I am repeatedly asked why I embraced forensic pathology; the answer is easy, and it is the same answer that many people give in relation to their jobs. It is the fascination of problem-solving – problems of a particular kind, to be sure, and as many as one wants to discover in every case. But one takes absolute priority, and that is the problem of identity. The question usually takes one of two forms:

1. What can we learn from the remains we have that will narrow the range of its possible identities? With investigation and effort, using many of the tools set out in this book, and often a bit of luck, this question may transform into:
2. Are these the remains of X, a particular named person?

Until there is a positive answer to the second question, the riddles surrounding the death will remain unanswered. Even more fundamentally, as Victoria's first State Coroner, Hal Hallenstein, observed, it is a hallmark of our civilization that we regard it as an affront, an indignity, an abrogation of our responsibilities, that a person could live amongst us, die and be buried without a name.

In one of my early cases as a forensic pathologist in the UK, skeletal remains of a young woman were found in the woods of a ducal estate in Oxfordshire. The only clothing present was a stocking tied around the cervical spine. One of the contributors to this book, Richard Neave, was responsible for creating the face that complemented the skull, a contribution that assisted in the identification of the deceased, who turned out to be a backpacker from Scandinavia. The identification led to the discovery of a whole pattern of the most serious criminality by an offender who targeted single, foreign, female backpackers.

My remarks thus far are biased from my own background. This book goes much further than pathology and also maps out the terrain of craniofacial identification in the living. Is this adult in fact X who went missing as a young adolescent? The study of the facial changes associated with ageing has recent origins and is well set out here.

One of the stunning features of this book is the range of disciplines represented amongst its contributors and the seniority and experience of that representation. It is not surprising, but it is to the great credit of the editors, that they have been able to summon the top people to the task. In so doing, they have rendered a substantial and enduring service to the science of human identification.

Stephen M Cordner MA MB BS BMedSc DipCrim
DMJ MRCPath FRCPA
Professor of Forensic Medicine, Monash University;
Director, Victorian Institute of Forensic Medicine,
Australia

Preface

Each year in Victoria, 6000 people are reported missing. This is in a State of only four million people. Despite investigation by a variety of agencies, approximately 1% of these missing persons continue to be unaccounted for in the long term. At the same time, significant numbers of decomposed human remains or skeletons are brought to the attention of the coroner, who has a duty to identify them. In countries with larger or more mobile populations, the problems are correspondingly more difficult.

The cultural background of modern-day Australia results in a high level of sensitivity regarding the disturbance of the remains of indigenous peoples. This same concern finds expression in many other countries that have experienced a high level of immigration in recent years. The investigation of human remains in such a setting can assume a political or social dimension far removed from ordinary scientific aspects of death investigation.

Concealment of the victims of homicide, or the disfigurement of their remains to thwart identification, is relatively uncommon. However, once a body has been discovered, the identification of the victim is an essential prerequisite to the conduct of any police investigation. In such a situation, the scientific challenge may be enormous, yet at the same time the tasks of the investigator must be conducted in a way that satisfy the needs of the courts and justice system.

This book attempts to bring together information on methods of human craniofacial identification and to describe the ways in which such methods may be integrated with other techniques for establishing identity. We anticipate that all those involved with forensic science, law enforcement and the justice system will find the material in this book of use. The specialist areas covered here will be of particular benefit to forensic pathologists, forensic odontologists and forensic anthropologists.

Part 1 deals with the scientific principles that underpin all approaches to craniofacial identification. The chapters emphasize the need for the strategic management of the scene or recovery of remains in order that the material recovered has maximum evidential value. Chapter 3 deals with the place of the autopsy and the role of the pathologist as co-ordinator of the activities of the other specialist investigators whose roles are covered in greater detail in Chapters 4, 5 and 6.

In Part 2, we examine the techniques used in craniofacial identification, with emphasis on specific methodologies. Chapters 11, 13 and 15 deal with issues that pertain also to identification of the living. These have ramifications for the analysis of surveillance video systems in criminal investigation and in the control of access to secure areas.

An understanding of the facial changes that accompany ageing is an essential prerequisite for finding and identifying the long-term teenage runaway or identifying the elderly person who may be a disoriented Alzheimer's sufferer. These issues are dealt with in Part 3, which describes the changing face.

The medico-legal context is central to many of the issues surrounding human identification, and these are covered in Part 4. Chapter 18 examines the reliability of commonly used facial approximation techniques, contrasting their usefulness as an aid to investigation with their evidential value in court. The other chapters in this section deal with the practical issues of giving evidence in court and the law relating to proof of identity.

The editors would particularly like to thank Professor C A Briggs for his help and advice, in addition to his own important written contributions.

J G Clement
D L Ranson
1998

Acknowledgements

Professor C A Briggs deserves a special mention in relation to this book. His advice and input have been tremendous. In addition to his own major contributions to this book, he stepped in and provided specialist anthropological and anatomical support on many occasions; for this, the authors are particularly grateful.

Thanks also go to: Aboriginal Affairs Victoria; Sherie Blackwell – Technical Officer, School of Dental Science; Patricia Bordbar – Dental Practitioner, for contributions and advice in regard to Chapter 1; Robyn Chau (make-up artist); Nathan Cochrane – Dental Student, School of Dental Science, University of Melbourne (model for illustrations); Kate Fletcher – Administration Assistant, School of Dental Science; Jacqueline Harris (model for illustrations); Trish Hartshorn – Administration Assistant, School of Dental Science; Jane Holden – Physicist and Engineer; SC Howard Hopper, Victorian Forensic Science Centre – Crime Scene Photography Unit and Victoria Police; Anne Humphreys (model for illustrations); Dr Hans Keur – Head of Radiology, Royal Dental Hospital of Melbourne; Sui Wei Kong Dental Student, School of Dental Science, University of Melbourne (model for illustrations); Christina Olsson-Jacques – Physicist, Australian Reference Laboratories; Alan Owen – Engineer, Royal Dental Hospital of Melbourne; Larissa Pogrebnyak (model for illustrations); Carmen Roberts – Victorian Institute of Forensic Medicine; Rob Sutherland – Radiographer, Royal Dental Hospital of Melbourne; Tiffany Tam – Dental Student, School of Dental Science, University of Melbourne (model for illustrations); Dr Walter Woods – Senior Lecturer, Department of Anatomy, University of Queensland.

PART 1

Principles

CHAPTER 1

Craniofacial identification

JG CLEMENT, DL RANSON

Importance of the living face for identification	3	Identification of the living	6
Visual identification of the corpse	4	Future developments	7
Mortuary and laboratory investigation of remains to		Legal context	7
establish identity	6	Conclusion	7

Importance of the living face for identification

Humans are highly social animals with an associated compunction to communicate. They have large brains, an innate inquisitiveness, a conscious awareness of self and a remarkable capacity to learn, reason and remember. In contrast with many other mammals, humans have poorly developed nasal structures and at best only a mediocre sense of smell. Perhaps as a compensation for their short noses and poor olfactory sense, humans have flattened faces over which a single embryonic sheet of mesoderm has become highly developed into a very sophisticated array of muscles of facial expression, which are inserted directly into the deep layers of the overlying skin. As a result, the range and subtlety of human facial expression far surpasses that found in any other genus or species. Humans need to be able to exchange complex thoughts and emotions in order to survive and flourish in co-operative groups and, given its unique structure, the human face operates as one of the principal conduits for communication between individuals.

The ability to distinguish friend from foe is also a particularly important skill for humans to develop. The killing of members of competitive groups of one's own kind is likely to have been prevalent since prehistory. In this setting, the ability to identify friends or individuals who pose no threat is essential.

Similarly, at birth and for a considerable time thereafter, humans are entirely dependent upon the support of their parents or other older members in their group in order to survive. The ability to recognize those who will be supportive and who will nurture them must therefore be an important survival skill in the youngest of infants. At the outset, these skills may not be subtle, but neither are the needs of such children. Quite how the very young come to recognize their adult supporters is still the subject of conjecture and research. However, since an infant will often be lying in different positions with respect to his or her care providers, the ability to recognize a particular face must be independent of the orientation of the person's features.

The recognition of a face is dependent upon two skills: first, the ability to store or encode the information gleaned from observation in memory; second, the ability to recall the stored information, which equates to recognition. As with most cognitive tasks, the ability to recognize faces increases markedly between birth and 10 years of age. It is likely that young children use different methods for encoding and recalling a face. Infants are thought not to be able to distinguish between scrambled and unscrambled faces or even notice the absence of certain features until they are 14–16 months old. It is therefore reasonable to infer that infants are similarly unlikely to discriminate between individuals on the basis of differences that are heavily dependent upon the internal configuration of the face. However, this poses a conundrum. How is the child, from a very young age, able to recognize his or her mother so clearly from within a group of women? In this context, it is also important to consider identification clues such as smell, sound and touch as well as direct visual information. In the adult world, similar parallels exist, in which gait, posture, clothing and voice all provide important ancillary clues for the determination of race, gender and individuality in addition to any features seen directly in the head and the face.

Perhaps the development of the ability to recognize faces in an adult way progresses akin to a child's speech development. To begin with, children may refer to all men as 'Daddy' and all four-legged animals as only a cat or a dog. Later, further development leads to a more accurate observation of the intrinsic characteristics of the animals concerned so that the child is able accurately to assign the correct name in each case. A similar trend is evident for the encoding and recognition of faces through childhood to the adult state, where reliance upon internal encoding comes to predominate over specific feature recognition. This is illustrated when someone shaves off a beard or moustache. Their friends are aware that a change has occurred, but they are quite uncertain of its exact nature. These recognition factors are extremely important both for assessing witness identification during police investigations and in evaluating evidence of identity that is presented in court. In all these areas, it is important to understand how faces are seen and recognized if people of different ages are to be questioned in a meaningful and valid way for the purpose of recalling a person who is being described from memory.

Studies to find those facial features that are more important for recognition have often been fraught with confounding contextual problems. Pose, orientation of features, expression and the nature of the encounter between observer and observed all exert an effect. Jones's (1979) survey asked subjects 'What facial features draw your glance and grab your attention?' The results were 'eyes' 62%, 'hair' 22%, 'mouth' 8% and 'other' 8%. Despite the obvious shortcoming that people do not always say what they mean or try to rationalize something that is really an unconscious act, this study provided answers that were closely similar to the results of other studies (Ellis *et al.*, 1980). Shepherd *et al.* (1978) asked subjects to describe a face that they had just seen and listed the following features in order of frequency of use: hair, eyes, nose, eyebrows, face shape, chin, lips, mouth, ears, face lines, complexion, forehead and cheeks.

Rhodes (1988) did not recognize the emphasis of the earlier studies on upper facial features and proposed a hierarchical system that attempted to describe

the manner in which faces are recalled. The first-order features, for example 'eyes', 'eyebrows' and 'mouth', can be characterized independently of other features. Second-order features, such as spatial relationships between first-order features and information concerning face shape, are essentially configurational. Third-order features, for example, age, weight, race and sex, complete the descriptors.

It may be erroneous to assume that all adults see people in the same way. In view of the enormous amount of information, both static and dynamic, available to an observer of a living face, compounded by the underlying psychological, emotional and cultural standpoint of the observer, it is likely that we all perceive people in different ways. Indeed, from our own experience, we are all aware that we can perceive the personal characteristics of a particular person in different ways at different times. A lover may have a different impression of the size of their partner's nose when they are together from the impression they have of it after they have 'split up', the impression in this situation depending particularly on the emotional state they are in when they make the observation!

People are better at recognizing individuals from within their own racial group. This may arise because the extensive pre-existing knowledge of one's own range of ethnic facial prototype allows due consideration of finer points of difference to be recognized. Inter-ethnic recognition performance is initially poorer, and this may reflect a temporary return to the recognition techniques of childhood in which external overall features such as 'hairstyle' temporarily assume a greater importance than does internal feature recognition, for example 'eye shape'.

Salient feature prominence is also different within particular ethnic groups (Laughery et al., 1988; O'Toole et al., 1994). Amongst Caucasians, 'hair type', 'eye shape', 'face shape' and 'skin texture' were the most salient features. For black Africans, the most important criteria were 'skin colour/texture', 'face shape', 'thickness of lips' and 'breadth of the nose'. Such differences in perception have obvious forensic connotations.

Visual identification of the corpse

In many parts of the world, the formal and legal identification of the dead by next-of-kin or others takes place in a coronial context. This is an inquisitorial system of great antiquity and, within the appropriate legislative framework, can exert considerable influence for improvements in society. These may range from important health and safety recommendations for the home and the workplace through to investigations of deaths in custody or cases of arson and fatal fires. Whatever the scope of the investigation, the vast majority are initiated by the death of a person.

With most of these deaths, the identity of the deceased is already known by virtue of the surrounding circumstances of the death. Legal confirmation of identity in these cases is simply a matter of observing the legal formalities rather than applying specialist medical procedures. In such cases, the pathologist investigating the death for the coroner duly sets about determining the medical cause, time and circumstances of death. For a minority of cases (in the Western world typically 0.1% of all coronial/medical examiner cases), the identity of the deceased initially remains in doubt, and this uncertainty needs to be removed. This is not a mere bureaucratic 'loose end' but gives cognisance of the fundamental human right to have an identity both in life and after death.

In many ways, the manner in which a society deals with its dead may reflect its attitude to the sanctity of life and the rights of the individual. During this century, there have been numerous notorious regimes that have terrorized, and even attempted to eradicate by institutionalized murder, sections of their own community. A strong, independent and outspoken coroner (or the equivalent) is an essential safeguard to such excesses. In a more pragmatic context, the identification of the dead is essential for the life of others to proceed and return to normal. The practical need for the expedient inheritance of property is a good example because, if the identity of the deceased should be problematic or prove to be insuperable, many others can suffer real hardship as a consequence.

One of the most emotionally difficult tasks that anyone may have to perform, in a formal legal setting, is that of identifying a body as that of someone whom they once knew. The person asked to undertake these duties is often a close relative, friend or workmate as these are the people who knew the deceased best in life.

No matter what the circumstances of the death, the identification of someone who was a friend or a relative is almost invariably a very stressful ordeal for the witness. Inevitably, some mistakes will be made, rarely some frauds will be perpetrated and, in some cases, bodies will be unrecognized and remain visually unidentifiable unless expert assistance is made available.

In the best of circumstances, the body that has to be identified will be fresh, intact, clean and unmutilated. A body arising from a recent drowning or drug overdose may be a good example. Even in the clean, bright, non-threatening environment such as is found in a modern mortuary, and with the support of an enlightened and sensitive staff, the family of the deceased might still find it difficult to identify the body. There are a variety of reasons why this may be so. The most obvious (and overstated) is 'denial' on the part of the next-of-kin, who just cannot accept that it is a member of their family who has died. However, a dead body may bear much less similarity to the person in life than might be first anticipated. The pallor of death, the unkempt hair or an unrecognizable hairstyle, the lack of expression, make-up or dentures, all make identification more difficult. In life, there is a rich but subtle exchange of signals by means of expressions or gestures between people, which mutually reinforce recognition. These exchanges are obviously entirely lacking, and that too is very disconcerting for someone who may previously never have seen a dead body.

In more difficult cases, bodies may have significant injuries and be disfigured. They may remain bloodstained from the events in which they were killed or may be so damaged that the general configuration of the body is lost. At some stage, a decision has to be made on the degree of psychological stress and trauma that may have to be inflicted on witnesses in order to achieve a 'visual identification'. The decision to proceed with a visual identification has to be balanced against the likelihood of a reliable outcome and the trauma inflicted upon the family.

Some cases are completely unrecognizable by any conventional criteria. Decomposition processes involving bloating of the body, blackening of the skin and loss of tissues such as eyes, skin, hair and nails interfere markedly with the likelihood of successful visual identification. The victim of a fatal fire often has no clothing, documents, jewellery, skin, hair or eye colour and may appear as an almost skeletonized body but with some internal organs intact and some of the extremities of the body burned away. It is useless to expect the family to attempt to identify such a body that has been so badly destroyed. Sometimes the family insist on viewing the body. Their reasons for wishing to do so are often their own, but advice from bereavement counsellors generally suggests that it is better for the family to view the body in a setting where they have been warned what to expect. In some cases, viewing the remains, no matter how disfigured or incomplete is essential before grieving and healing can commence. The role of the identification expert is obviously paramount in such cases. After the trauma of the first few days surrounding the death or the discovery of the body have subsided, all those concerned with investigating the death and supporting the next-of-kin have to be entirely confident about the certainty of the identity of the deceased.

Where foul play is suspected, it is essential to establish the identity of the deceased using the strictest possible criteria. Murder is one of the most serious offences and, in some jurisdictions, to be found guilty may lead to the death penalty. Unequivocal identification of the victim is of almost paramount importance in such cases, and identity may have to be linked to levels of certainty that amount to proof 'beyond reasonable doubt' rather than only 'on the balance of probability'.

In order for the maximum amount of information pertaining to identity to be gleaned from a scene, it is very important that a rigorously methodological approach be adopted for the investigation. The security of the scene, the order in which it is processed and the choice of persons requested to attend and assist all have a potentially vital influence on the success or failure of the investigation. It is important that any investigating authorities think before they act or else the important evidential value of certain features in a scene may go unrecognized. It is equally important to establish, as close as possible to the outset of any multidisciplinary investigation, exactly what needs to be discovered or corroborated, perhaps at the expense of other evidence of lesser importance. A conference between coroner, police, pathologist, anthropologist and odontologist at the beginning of the investigation can be enormously beneficial to its efficient progress later on. It serves many purposes other than the mere pooling of expertise, the most important of which may be the sense of a tangible commitment to a team approach in which all feel valued and motivated as well as better informed.

A body may have lain undiscovered for many years, yet as soon as it is found there is often an almost frenzied haste to recover the remains and begin or rekindle an investigation. This enthusiasm is understandable. However, enthusiasm is no substitute for method, and sometimes when an investigation is undertaken in too hasty a fashion or in the absence of expert advice, much important information is never fully recovered and in some cases physical evidence will be lost. Chapters 2 and 5 emphasize a more considered 'archaeological' approach to the recovery and assessment of remains. Experience has shown that the small amount of additional time expended at the scene necessary for its fullest investigation is repaid over and over again during the course of the investigation.

Mortuary and laboratory investigation of remains to establish identity

'A sound knowledge of human anatomy is never superfluous'. This statement is never more valid than in the context of a forensic autopsy. The expert, be they an anthropologist, pathologist or odontologist, have to be the master of the anatomy relevant to their particular disciplines. When completely unidentified skeletal remains are studied, it is frequently the case that animal bones or teeth are included with any human counterparts. These non-human remains have to be identified so that they can be excluded from the investigation process. Similarly, obtaining information on race, gender and age from the skull is often possible, but not in the absence of a great deal of experience on the part of the investigator. It takes a long time to accumulate enough experience to appreciate the range of human variability and to use that knowledge in the carefully considered manner that will convince a jury. Chapters 3, 4, 5 and 6 describe the principles underpinning the forensic autopsy and the anatomical basis of the anthropological and odontological assessment of the craniofacial complex. All of these principles find usage in the establishment of identity by the comparative process of craniofacial superimposition, in which images of the skull of an unknown person are compared with corresponding photographs or radiographs of a known person in life. This fastidious technique and its limitations are described in Chapter 12.

Autopsy procedures need to be varied according to the state of the body, the presumed manner of the person's death and an appreciation that, in a particular case, establishing identity is an issue. On occasions, following the establishment of identity, the pathologist wishes to retain the remains until the case is brought to court. This may conflict with the wishes of the family to bury or cremate the remains of their next-of-kin as soon as possible. Modern dental materials now make the construction of very accurate replicas of skeletal remains (including osseous injuries) entirely feasible. These valuable *aides-mémoire* for the pathologist allow early reconciliation of the conflicting need to retain evidence and the family's need to observe the appropriate funeral rites and to grieve. A description of these and other reconstruction techniques is found in Chapter 7.

Identification of the living

Fortunately, not all those who need to be identified have to be viewed as corpses. One of the greatest social problems of the late twentieth century is the huge and rapidly increasing number of adolescents who leave their families to become 'street kids'. A less well known problem is that of teenage (or younger) 'throwaways', whose families have not only rejected them but also ejected them from their home. The stark reality is that there are no grades to homelessness, irrespective of how it has arisen. The rigours of life without housing or adequate income often lead the victim into petty crime, health problems and substance abuse. The hopelessness of the homeless is reflected in high levels of licit and illicit drug abuse in teenage runaways. Drug addiction in turn amplifies the problems of low income and leads to further crime in order to support expensive habits.

For those charged with locating 'runaways' or 'throwaways', it is important to understand just how dramatically facial features can be altered by a combination of the normal processes of maturation and with the adverse effects of 'living rough'. Chapters 11 and 16 provide a basis for understanding the normal changes that are experienced by children as they progress to maturity and suggests methods by which some of the physical changes to the head and face can be recorded to chronicle change.

In parallel with the problems of lost or missing teenagers, it is also predicted that there will soon be an substantial rise in the number of older people affected by some form of dementia. Many of these people can appear deceptively purposeful, yet they may have no idea where they are or what they are doing. Other people in these age groups require medication at regular intervals, without which they may quickly become severely unwell. If they are already disoriented in time and place, this compounds the problem. The ability for searchers to predict how an adult person's appearance may have altered with time will become increasingly important in the search to locate them. Chapter 17 describes a classical artistic view of ageing of adults, but most people do not possess such insights or talents. There is therefore an urgent need to develop automated or semi-automated systems that can be operated by people with a modest degree of training that are able to predict how faces may change over time. This problem applies equally to both the young and to old missing persons, but the solutions to predict the changes to the face wrought by age in each case are likely to be somewhat different.

Future developments

Despite the fact that most portrait pictures used to identify missing persons will be displayed in a two-dimensional format for years to come, it can be appreciated that they represent only a single viewpoint of what is in reality a changing three-dimensional object, in this case the head. Despite the limitations of two-dimensional images, it is likely that only the really valid facial ageing systems will, in effect, create a virtual or physical three-dimensional model in the background from which appro-

priate two-dimensional views can be extracted after manipulation of the model. Again, the classical approach to creating a three-dimensional model of a face has been to use a combination of anatomical knowledge and sculpting techniques. An account of this approach is given in Chapter 14. This technique suffers from the same drawbacks as artistic portraiture. It requires a high level of skill and a great deal of knowledge. The success of forensic art, both portraiture and sculpting, is discussed in the context of a massive homicide investigation in Chapter 18. The results are not encouraging.

The explosion in information technology and the availability of formidable quantities of computer power at modest cost has suddenly offered an alternative way in which to construct and manipulate models of heads and faces. Chapter 13 considers the essential prerequisite of this process, which is the quantification of facial shape and form. Implicit in this work is the concept that some form of image of the craniofacial complex needs to be captured and recorded, either prior to or simultaneously with the determination of its shape and form. This approach is further extended in Chapter 15, where the computer modelling of facial form is discussed. Predictions on the future development and use of this technology are fraught with danger, but it seems likely that these developments will have application in security systems and for the identification of criminals whose images have been captured on security video.

Legal context

This last example serves as an important reminder not to lose sight of the legal context in which the pathologist, anthropologist, odontologist, engineer and scientist with a role in human identification have to work. The best research and the most thorough investigation may founder in court if insufficient consideration is given to the reporting and presentation of findings. An appreciation of their true evidential potential has to be developed, and the relationship between 'Identity' and the law has to be fully understood. These medico-legal issues are complex, but they are the essential framework in which the forensic investigator has elected to work. Chapters 19 and 20 deal with these issues.

Conclusion

Despite all our scientific endeavours, understanding how we recognize a face remains largely elusive. Computer-aided three-dimensional reconstruction of the head is becoming increasingly sophisticated, and we are able to record and reproduce more and more detail of facial form. Yet the value of this increased precision and rendering of fine detail is obscure. Traditionally, the courts have been reluctant to embrace new technologies that are outside the ordinary experiences of the 'man in the street'. Indeed, the recognition of an individual by an eyewitness is an exception to the rule prohibiting ordinary witnesses of fact from giving opinion evidence. In reality, all such statements of identification are matters of personal opinion, yet courts accept that, in matters of human identification from direct facial recognition, we are all experts.

While facial recognition-based identification of individuals by eyewitnesses can be mistaken, people can, most of the time, identify each other from only a very limited set of data. Traditional party games such as 'blind man's bluff' have long exploited this skill. Coarse, low-resolution, high-contrast images of famous historical figures are instantly recognizable, yet it is hard to explain how we have been able to identify them. There is a strange irony to all this. While we struggle to obtain more and more detail and accuracy in the scientific rendering of the human face, it is still not clear whether the increased information we can provide leads to any improvement in the accuracy of facial recognition. In the end we still have to balance science, art and human experience in order to make the best use of the techniques currently available for human identification.

References and further reading

Bass WM, Birkby WH. 1978: Exhumation: the method could make the difference. *FBI Law Enforcement Bulletin* **47**, 6–11.

Cannon J. 1985: Head posture – an historical review of the literature. *Australian Orthodontic Journal* **9**(2), 234–7.

Christie DFM, Ellis HD. 1981: Photofit constructions versus verbal descriptions of faces. *Journal of Applied Psychology* **66**(3), 358–63.

Davies G. 1983: The recognition of persons from drawings and photographs. *Human Learning* **2**, 237–49.

Davies G. 1986: Capturing likeness in eyewitness composites: the police artist and his rivals. *Medicine, Science and the Law* **26**(4), 283–90.

Davies G, Little M. 1990: Drawing on memory: exploring the expertise of a police artist. *Medicine, Science and the Law* **30**(4), 345–53.

Davies G, Shepherd JW, Ellis HD. 1978: Remembering faces: acknowledging our limitations. *Journal of the Forensic Science Society* **18**(1–2), 19–24.

Davies G, Ellis HD. Shepherd JW (eds) 1981: *Perceiving and remembering faces*. London: Academic Press.

De Haan E, Newcombe F. 1991: What makes faces familiar? *New Scientist* 9 Feb, 39–42.

Ellis HD. 1981: Theoretical aspects of face recognition. In Davies, GM, Ellis HD, Shepherd JW (eds). *Perceiving and remembering faces*. London: Academic Press. 172–97.

Ellis HD, Shepherd JW, Davies GM. 1980: The deterioration of verbal description of faces over different delay intervals. *Journal of Police Science and Administration* **8**, 101–106.

Gombrich EH, Hochberg J, Black M. *Art, perception, and reality*. Baltimore: Johns Hopkins University Press.

Harmon LD, Hunt WF. 1977: Automatic recognition of human face profiles. *Computer Graphics and Image Processing* **6**, 135–56.

Jones B. 1979: Lateral asymmetry in testing long-term memory for faces. *Cortex* **15**(2), 183–6.

Laughery KR, Fowler RH. 1980: Sketch artist and identi-kit procedures for recalling faces. *Journal of Applied Psychology* **65**(3), 307–16.

Laughery KR, Jensen DG, Wogalter MS. 1988: Response bias with prototypic faces. In Gruneberg MM, Morris PE, Sykes RN. (eds). *Practical aspects of memory: current research and issues*. New York: John Wiley & Sons, 568.

Morse D, Dailey RC, Stoutamire J, Duncan J. 1984: Forensic archaeology. In Rathbun TA, Buikstra JE. (eds). *Human identification: case studies in forensic anthropology*. Springfield: Charles C Thomas, 53–64.

O'Toole AJ, Deffenbacher KA, Valentin D, Herve A. 1994: Structural aspects of face recognition and the other-race effect. *Memory and Cognition* **22**(2), 2208–224.

Rhodes G. 1988: Looking at faces: first-order and second-order features as determinants of facial appearance. *Perception* **17**(1), 43–63.

Saunders DM, Vidmar N, Hewitt EC. 1983: Eyewitness testimony and the discrediting effect. In Lloyd-Bostock SMA, Clifford BR (eds). *Evaluating witness evidence*. Chichester: John Wiley.

Sergent J. 1984: An investigation into component and configurational processes underlying face perception. *British Journal of Psychology* **75**, 221–42.

Shepherd JW, Deregowski JB. 1981: Races and faces: a comparison of the responses of Africans and Europeans to faces of the same and different races. *British Journal of Social Psychology* **20**, 125–33.

Shepherd JW, Davies GM, Ellis HD. 1978: How best shall a face be described? In Gruneberg MM, Morris PE, Sykes RN (eds). *Practical aspects of memory*. London: Academic Press.

Solow B, Tallgren A. 1976: Head posture and craniofacial morphology. *American Journal of Physical Anthropology* **44**, 417–36.

Wolf DJ. 1986: Forensic anthropology scene investigations. In Reichs KJ (ed.) *Forensic osteology*. Springfield: Charles C. Thomas, 3–23.

CHAPTER 2

Management of the scene and forensic evidence

MA RAYMOND, WJ ASHLEY

General considerations	9	Recording of crime scenes	13
Purpose of scientific evidence	10	Searching techniques	15
Exchange of evidence	10	Collection of evidence	16
Scientific approach	11	Safety	18
Initial assessment of the scene	11	Case management	19
Security and scene preservation	12	Specialized scene examination	19
Initial examination	13		

General considerations

A 'missing person' is usually classified by the layperson as an individual whose whereabouts are of concern to those 'near and dear' to them. The 'disappearance' is generally, but not always, one of design.

This section deals primarily with those scenes where there is no body associated with the scene or, if there is, it is no longer in a state in which it is easily recognizable. The former case usually results from a distress call from a relative, friend or neighbour who has tried to telephone or who has visited the location (usually a dwelling place) and is concerned by the apparent absence of that person. There are sometimes indications that not everything is as it should be as there may be a build-up of newspapers, mail, 'junk' mail and milk bottles, or clothing on washing lines; furniture or valuables may have been disturbed or are clearly missing, or the family car may be missing. A further clue to foul play may be the presence of blood, which is manifest as a pool or tiny droplets on various surfaces or as tiny isolated stains which themselves indicate attempted deliberate removal.

Those cases in which the body is no longer recognizable relate to:

- those partially preserved bodies or skeletal remains that are discovered or unearthed accidentally or in the course of an investigation;
- significant facial and/or body disfigurement as a direct result of a vehicular, aviation or boating accident (the disfigurement may be due to the accident itself, to a fire resulting from the incident or even to long-term water immersion);
- a bombing incident;
- a natural or man-made disaster such as a severe bush fire or an earthquake.

Whether the 'missing person' incident is deemed to be accidental or deliberate is not initially important in the context of the scene. Either scenario should be treated within the rules of crime scene investigation and all it entails. If foul play is suspected, it is then of paramount importance that the body be located. The first stage of an investigation may be the systematic interviewing of neighbours and the sifting of local hospital admittance registers. Where those obvious routes of enquiry are unsuccessful, it may become necessary to use alternative methods of location of the body, some of which are simple, others technologically very complex. This means that the location of the possible scene(s) must be established.

A 'crime scene' is the term used to define a location that is associated with a suspicion of criminality. Horswell, in *Expert Evidence* (1993), defined it as 'any venue that has the potential to reveal evidence of the commission of an offence or to rule out the commission of an offence'. This is because crime scenes and those directly instrumental in their creation reflect both the trauma of the incident and (to some degree) the associated passage of time both during and after the events that gave rise to the scene. Consequently, analysis of any relevant material associated in any way with the event may reveal a wealth of significant information.

Physical evidence in relation to the investigation of a crime or an incident could be said to embrace any or all objects and articles, tangible or latent, living or inanimate, solid or liquid, that have a relationship with or pertain to a crime or incident. Further definitions of evidence come from the Federal Bureau of Investigation *Handbook of Forensic Science* (1990):

1. that which is legally submitted to a competent tribunal (be it a coroner or a criminal court) as a means of ascertaining the truth of any alleged matter of fact under investigation before it;
2. anything which a suspect leaves at a crime scene or takes from the scene or which may be otherwise connected with the crime.

Where there are allegations of criminality, the value of that evidence is determined by how useful it is in verifying whether a crime has indeed been committed and, if so, the extent to which it implicates the person or persons responsible and/or exonerates the innocent.

To utilize the full potential of evidence, the police investigators, crime scene examiners, scientists, pathologists, odontologists, anthropologists, etc. must produce a set of facts, and informed opinions deduced from those facts, which make it unreasonable to believe any conclusion other than what is presented by the physical, chemical, biological, odontological, anthropological and pathological evidence. It is therefore incumbent on those involved to ensure the quality of the evidence recorded, collected, stored and analysed, and the opinions derived therefrom.

The management of evidence from its initial location to its examination and the presentation of evidence to a court of law is paramount and should not be undermined or neglected owing to a lack of experience or resource constraints. The purpose of this chapter is to identify the objectives and procedures of evidence management as applied to an incident scene, while highlighting specific or advanced methods that may assist in that process in relation to 'missing persons'.

Purpose of scientific evidence

The purpose of scientific evidence collection and examination broadly includes the following:

- the identification of the missing person (fingerprints, DNA typing, odontological comparisons);
- the association of biological (family DNA comparisons, anatomical features, facial reconstruction) or physical (jewellery, clothing, identity documents) attributes, traits or links;
- dating of the grave site or contents;
- the sexing or ageing of the bones or body;
- the development or linkage of similar *modi operandi* concerning the manner of death or disposal of the body/skeletal remains;
- the identification of suspects;
- the elimination of suspects;
- provision of information to the investigator and to the judicial/coronial system;
- reconstruction of the scene.

Exchange of evidence

When two or more objects come into contact, there will frequently be a transfer of small amounts of material from one object to the other. Some of the material transferred may be very small, as is often the case when fabric comes into contact with rough surfaces. On the other hand, some physical evidence may be macroscopic, such as shoe or fingerprint impressions.

The evidence may have been removed by a cautious criminal, inadvertently by well-meaning individuals entering and walking through the scene or, in the case of the discovery of skeletal remains or a decomposing body in the bush, by the passage of time. This loss of evidence must clearly be minimized wherever possible by the correct management of the scene and the potential exhibits located at the scene. As stated earlier, there is a presumption based on the observations of Locard that people will always leave something of themselves or their immediate environment at a crime scene and, in doing so, take away part of that scene with them (Horswell, 1993). This may be fibres, blood, shoe or tyre marks or fingerprint impressions. This so-called exchange principle has been well stated by Nicholls (1956):

> When any two objects come into contact there is always a transference of material from each object onto the other, such a transference may be large or small, it may be readily detectable or it may be very difficult to detect, nevertheless it occurs and it is the business of the scientist to find and prove the transference wherever possible, however small this may be.

Application of this principle often allows the scene examiner, at least in part, to reconstruct or identify the missing person and/or to reconstruct the scene itself. The actual degree of transference is subject to one or all of the following:

- the degree of force or pressure applied between the two objects;
- the nature of the contact, i.e. scrub, smear, brushing action, etc.;
- the types of surface;
- the duration of the contact interchange;
- the type of fabric;
- the amount of time elapsed since the contact;
- the movement history of the object bearing the transferred material: washed, dried, shaken, etc.

It must be remembered that not all evidence is obvious to the naked eye and therefore careful examination and the use of various physical, photoluminescence and chemiluminescence techniques may be required to assist in the identification and subsequent collection of latent evidentiary items. Physical techniques include the use of fingerprint powders, a Dust Lifting Kit (DLK), as marketed by Foster and Freeman (UK) for dustmark impressions, and high-contrast film, infra-red and ultra-violet film to enhance images of latent material (Gibson, 1978; Krauss and Warlen, 1985). There are also a large number of chemical enhancement techniques to deal with blood and other material impressions at the scene and in the laboratory (Raymond, 1993). Leuco-crystal violet, amido black and luminol are popular chemicals for enhancing trace amounts of blood (Lake and Ganas, 1995). Potassium and sodium thiocyanates, as well as Bromophenol Blue and diaminobenzidene, are common chemicals used for the enhancement of latent impressions containing iron and mineral deposits (Bodziak, 1990; Brundage, 1994; Fischer, 1994; Shor, 1994).

Scientific approach

In order to process a scene efficiently and to maximize the recovery of evidence associated with the scene, the examiner must be continually mindful of the need to approach the scene or body in an ordered, structured, informed, scientific manner.

This scientific approach means that the examiner should be able to identify and understand what physical evidence is and the ramifications of that evidence in terms of any subsequent biological, chemical, pathological, odontological, botanical or entomological analysis. The examiner must know how to secure, preserve, record, collect and, where appropriate, examine and interpret the potential evidence.

To find and understand the value of scientific evidence often requires patience and thoroughness, and failure to exercise these qualities may lead to:

- inadequate collection of evidence at the scene;
- inadequate sampling of evidence;
- destruction of evidence at the scene owing to carelessness;
- preconceived ideas;
- a lack of communication between the coroner, the investigator, the scientist and the crime scene examiner.

Thus the examination of an incident scene and the subsequent recording and collection of relevant physical evidence requires skill and knowledge. The manner in which a scene is examined may be a critical factor in determining the success of an investigation.

As physical evidence or so-called identification science has increasingly become a powerful aid to missing person identification, the judicial system is placing more emphasis on forensic examinations and results. Accordingly, the manner in which evidence is recorded, preserved and collected, along with the relevant examinations and observations, must be able to be rigorously tested in a court of law.

A systematic approach to the examination of a scene should ensure:

- an efficient and thorough examination;
- orderly photography and note-taking;
- increased credibility as an expert witness.

Initial assessment of the scene

Prior to attending the scene of a missing person or unidentified deceased, the respective scene examiner, be they a crime scene specialist, pathologist or anthropologist, should receive from the investigator the best possible information relating to the scene or incident. Although prompt attendance will ensure preservation of the scene, time spent planning and organizing resources will allow and promote a more efficient examination of the location of interest. A scene examiner should consider the following:

- which specialist personnel may be required (photographer, pathologist, odontologist, biologist, geologist, fingerprint examiner, etc.);
- what equipment may be required, including lighting or extra-heavy or specialist equipment, such as manual or mechanical sifting equipment and soil probes;
- what transport is necessary, for instance a four-wheel drive vehicle or air transport for remote locations.

On arrival at the crime scene, the examiner must make contact with the police officer or investigator in charge of the investigation and ascertain the following information:

1. whether the scene has been properly secured and controlled;
2. what was thought to have happened (what scenario has been given);
3. when and where it happened;
4. whether there is a suspect;
5. who has entered the crime scene;
6. what is known about the missing person or identified deceased.

Obtaining more detail at the outset will make it easier for the scene examiner to determine what is required regarding the scene examination and what the anticipated level of contamination might be. It is also very important not to accept the information given by the investigator or witnesses at face value. A good scene examiner will weigh the information against the evidence that presents itself at the scene and later in the laboratory. If there is any conflicting evidence, this must be explained and recorded in the normal manner. It is the duty of a scene examiner to be objective and impartial in the all facets of his or her work and to report accordingly.

If the crime scene is very large, involves multiple deaths, has political ramifications, is a disaster situation or may provide perceived conflicts of interest (e.g. the 1988 attack on Pan Am flight 103 over Lockerbie), the scene examiner must ensure that an informed scene co-ordinator is appointed. This protocol is enacted in a number of jurisdictions, thus freeing the crime scene examiner to go about the tasks required of him or her. The scene co-ordinator should in no way interfere with the scene examination but be supportive of the team and act as an interface to the investigator(s) and other interested parties (coroner, government ministers, etc).

Security and scene preservation

It is vitally important that the scene be secured with the appropriate tape or barriers at the earliest opportunity. The extent of the scene should be judged from the furthest piece of potential evidence. Naturally, with disasters such as Lockerbie, the securing of the scene is challenging, not only because of its size but also in the magnitude of the resources to ensure that all available evidence, body parts and property are secured, thereby ensuring correct recording and collection for the purpose of identifi-

cation (Knox, 1990). A police member should guard the crime scene and maintain a duty log-sheet of those who enter the scene and their reasons for being present.

The scene examiner should also assume control of the examination of that scene and plan the method of examination as well as who should be allowed into the scene. As previously identified in 'Initial assessment of the scene', other persons or services with specific tasks or expertise may require entry to the crime scene before, during and after the examination of the scene by the crime scene investigator. These people may include the officer in charge of the investigation, the pathologist, the anthropologist, ambulance personnel, fingerprint examiners, the coroner, biologists and so on. However, it is important that the number of personnel entering the scene be kept to a minimum.

The methods commonly used for securing incident scenes include:

- posting guards;
- crime scene tape;
- the strategic placing of vehicles;
- barriers.

In applying any or all of the above, designated safe-walk areas should be clearly marked. Securing a scene either overnight or for a length of time may be necessary if the result of a post mortem may influence the direction of further scene examination. Similarly, the examination of a crime scene is best performed in daylight, and every attempt should be made to search in daylight hours. Naturally, for reasons beyond the control of the examining team, this may not always be possible; therefore the examiner should have included additional lighting as part of

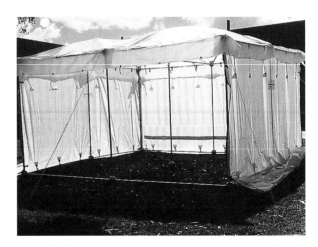

Fig. 2.1 Shows a purpose-built 'forensic' tent for use in exhumations or inclement weather

the contingency when making the initial assessment of the crime scene.

Security of exhibits or evidence is just as vital. A number of crime or forensic laboratories utilize specially designed forensic tents to shield and protect evidence from inclement weather, the public and the media. Forensic tents are designed to cover a cadaver or larger areas of interest. These tents are obviously also useful for exhumations (Fig. 2.1).

Initial examination

This is the planning stage of the searching process. A general survey of the scene is essential in developing a systematic approach. The examiner should enter the scene from the same route used to evacuate people, bearing in mind that the suspect may have also used the same exit point. At this stage, it is advised not to touch or disturb anything but to formulate a plan of action regarding the full and proper examination of the scene. The plan for the scene search should be methodical and systematic and adopted after consideration of:

1. the objectives of the search – what is to be sought;
2. the known facts;
3. any ambiguities in witness accounts;
4. which personnel are present and their role at the scene.

At this preliminary stage, one must also take account of other general factors that may influence the examination, such as weather conditions, time constraints, lighting, search patterns, geography/demography, personnel required and any safety precautions that may be necessary in the context of the scene. Other primary considerations include the location of the point of entry and exit, and the subsequent evaluation of any tool marks, shoe sole impressions, fingerprints, tyre marks and trace material. Other than the 'contained' crime scene area, the 'outer' region of the crime scene should also be examined for shoe sole impressions, abandoned weapons, cigarette butts, etc.

The scope, direction and plan of the search must be communicated to all relevant parties by the examiner. It must be remembered that these are considerations only, as hard-and-fast rules applicable to every scene do not exist. A flexible nature is a healthy aid to every person associated with scene and scene material examination and analysis.

In dealing with unrecognizable bodies, skeletal remains or missing persons, the scene examiner must consider every piece of possible evidence as having a potential bearing on the reconstruction of events. Soil and foliage disturbance, bloodstain patterns and insect populations may all have some part to play in scene reconstruction.

Recording of crime scenes

The recording of crime scenes is an important task and one that must be accomplished using thought, thoroughness and a planned approach. There are several ways in which a scene may be recorded:

- photographs;
- video;
- notes (narrative description);
- sketches and plans.

PHOTOGRAPHS

Scenes will not remain undisturbed for very long (if not already contaminated), so the objective of scene photography is to record the scene in a condition as near as possible to its original state. Police, ambulance personnel, witnesses and the public in general may have contaminated the scene. Identification, isolation and cordoning off the scene are imperative if the scene is to be recorded and examined in anything approaching a near-pristine condition. The photographing of a scene should be one of the first objectives of the scene examiner. As already explained, it is prudent, however, for the scene examiner to conduct a preliminary survey of the scene. This will help in determining which photographs will be required and their possible sequence. It is important to note that no reconstruction of evidence for photographic recording is permitted.

Format for exterior crime scene photography

1. Photographically capture the location of the scene from a distance and include a landmark such as a street sign in the frame. Aerial photography may be necessary to do this adequately.
2. Take medium-distance photographs to record the relative positions of closely related items. Ensure that the photographs overlap each other to maintain photographic continuity.
3. Take close-up photographs of individual items of evidence. It may be necessary to duplicate photographs with a measuring tape in one of the pairs of photographs.

Aerial photography on its own or coupled with infra-red imaging may be useful in the possible identification of a burial or suspect grave site (Fig. 2.2).

Format for interior crime scene photography

1. Photographically establish the position of the building.
2. Photograph rooms and other interior areas from designated observation points, using a wide-angle lens if necessary. Show the relative position of all items within the area.
3. Take medium-distance photographs of evidence using standard lenses.
4. Take close-up photographs of individual items of evidence.

The photographs must include, where relevant, any footprints, tyre tracks or tool marks (prior to casting), witness viewpoints, detailed photographs of the deceased and specifically any injuries, weapons, trace material, article damage and potential evidence revealed during the scene examination process. Further photographs depicting examinations and results will be required at the scene and also back in the laboratory.

VIDEO

The procedure for video recording is similar to that for still photography. Video recording of the scene should be completed after the preliminary examination by the scene examiner and after completion of the initial still photography. The use of video recording is gaining importance, particularly with re-enactments and the ability to reconstruct events using digital imaging technology via the video format.

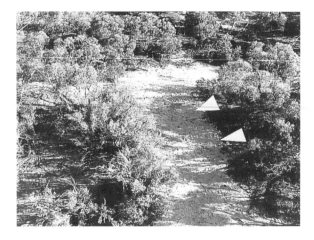

Fig. 2.2 Aerial photographs showing changes in soil denoting a possible grave site

For large areas, this format can be coupled to a global positioning system (GPS) mounted in a helicopter or fixed-wing aircraft, such that each area and item of interest is recorded and positioned. This procedure has the potential to drastically reduce the search time. The record/position procedure can be repeated at a later date, if necessary, to show any changes in vegetation and growth. These changes may warrant further investigation.

NOTE-TAKING

Comprehensive notes, describing the scene and the scene examiner's actions, are made as a matter of course. A narrative description of a scene can be used to complete a report or statement and refresh the scene examiner's memory during judicial proceedings. Therefore the notes should be made contemporaneously and be an accurate account of the scene and its examination. They should include:

- date, time and location of the scene/search;
- weather and lighting conditions;
- identity of other personnel participating in the search or examination, including the investigating officer;
- details of briefings with other personnel present;
- general conditions of the scene;
- specific conditions of the scene;
- condition, type and position of any potential evidence found, collected or received;
- continuity details in relation to the movement of any potential evidence.

Notes should be comprehensive and succinct, and should follow the logical sequence of the scene examination. Any discontinuity in the notes should be explained and dates and times of examination and continuity details included.

Environmental factors may play an important part in the investigation process. Such factors as lighting (on or off), street lighting, general security, positions of blinds, windows and locks, heaters, electric blankets or timers, television status, newspapers (noting the lastest edition), clocks (stopped, fast or slow), drugs and prescribed medication (Horswell, 1993) may all be relevant to a particular event. Naturally, the notes may include sketches or plans.

SKETCHES, PLANS AND MAPS

A scene sketch is a hand-made pictorial representation of of the scene and its contents (Fig. 2.3).

It is useful in clarifying investigative data and making the locality easier to understand by eliminating unnecessary detail. It also materially assists in

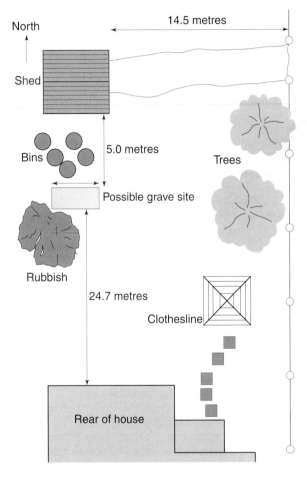

Premises at Lot 5 Wilson Rd, Yarrambat
Sketch prepared by Sgt. 23456 of the C.S.S. on 5/5/94

North

14.5 metres

Shed

Bins

5.0 metres

Trees

Possible grave site

Rubbish

24.7 metres

Clothesline

Rear of house

Fig. 2.3 Sketch of a crime scene

the reconstruction and interpretation of the chain of events that took place in the commission of an incident. A good crime scene sketch will complement and augment photographs that provide useful visual evidence but not a perspective of the evidence. A sketch does not replace either photographs at the scene or a detailed textual description of evidence. If the area of interest is a room in a house, the reconstruction of events may require the examiner to make measurements of the room and measurements of the items and trace material (such as blood stains) on surfaces within the room. To make any type of quantitative reconstruction analysis requires a mathematical framework. This framework must allow the practitioner to describe the position of the material of interest in three-dimensional space. This may be accomplished by the establishment of a datum point and a system of co-ordinates (Morse *et al.*, 1976). Sketches should be used to show:

- dimensions of rooms, furniture, doors and windows;
- distances from and to apparently relevant objects;
- distances between objects. These distances should be measured on two axes from non-moveable items such as walls or floors.

When preparing a sketch of a scene (either external or internal) and incorporating measurements, the following protocol should be adopted:

1. The contents of the sketch plan should be determined.
2. The method for recording and measuring the scene should be determined.
3. Due north should be noted using a compass and be marked on the sketch.
4. Two immovable points, such as a wall or floor, should be 'fixed' as reference points for any subsequent measurements.
5. The overall dimensions (if a room) and the position (and, in certain cases, dimensions) of relevant items should be systematically recorded.
6. The positions of all items of interest should be documented prior to their removal.
7. A notation that the sketch is not to scale should be included.
8. The creator of a sketch should initial or endorse the sketch with his or her name, the date and the time.

Searching techniques

The method of searching will depend on the scene, the circumstances and the given conditions. The scene examiner will need to plan the method of searching and adhere to it closely. If the examiner is disturbed during the searching phase, this must be noted and the source of distraction dealt with later. There are a number of different methods for searching, including:

- line searching;
- zonal searching (which is particularly useful where the evidence is fragmented, for example, at the scene of an explosion);
- grid searching;
- spiral searching (in particular, where the terrain is difficult to negotiate);
- strip searching.

In all of the above, the examiner must fully brief searchers on items of interest that may have some bearing on the case. The examiner must also control the search, stopping it when something of interest is located and having that item evaluated, photographed and collected. The ability of the examiner to maintain enthusiasm amongst searchers and keep them up to date with the progress of the case is important in relation to morale and effective searching.

Line search

In planning a line search (Fig. 2.4a):

- determine the area to be searched;
- position searchers according to the terrain in order not to overlook any items of potential interest (Fig. 2.4a).

Zonal search

This is most appropriate for explosion scenes or fragmentation of evidence. With this type of search (Fig. 2.4b):

- divide the total into zones;
- use sufficient staff to cover the zones.

Grid search

- Divide the area into grids.
- Search each grid individually (Fig. 2.4c).

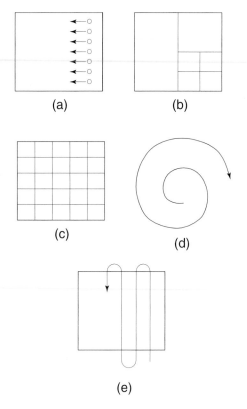

(a)   (b)

(c)

(d)

(e)

Fig. 2.4 (a) Line searching method. (b) Zonal searching method. (c) Grid method of searching. (d) Spiral search method. (e) Strip method of searching

Spiral search

- Start at the point of obvious evidential interest and work outwards (Fig. 2.4d).

Strip search

- Commence at a predetermined point.
- Set the width of the strip segment.
- Search each segment in turn. (Fig. 2.4e).

These search types are self-explanatory but are necessary as they provide a structured search format and minimize the possibility of leaving areas unexplored.

Collection of evidence

The collection of evidence is an important phase of a scene examiner's work. Any items that may afford evidence of the identity of missing persons or lead to the successful conclusion of an investigation should be collected from the scene. When in doubt, an item should be collected as its relevance may only become known sometime in the future. Consequently, it is better to collect too much than too little. An irrelevant item may be discarded, but a relevant item that has not been collected is lost. A team comprising of the correct balance of experts should, however, minimize the amount of extraneous material collected.

After the general survey of the scene, the sequence in which areas should be searched and evidence collected should be apparent. The collection protocol is generally as follows:

1. All evidence should be fully described and photographed *in situ* prior to collection.
2. All evidence must be collected legally in order to be admissible at any subsequent judicial proceeding. A number of Statute and Common Law powers generally apply to the collection of evidence within a given jurisdiction and, as such, the scene examiner must be conversant with those powers and the implications for the legality of the evidence collected. The proper collection and labelling of evidence will ensure continuity.
3. All evidence must be properly handled and packaged to minimize contamination and/or destruction.

PRIORITY OF COLLECTION

The following elements should always be given priority where applicable:

- any potential evidence that is in danger of being affected or destroyed by wind, rain, vehicles or people, should be collected immediately or protected in the most suitable manner;
- any potential evidence that will enable 'safe' access to a body or to any critical area of a crime scene; for example entry or exit points and paths;
- those critical scene areas that may render the most evidence or, once processed, enable the removal of a body;
- any area that may give a quick indication of the identity of the deceased or assailant(s);
- any material that will, when processed, obviate the need for guards or crime scene tape, or will once again allow free traffic movement.

In determining the manner and sequence of the collection of potential evidence, consideration must be given to the possible accidental destruction of that evidence and therefore to which approach is likely to yield the best information. Consultation with other experts in different fields (e.g. fingerprint examiners, pathologists and biologists) as to the sequence and method of collection is necessary to ensure the best results. For example:

- Polished floors need to be examined first with oblique lighting to locate latent shoe impressions, if any.
- Trace material should be collected prior to dusting for fingerprints.
- Bloodstains, if any, may need to be interpreted in relation to other objects (see Bloodstain pattern interpretation below) and collected prior to fingerprinting.
- Larger objects should be searched for and collected prior to smaller objects.

A systematic approach to the collection of evidence will ensure that all the evidence *is* collected. All the items should be labelled at the time of collection either by description, numerical sequence or both in order to maintain continuity. In the case of large or complex crime scenes, consideration should be given to a master log of exhibits or the employment of an exhibit officer.

SAMPLING

Sample types fall into three basic categories:

1. the suspect, questioned or evidence sample;
2. the control sample;
3. the reference sample.

The potential evidence collected from the scene that requires identification and future comparison is termed the suspect, questioned or evidence sample.

The control samples provide background or contamination information about the substrate from which the questioned sample was taken. For example, where a blood sample is collected from an oily garage floor, the blood is the questioned sample and the sample of the oil on the floor adjacent to it is the so-called control sample. Reference samples are known standards against which the suspect sample may be compared. For instance, a blood sample taken from a suspect or complainant is a reference sample, which may then be compared against a blood (questioned sample) stain on the victim's clothing. The composition of soil on the shoes of the unidentified deceased may be compared with surface soil samples (standards) from the area in which the deceased was found.

The amount or size of sample taken depends on the circumstances. Generally, the scene investigator will err on the side of caution by collecting rather more than is thought to be required.

LABELLING

All items should be labelled at the time of collection, usually by description and numerical sequence. Correct labelling allows the identification of the exhibit right through to its presentation in a court of law if necessary and allows every practitioner along the continuity chain meaningfully to establish the source of this exhibit.

Labels should be brief in narrative, indicating item, location, time and date, and the name of the person collecting the item. The label should be securely affixed to the container or package that contains the potential exhibit. Some jurisdictions label the actual exhibit itself, insofar as this is practical.

PACKAGING

The packaging and transportation of articles is equally as important as the location and recording of items of interest. The collection of articles and their proper storage in the most suitable medium will minimize the potential for contamination, loss or breakage (Bass and Birkby, 1978). This should then minimize subsequent debate in any subsequent legal proceedings, should they arise. Each article and its moisture content (wet or dry) has to be considered. The use of paper bags is a preferred option of scene examiners and those who are to undertake future examinations and analyses. The paper bag allows the evidence to 'breathe' and prevents sweating and subsequent loss of evidence in certain instances (for example, biological fluid-stained clothing or footwear). Plastic bags are also useful in many

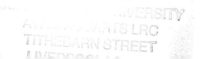

circumstances but should never be used to contain wet items. Should this occur, the timely removal of the evidence in order to allow it to breathe and dry out is critical. The dried evidence should then be stored and sealed in a paper bag. Failure to undertake this simple task will cause mould or fungal growth, possibly destroying any latent or microscopic biological evidence present.

Skeletal remains are usually damp or have been affected by their environment, making them subject to breakage or deterioration. Bones should be collected and packaged with care, ensuring that there is no or very little separation of the bones or parts of the skeletal structure. If bones or remains are brittle, consideration should be given to sealing or encasing them in an appropriate medium; for example, with appropriate consultation, jaws, teeth or dental work may be glued together to make subsequent cadaver dental record comparison easier. The set of bones or remains should be collected intact, where possible, by incorporating the surrounding substrate material (Fig. 2.5).

This will allow for a greater appreciation of the positioning of the body and changes in soil and substrate material around the body or remains, and give the examiner the opportunity to continue his or her work in a more clinical environment. Body bags or strongly constructed boxes are an ideal method of packaging the evidence. If skeletal remains have been scattered and appear fragile, cushioning of the bones with cotton wool or another appropriate medium is most desirable.

It is very important to ensure that all wet articles are dried prior to packaging for subsequent examination. Exemptions to this rule include those evidence items which may have been contaminated with a flammable liquid that needs to be identified by chemical analysis in the laboratory. Special non-

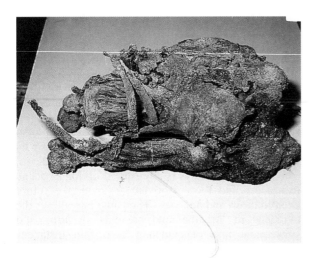

Fig. 2.5   Remains and substrate material from burial site

permeable bags manufactured from polyvinylidine chloride or glass jars with vapour tight seals are suitable containers for this type of evidence.

Appendix II identifies some of the various types of evidence likely to be encountered and the most appropriate packaging container for each type. The list includes some information found in the FBI *Handbook of Forensic Science* (1990).

Safety

Owing to the wide range of potentially dangerous crime scenes attended, personal safety is paramount, and the need to use proper and approved safety equipment cannot be overemphasized. Biological and chemical hazards are always present when dealing with scenes of the nature described where there may be putrefied flesh or copious volumes of blood.

Clearly, a scene where biological fluid or tissue has been spilt represents an occupational health and safety issue. The incidence of blood-related viruses, notably, the human immunodeficiency (HIV) and hepatitis B (HBV) and hepatitis C (HCV) viruses, is on the increase.

All three viruses remain active in liquid and stain form for a period of time. Literature suggests that the HIV virus survives up to a few days in stain form but a few weeks in liquid form. Hepatitis B, however, survives even in stain form for a matter of months, whereas the more labile HCV is inactivated by the drying process in a matter of days.

The only way any of these viruses can be contracted is via the mucous membranes, for example the mouth, eyes or nose, or directly through the bloodstream itself. Transmission via the mucous membranes may be through accidental contact with dried blood or tissue adhering to or becoming dislodged from the ceiling of a stained room at a scene, or the roof of a car during the sampling or measuring process. Safety glasses or goggles and standard gloves, face masks and other protective clothing should be worn whenever appropriate.

The penetration or entry of viruses directly into the bloodstream presents a more probable mode of transmission. It is relatively easy to accidentally pierce the skin through a glove when using a pair of dividers to make measurements during a bloodstain pattern examination, for example. Consequently, it is recommended that magnifying eyepieces with graticules be used in place of dividers for such examinations.

Pins or needles are not uncommonly 'hidden' or lodged in carpets and clothing. Hypodermic needles may have been left in positions not obvious to the examiner and represent a hazard during any searching process. Examiners trying to exhume the remains of a body may well encounter fragments of bone, glass or metal. It is imperative that practitioners at the scene promptly cover any cuts on their hands with non-perforated dressings and wear gloves appropriate to the task at hand.

Disinfectants that are known to deactivate bacteria and viruses should be used routinely on any part of the body that may have contacted biological material, and a solution of sodium hypochlorite should be used to sanitize instrumentation that cannot be placed in an autoclave. Hepatitis B immunization is available and should be considered by all personnel designated for crime scene attendance. In the event that an examiner pierces his or her skin with a sharp object like a pin, immediate medical advice should be sought.

Case management

The management of evidence does not stop at the scene. The scene examiner or specialist assisting at the scene must ensure that full communication continues, particularly with those entrusted with the responsibility of examining and analysing the evidence further in a laboratory or mortuary. As mentioned in the section on the preservation of potential exhibits, the examiner must ensure that all exhibits collected are correctly dried and secured in the appropriate containers.

The specialists should be made aware of the scene scenario so that the relevance of particular exhibits is apparent. Such consultation will allow the priority of examination to be determined as a single item may require examination by more than one specialist service. In major incidents, a conference between all investigators, including scientists, crime scene examiners, the coroner, pathologists, odontologists and anatomists (where required), should be organized. Such a meeting enables investigators to resolve any ambiguities, set priorities, minimize the number of items that need further examination and give all the specialists a clear direction as to their role in the investigation.

A final component of case management is the production of reports or statements reflecting the findings of the examination. Some reports or statements may simply be descriptive and factual while others may contain opinion evidence relating to a specific part of the examination, be it the scene or subsequent examination in the laboratory. The correct presentation of the evidence (descriptive reports, diagrams, charts or models) is paramount. This enables the trier-of-fact to weigh the evidence objectively.

Specialized scene examination

It is not intended that the full gamut of specialized scene examination and reconstruction be addressed here as a number of areas are considered in some form in other chapters of this book. Consequently, only selected areas are described below.

BLOODSTAIN PATTERN INTERPRETATION

Where blood is detected at a scene in the absence of a body, a number of deductions may be made to assist the investigator in the reconstruction of the scene. It may be that there are only traces of blood that will require enhancement, as described above. Alternatively, there may be patterns of bloodstains that themselves tell a story.

The colour of the stains, their shape, size and distribution, can be used to indicate whether foul play may have occurred. In addition, the patterns of stains can be used to indicate to investigators the type of weapon used, the types of injury sustained, the likelihood of and distribution of bloodstains on a suspect and whether or not a clean-up was attempted by individuals associated either directly or indirectly with the assault. Furthermore, subsequent protein or DNA profiling of any questioned blood, body fluid or cellular material using the family of the missing person as the points of genetic reference may give a very strong indication of the source of the material.

The physical reconstruction of the scene is clearly a function of the volume of blood spilt, the surfaces upon which the blood has been deposited and the patterns themselves. The volume of spilt blood associated with the scene of an assault obviously varies with the nature of the crime and can vary in volume from microlitres to litres. This volume clearly depends on the type of wound(s) to the victim(s) and the position of each wound in relation to clothing or bedding that not only absorbs the blood but is also easily removed from the scene.

Information may be gathered from the scene itself and from any bloodstained clothing located at the scene or subsequently on the body (Eckert and James, 1989; MacDonell, 1993), regarding:

- the origin(s) of the bloodstains;
- the distance between the target surface(s) and origin(s) at the time the blood was shed;
- the position and subsequent movement of the complainant/victim, the assailant and/or the objects at the time that the blood was shed;
- the type and direction of the impact(s) that produced the bloodstains;

- the minimum number of blows and/or shots and the possible type of weapon used;
- the order of deposition (of different stain patterns);
- the anticipated damage to the victim;
- evidence of any deliberate removal of bloodstains;
- correlation with the subsequent post mortem and/or serological or DNA typing results in the case of multiple bleeders;
- tangible support for or disagreement with re-enactments by the suspect(s).

In the absence of the body, it may also be necessary to identify the species of the stains as being either human or animal. Therefore presumptive testing and sampling at the scene should be followed by laboratory analysis.

Examination and analysis of both the physical characteristics and genetic markers of the clothing of the deceased and the suspect, if and when apprehended, may greatly assist in establishing culpability.

SOILS/BOTANICAL MATERIAL

It is sometimes the case that a buried body is accidentally exhumed by the action of a digging dog or excavating machinery. Sometimes it is not known, until the discovery of the body, that the deceased was actually missing. This may also be the case where bodies left on the surface have been covered by vegetation. The clearing of a site may reveal the scattered remains of a human body (Fig. 2.6).

In those cases where foul play is suspected, it is imperative that the soil and vegetation be sampled in a way that the former accurately reflects both the composition in the grave at various depths and adjacent to the site, and the latter the surrounding flora. It may become necessary at a later stage to compare

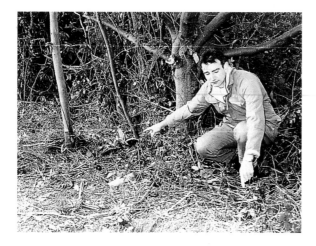

Fig. 2.6 An area of scattered remains and undergrowth

soil and/or vegetation detected on the footwear or clothing, or in or on the vehicle of the suspect with the soil and/or vegetation from the scene(s). It should be remembered that the flora associated with the scene changes with seasonal variation, and any sampling for comparison purposes should be carried out with that variable in mind (Fig. 2.7).

Many victims of crime are disposed of by burial. Consequently, the discovery and exhumation of remains present a number of variables that have to be considered by forensic examiners. Investigators may want to establish the time interval since death. Therefore all possible events that may have had an impact on the evidence have to be considered, and scene examinations therefore cannot be hurried: they must be thoroughly planned. Studies by Rodriguez and Bass (1985) showed that depth, moisture, heat (soil temperatures) and insects affect the decomposition of human remains. The greater the depth, the slower the decomposition. Bodies buried less than 30 cm below the surface will often be attacked by carrion insects that greatly influence the process of decomposition. With shallow graves, consideration has to be given to animal predation, where the cadaver is attacked by rodents, leaving post mortem markings that could be identified as lesions, wounds, etc.

The examiner must also be mindful of any impression that the body or face of the deceased may have left on the soft substrate prior to decomposition. Facial features or other characteristics may be evident in the soil or ice, and appropriate recording and casting of those indentations may help in the identification process.

The ruins of Pompeii provide an excellent example of a site where the surrounding substrate material has preserved features of interest. Pompeii and many of its inhabitants were covered in hot ash and lava when Mount Vesuvius erupted in AD 79. Altogether, approximately 2000 people perished and some were later found embedded in the ashes. These ashes formed a 'plaster mould' that preserved the body outlines many centuries after the body itself had mouldered into dust. The careful injection of filler material through such a mould should allow the bodies to be reconstructed such that identifiable features would be visible.

VISUAL LOCATION OF THE BODY

In those instances where it is necessary to locate a body, the soil and, to a lesser extent, the vegetation, may provide a clue to its location. The following characteristics are useful indicators:

1. The mixing of different soils, such as top soil with subterranean soil, will usually be obvious

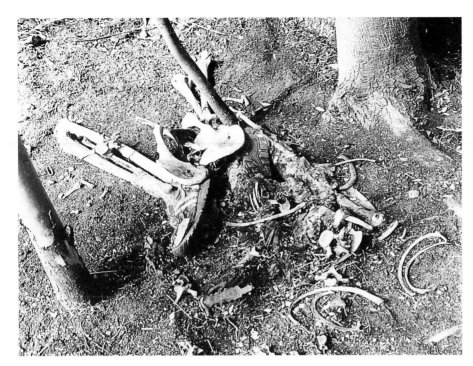

Fig. 2.7 Shows the remains once the undergrowth had been cleared

for a few days at least (depending on the weather). The difference may be obvious as either a colour, size or dampness variation or a combination of these and may be most noticeable from the air.

2. Disturbed vegetation over the area of the grave site caused by the excavation of soil may be evident. The flora is simply damaged by the process and naturally dries out. A botanist may also be able to estimate how long the vegetation has been damaged from observations of the height, distribution and depth of root systems involved at the sites (Boyd, 1979). The deeper the grave site, the greater the impact on the vegetation. Shallow grave sites will, over a period of time, show the reverse of damage by regrowth of the vegetation.

3. There may be 'crop marks', so-called because crops and grasses appear to flourish in the vicinity of shallow grave sites. The organic material of the human body acts as a natural fertilizer (Rodriguez and Bass, 1985). These changes in vegetation and the environment may be identified by aerial surveillance or from thermal imaging of a region using sophisticated methods of thermography.

4. The area over the grave site may become concave relative to the surrounding soil. It may take a matter of months before the concave nature of the excavation is obvious to the naked eye.

5. Dead insects and pupae located in the grave subsoil, and also any live maggots present, may enable an entomologist to glean information about the age of the grave (Kashyap and Pillay, 1989; McKeown, 1991). The life cycles of the carrion insects may actually assist in determining a time of death.

6. Damaged fibres may assist an appropriately skilled expert to estimate a time of death (Morse and Dailey, 1985).

PHYSICAL OR CHEMICAL LOCATION OF THE BODY

1. A long metal probe may indicate that the soil is less compacted than the surrounding area, signifying that the soil has recently been disturbed. Sometimes the disturbed soil remains uncompacted for many years (Bradley, 1991).

2. A metal detector may be used to show the presence of metal associated with the body (jewellery or keys, for example).

3. A probe may be used to test soil pH at various depths. Acids are produced from the breakdown of sugars and carbohydrates present in organic matter. As the decomposition process continues, the breakdown of albuminous tissues results in a high concentration of an alkaline substance (Imaizumi, 1974). The pH can be monitored simply by using litmus paper or a field pH meter. (In addition, lime may have been used in a misguided attempt to accelerate the decomposition

process. Lime will leave the soil strongly alkaline.) (Fig. 2.8.)

Other techniques include gas sensors, particularly for methane gas (formed by decomposition of the body), and remote sensing, both of which have occasionally proved successful (Krogman and Iscan, 1986). The decomposition of tissue forms various gases, including ammonia, hydrogen, hydrogen sulphide, hydrogen phosphide and methane (Boyd, 1979).

There are also a growing number of instrumental methods available for the detection of subsurface variation. These include resistivity meters, induced polarization, subsurface interface radar, nuclear densitometry, seismic exploration and magnetic surveying equipment such as the differential fluxgate gradiometer, the proton magnetometer and the proton gradiometer.

PHOTOGRAMMETRY

Photogrammetry is essentially the process of taking stereoscopic scene photographs that are then used to draw scaled plans. In providing evidence in cases involving homicides, missing persons, industrial accidents and disasters, plans are required which accurately and objectively record the incident area. Importance is therefore placed on the survey or plan and any associated notes. The use of a measuring tape is still practised today and is very time-consuming; its limitation is that only points of apparent interest at the time are recorded. Later reviewing of evidence or information may suggest unrecorded items of interest or be lost as a result of environmental or contaminant issues. Photogrammetry provides a method of providing accurate measurements that encompass the entire defined area or incident. Photogrammetry gives the examiner a method of obtaining a realistic spatial image of an incident or an object in which the exact relative positions of evidence germane to the scene are clearly and accurately documented (Snowden, 1980; Stegner, 1986; Coroneos, 1991). This method allows the scene to be recorded in the shortest possible time with limited disturbance to the items of interest. This is very important when dealing with traffic accidents or disasters such as aircraft crashes.

A further advantage of photogrammetry is that it limits the requirement for an examiner to enter the scene to record it. This is no more evident than in a scene where entry will destroy evidence or where there are inherent dangers to the examiner. Accurate measurements of key items are made and the data collated to give a two- or three-dimensional plot of the area from the stereo photographic images. The stereo photographs have great demonstrative value as well as high information content and can be stored

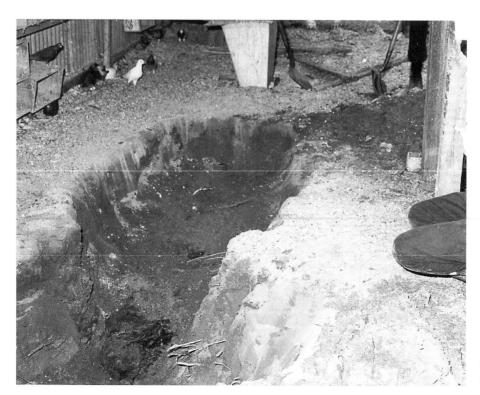

Fig. 2.8 Human remains buried in a chicken coop highlighted problems in reading the pH levels of the soils

indefinitely for future use. The use of the plotted diagram then supplements photographic and descriptive note evidence.

An example of a plotted diagram from a stereo photogrammetric image is presented. This system should be used for major incidents and any scene that may later require dimensional analysis to assist interpretation.

Photogrammetry of crime scenes from either an aerial or terrestrial perspective shows clear advantages over more traditional methods of recording and measuring scenes (Fig. 2.9).

THERMAL IMAGING

The expensive remote sensing or thermal imaging technique requires that infra-red photographs be taken from aircraft, preferably in the early hours of the morning, when the heat differential between that generated by the decomposing body and its cool surrounds is at a maximum. An experiment that monitored the heat change associated with freshly butchered sheep buried at different depths and at different times was carried out by the Victoria Forensic Science Centre, Victoria, Australia (Knight and Mur-

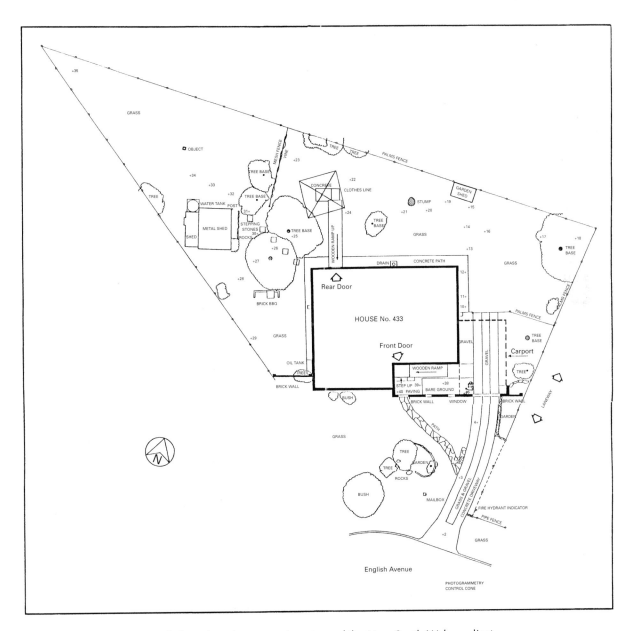

Fig. 2.9 Photogrammetrical plan of a crime scene (courtesy of the New South Wales police)

rihy, 1993). A thermographic video camera was mounted in a helicopter and images recorded over a period of 4 weeks. It was possible to distinguish each grave site, but the heat emitted over the assessment period decreased to a point at which it was no longer easily detected.

A commercial system known as FLIR (Forward Looking Infra-red) has been used by the Royal Canadian Mounted Police for a number of years (Saunders, 1990). The use of the system to search for missing persons has reduced the need for human resources and time commitments, particularly where the terrain is rugged and extensive. Current systems are very sensitive and can identify tracks, motor vehicle exhaust heat, engine heat and the movement of individuals.

In cases of questioned human identification, the value of the complete and accurate recovery of human remains cannot be overemphasized. In this chapter, the critical importance of managing the collection, documentation, transportation, storage and examination of remains is highlighted from both a scientific and a legal perspective. In cases of suspected homicide, the identification of the victim is of paramount importance. For identification of human remains to be established, some legal process is nearly always involved. It therefore follows that the quality of the scientific investigation must be mirrored by a management process that meets the evidential, documentary and legal requirements of the jurisdiction responsible for establishing identity. In practice, the management of a scene of discovery of human remains often involves compromises. However, the scientist must always endeavour to take the legal issues into account when scene management and processes are being determined.

References

Bass WM, Birkby WH. 1978: Exhumation: the method could make the difference. *FBI Law Enforcement Bulletin* **47**(7), 6–11.

Bodziak W. 1990: *Footwear impression evidence.* New York: Elsevier Science.

Boyd RM. 1979: Buried body cases. *FBI Law Enforcement Bulletin* **48**(2), 1–7.

Bradley SJ. 1991: Skeletons in the closet. *Australia Police Journal* Jul–Sept, 84–93.

Brundage DJ. 1994: Ammonium thiocyanate: a successful technique for dusty footwear impressions. FBI International Symposium on Footwear Evidence, Quantico, VA (unpublished).

Coroneos C. 1991: Photogrammetry may revolutionise the way archeological sites are recorded. *Victoria Archeological Society Newsletter,* Melbourne, Australia.

Eckert WG, James SH. 1989: *Interpretation of bloodstain evidence at crime scenes.* Amsterdam: Elsevier Science.

Federal Bureau of Investigation. 1990: *Handbook of forensic science.* Washington, DC: FBI.

Fischer JF. 1994: An aqueous leucocrystal violet enhancing reagent for blood impressions. *FBI International Symposium on Footwear Evidence,* Quantico, VA (unpublished).

Gibson HL. 1978: *Photography by infra-red.* New York: Wiley Interscience.

Horswell J. 1993: Crime scene examination. In Freckelton I, Selby H. (eds) *Expert evidence.* Melbourne: Law Book Company, ch. 98.

Imaizumi M. 1974: Locating buried bodies. *FBI Law Enforcement Bulletin* **43**(8), 2–5.

Kashyap VK, Pillay VV. 1989: Insects and crime investigation. What is forensic entomology? *International Criminal Police Review* Mar/Apr, 12–16.

Knight R, Murrihy P. 1993: *Thermal imaging.* Victoria Forensic Science Centre, Victoria (unpublished).

Knox W. 1990: Lockerbie: the grim search continues. *Australian Police Journal* **39**, 8–11.

Krauss TC, Warlen SC. 1985: The forensic use of reflective ultraviolet photography. *Journal of Forensic Sciences* **18**, 296–302.

Krogman WM, Iscan MY. 1986: *The human skeleton in forensic medicine.* Springfield IL: Charles C. Thomas.

Lake S, Ganas J. 1995: Optical enhancement of leucocrystal violet treated impressions in blood. *Australian & New Zealand Forensic Science Society Meeting, Auckland* (unpublished).

MacDonell HL. 1993: *Bloodstain patterns.* New York: Laboratory of Forensic Science.

McKeown P. 1991: Bugs and bodies or the entomological sleuth. *Royal Canadian Mounted Police Gazette* **53**(11), 10–14.

Morse D, Dailey RC. 1985: The degree of deterioration of associated death scene material. *Journal of Forensic Sciences* **30**, 119–127.

Morse D, Crusoe D, Smith HG. 1976: Forensic archaeology. *Journal of Forensic Sciences* **21**, 323–332.

Nicholls LC. 1956: *The scientific investigation of crime.* London: Butterworths.

Raymond MA. 1993: Forensic biology. In Freckelton I, Selby H. (eds) *Expert evidence,* Melbourne: Law Book Company, ch. 81.

Rodriguez WC, Bass WM. 1985: Decomposition of buried bodies and methods that may aid in their location. *Journal of Forensic Sciences* **30**(3), 836–852.

Saunders G. 1990: RCMP adopts FLIR. An airborne innovation in thermal imaging. *RCMP Gazette* **52**(10), 1–7.

Shor Y. 1994: Improved chemical reagents for the enhancement of footwear marks. FBI International Symposium on Footwear Evidence, Quantico, VA (unpublished).

Snowden J. 1980: *The use of terrestrial photogrammetry by the New South Wales Police Force,* Sydney (unpublished).

Stegner G. 1986: *Use of the wild aviolyt BC2 analytical restitution system for photogrammetric records of road accidents.* Switzerland: Wild Heerbrugg.

CHAPTER 3

The autopsy in human identification

DL RANSON

Introduction	25	Autopsy	29
Role of the forensic pathologist	25	Post-autopsy procedures	35
Skills	26		

Introduction

Compared with other medical or pathology tests, the autopsy is a very expensive investigative procedure. In most jurisdictions, the person performing autopsies is a medical specialist who has a high level of training and expertise in anatomical pathology or histopathology. The autopsy is perhaps best considered as a highly detailed, all-encompassing pathology test that surveys the body for the presence and stage of disease. It could also be considered to be the most comprehensive type of medical examination or procedure ever performed on an individual. Because the autopsy is a 'one-off' procedure, and is followed by the body being disposed of by burial or cremation, it is difficult or impossible to repeat parts of the procedure if mistakes or omissions are made.

There are a variety of autopsy procedures and techniques that can assist with human identification. In examinations of unidentified bodies or unknown human remains, the pathologist usually acts as the co-ordinator and team leader of the medical, dental, anthropological and scientific units involved in determining the identity of the deceased. In addition to taking on the role of co-ordinator, the pathologist can provide direct information on the morphology and individual physical characteristics of a body that goes far beyond the features used in ordinary visual identification by facial recognition. In many cases, the pathologist can provide evidence of physical characteristics, marks (such as scars and tattoos), disease and prior surgical and medical treatment. These observations may provide useful corroborative information in matters of questioned human identity.

Role of the forensic pathologist

In order to understand the place of the autopsy in human identification, it is necessary to understand the development of death investigation systems and the role played by forensic pathologists, coroners and medical examiners. The office of 'coroner' has its roots in Norman times, when death investigation was associated with important political and financial considerations. Coroners were associated with the collection of a number of fines and taxes that could be levied by the Crown in association with certain types of death. An example of this was the Deodand, a tax based on the financial value of the implement or object that had caused a person's unnatural death. For example, if a person were run over by a cart, the cart or its value was forfeited to the Crown as a tax, and the coroner was responsible for ensuring that the tax was paid.

Another role of the coroner was to ensure that a local community paid the fine of presentment of Englishry. This fine was imposed by the Norman invaders probably to protect them from retaliation by the conquered English. If a dead body was found, the community had to prove that the body was English rather than Norman. If a coroner found that a deceased person was not of English blood, a heavy fine would be levied. This latter role is perhaps the origin of the involvement of coroners in the processes of human identification. Today, the identification of deceased persons is the first of the duties of coroners, and if the identity of a body is unknown or uncertain, the death must be referred to the coroner for investigation. In some modern jurisdictions, the office of coroner has been superseded by that of medical examiner, who is for the most part a forensic pathologist who carries out the medical and allied scientific investigative functions that were part of coroners' jurisdictions.

Forensic pathologists are recruited from the medical profession, generally from amongst pathology specialists who practise in the field of anatomical pathology or histopathology. The principles of pathology applied in the work of the forensic pathologist are the same as those applied by clinical pathologists; however, there is a considerable difference in the nature of the work performed and in the mental and analytical processes applied. While the clinical pathologist is contributing directly or indirectly to the medical care given to patients, the forensic pathologist's focus is the end-point of forensic investigations, which are part of the judicial process. As a result, the information produced by forensic pathologists is usually presented to a criminal or coroner's court rather than to medical staff on a hospital ward round.

Skills

Because of their training, forensic pathologists gain a variety of specialist skills that they apply in their work. The basis of these skills is completion of a medical course, including an appropriate clinical internship and often a variety of other clinical appointments. As a result, the skills of a forensic pathologist cover a wide variety of subdisciplines in medicine and particularly subspecialties within pathology. These can be divided into clinical, pathological and legal areas, together with general skills in communication as a witness.

CLINICAL SKILLS

Forensic pathologists are first and foremost medical practitioners. They have undergone a full undergraduate training course of 5–7 years, which has included both preclinical and clinical studies. All forensic pathologists have spent at least 1 year, and in some cases several years, working in clinical medicine within a hospital setting. Some will have spent a considerable time working in other clinical specialty areas within a hospital, or in some cases in general practice, and their knowledge in these clinical areas may be considerable. The identification of deceased persons often relies in part on the identification of specific medical features at autopsy, such as evidence of particular surgical procedures or the effects of the use of certain drugs and other medical treatments.

FORENSIC PATHOLOGY SKILLS

As mentioned above, forensic pathology involves the application of basic pathology disciplines in the forensic or medico-legal setting. The pathological skills involved in forensic pathology can be divided into a number of areas: anatomical pathology, neuropathology, cytopathology, haematology, microbiology, immunology, molecular biology, and chemical pathology and toxicology. We will look at these in turn.

Anatomical pathology

Various descriptive terms are applied to the skills encompassed within anatomical pathology. There are indeed distinct semantic differences between these terms but, for most practical purposes, the type of professional specialization and skill involved is the same. Some of these terms include anatomical pathology, histopathology, surgical pathology and morbid anatomy. Pathologists practising in these areas have skills in the macroscopic or naked-eye examination of diseased organs and tissues, and in the microscopic examination of human organs and tissues.

Microscopic pathology examination forms the bulk of the work of anatomical pathologists in a hospital setting. Pieces of human tissue, removed either at surgery or in sampling techniques such as biopsies, are processed in the laboratory. Thin sections are cut, placed on to glass microscope slides and stained in order to reveal the nature of their cellular components. These sections of tissue are then examined under a microscope by a pathologist for the purpose of identifying whether there are any abnormalities present in the tissue, and if there are, what type of disease is involved.

In addition to this surgical pathology work, the anatomical pathologist also performs autopsies in a hospital setting where consent has been obtained from families and next-of-kin.

Most forensic pathologists have completed full anatomical or surgical pathology training and are therefore experienced in the performance of hospital autopsies as well as forensic pathology autopsies. In addition, they are skilled in the areas of microscopy of human tissues (histology) and identification within those tissues of various types of human disease. This surgical pathology training gives the pathologist experience of a variety of other medical specialties. Histological techniques can be used to identify disease and microscopic anatomical anomalies that can assist in the process of human identification. Histology of tissues can be of use even where the body is very badly decomposed, as the microscopic tissue architecture is often preserved in such cases. Examination of the reticulin architecture of decomposed tissues can distinguish between ovarian and testicular tissues and thus assist with the identification of gender.

Neuropathology

Neuropathology is a discrete subspecialty within anatomical pathology. A neuropathologist is usually an anatomical pathologist who specializes in the organs and tissues that comprise the central nervous system, peripheral nervous system and muscles. In a hospital setting, neuropathology staff are involved with the clinical disciplines of neurosurgery and neurology. Neuropathologists deal with diseases of the brain, the spinal cord, the peripheral nerves and the muscles of the body. A large part of the work of neurosurgeons is management of trauma to the head and central nervous system. Neuropathologists also deal with traumatic damage to the skull and tissues of the central nervous system.

The skills of neuropathology have a particular relevance for forensic pathology with regard to the processes involved in head injuries and the significance these have in relation to problems in craniofacial identification. A forensic neuropathologist may be able to identify evidence of previous head injury as well as diseases that may have resulted in the individual presenting to medical practitioners during life with conditions that may have required the taking of cranial radiographs. Such radiographs may be of use as reference ante mortem records, with which post mortem radiographs can be compared.

Cytopathology

The processes for identifying diseases of the body includes the examination of whole organs, specific tissues and the cells that go to make up those tissues. The histopathologist or anatomical pathologist, who examines microscopic sections of tissues under the microscope, looks at tissues of the body where the cells are arranged in their normal anatomical configuration. Cytopathologists examine the cells of the body in isolation or in small clumps where the cells do not form part of an intact tissue structure. The cells are obtained through a variety of sampling processes: scraping of the surface of tissues, as in examination of the cervix, or neck of the uterus; aspirating fluids from various parts of the body; or aspirating solid tissue masses.

The role of cytopathology within forensic pathology is limited. However, a wide variety of cytological techniques are employed within forensic pathology, and some tests for drowning and for the identification of spermatozoa employ procedures similar to those used in cytopathology.

Haematology

Haematology involves the diagnosis and treatment of diseases of the blood and includes the examination of peripheral blood and the blood precursor cells found in the bone marrow. Blood and bone marrow can be examined using techniques similar to those of cytopathology.

While the clinical aspects of haematology do not impinge greatly on the work of the forensic pathologist, many principles of human identification involve the analysis of blood. Blood group data as well as other serological typing can be obtained from fluids and tissues removed at autopsy. If samples of blood cannot be obtained or the blood is of poor preservation and quality, other tissues can be used for blood grouping. Fingernails and muscle tissue may be particularly useful in this respect. The determination of blood group in forensic science and forensic medicine is just one example of the use of haematology laboratory techniques and procedures in human identification.

Microbiology

Microbiology is the branch of pathology that deals with the identification of disease-causing microorganisms. Bacteria, viruses and fungi are just some of the agents that are dealt with by a microbiologist. Like other pathologists, microbiologists deal with samples taken from the human body, but their work can additionally involve the analysis of specimens taken from the environment. These samples are examined to determine which micro-organisms are present, and the organisms are often tested to see whether they are sensitive or resistant to antibiotics and other drugs.

While microbiology has limited application in the field of forensic pathology, all forensic pathologists understand basic microbiology principles and incorporate the results of microbiological testing into their medico-legal reports. Microbiological diseases play a part in a number of deaths investigated by forensic pathologists. Some of the individuals whose deaths form the subject of forensic pathological investigation have lifestyles that involve current or previous infection with particular agents. A good example of this is death associated with overdose of intravenous drugs, where there is often prior infection with hepatitis B, hepatitis C or HIV. In some cases, the detection of infectious disease processes at autopsy may provide corroborative information that can assist in human identification.

Immunology

Immunology has emerged in recent years as a key discipline within pathology. Immunological principles are applied in many of the other branches of pathology, including microbiology, haematology and anatomical pathology. Immunology has grown as a division of pathology and is now recognized as a major subspecialty. Immunologists study and test the function of the body's immune system and the diseases that are specifically associated with immune system dysfunction.

From the perspective of forensic pathology, many of the techniques of immunology are used in the forensic testing processes. The serological and blood grouping tests that are a feature of forensic science and forensic medicine are based on immunological principles. Specific immunological markers for human and animal antigens can help in distinguishing animal and human tissues in deaths where only small body fragments are recovered. In some difficult forensic pathology cases involving the identification of biological material and drugs, professional immunological expertise may be required.

Molecular biology

The use of molecular biology techniques to identify individuals has transformed identification methods in forensic science in recent years. These techniques have now become part of the routine services offered by forensic science laboratories. While they are still employed largely in the identification of living suspects from trace biological material left at the scene of the crime, their role in the identification of human remains is no less important. One of the difficulties with these techniques in identifying human remains is that the samples required for testing need to be fresh so that the DNA can be extracted. However, in recent years, variations on the original processes have resulted in molecular biology techniques being utilized even where decomposition has commenced. Of course, if the soft tissues of the body have been removed or are grossly decomposed, other techniques need to be employed. Nowadays, dry skeletal remains can yield sufficient material to allow molecular biology techniques to be employed. Similarly, dried tissues that have not been subject to decomposition, such as hair and nails, can be very useful. In old unsolved identification cases that occurred before molecular biological techniques were available, it is possible to test the tissue on the glass slides used for microscopy. Even where no original biological material from a suspected individual is available for comparison with the unidentified human remains, it is now possible to use blood samples from parents, siblings and offspring for comparison purposes.

Chemical pathology and toxicology

Chemical pathology, sometimes referred to as medical biochemistry, also encompasses the field of toxicology. There are chemical pathologists who specialize in the area of toxicology, but most doctors working in chemical pathology deal principally with the biochemical testing of human samples.

The field of toxicology uses many of the techniques of analysis that are found in the chemical pathology laboratory. The toxicologist does not generally measure natural body substances but analyses human tissues for the presence of drugs and other chemical agents that may have been taken into the body.

From the perspective of forensic pathology, chemical pathology and toxicology is an important related discipline. Toxicological analysis is a routine part of many forensic autopsies. Homicides, suicides and motor vehicle accidents are perhaps the most common cases in which drug analysis is involved. However, there is a wide variety of apparently accidental deaths, including those associated with work and recreation, in which toxicology and drug analysis are important in analysing the circumstances of the death.

Toxicological testing of human remains may provide useful information that can assist in the determination of identity. The presence of routine prescribed medication may provide corroborative evidence of identity, especially when the matter in question is the identity of each of a group of deceased individuals whose medical records are known. An example of this can be seen in the case of a small number of individuals who were burnt beyond visual recognition during the course of a fire in a long-stay hospital. Dental records provided identification of most of the dead bodies. However, in the case of two individuals whose cranial structures had been largely destroyed, identification was obtained from toxicology analyses that confirmed the presence of their routine medication.

LEGAL SKILLS

The knowledge that distinguishes forensic pathologists from their clinical colleagues is their understanding of legal process, medical law, court procedures and their rules of evidence. While doctors who engage in civil injuries work are also familiar with court processes, the remainder of the medical profession has little contact with the legal system and consequently has little knowledge of the legal principles involved in civil and criminal cases. Many forensic pathologists have gained their knowledge of the legal system through long experience of working with it. Most forensic pathologists agree that a sound knowledge of the legal principles that underlie their forensic work is of value in improving the quality of the service they provide for the legal system. In general, the legal profession also is more comfortable dealing with those medical practitioners who are familiar with, and regularly participate in, the legal process.

COMMUNICATION SKILLS

The main skill that forensic practitioners have in relation to their knowledge of the legal process is the ability to communicate medical fact and opinion, within the confines of the laws of evidence, to a tribunal composed largely of lay people. Medical practitioners are becoming increasingly better trained in the skills of communication, at both undergraduate and postgraduate levels. However, the skills they are taught relate largely to communicating with patients and with scientific and medical colleagues. These communication skills, while important and relevant, do not take into account the rules of evidence and legal procedure that constrain the way in which forensic medical practitioners communicate their findings to a court. A fundamental understanding of the legal process and the law of evidence can make all the difference in communicating matters of scientific fact and opinion during judicial proceedings. This area is covered in more detail in Chapter 19.

Forensic medical practitioners' communication skills are not confined to oral performance. Written communication is a feature of medico-legal work, and the formulation of appropriate medico-legal reports that meet the needs of the legal system is a basic task performed by the forensic pathologist. Medico-legal reports differ from ordinary medical reports in a variety of ways. Medico-legal reports do not have a fixed format but vary in their style and design according to their legal purpose. However, there is a basic structure to such reports, which can assist in their use by the justice system (see Appendix VII). The forensic pathologist, by training and experience, is usually well versed in the compilation of appropriate medico-legal reports.

Autopsy

The information that can be obtained by an autopsy is required by many different investigatory agencies and, as a result, the procedure has many purposes. The priority given to any specific purpose will vary according to the circumstances of the death so that, for example in the case of mass disasters, the issues of human identification and the reconstruction of the events leading to the death will be paramount.

For practical purposes, autopsies can be divided into two main groups: first, those performed for clinical medical reasons, and second, those performed for medico-legal reasons. The general pathological procedures of both of these autopsy types are the same; however, the emphasis placed on particular components of the autopsy differs. The issue of human identification is a good example of this difference. Identification of a deceased person is rarely an issue in autopsies performed for clinical medical purposes, whereas it is an essential element of medico-legal autopsies, with important ramifications for the coronial, criminal and civil justice systems.

The goals and aims of autopsies have differed over the centuries. Nowadays, however, there is considerable uniformity of purpose, most pathologists agreeing on the value of the procedure to medical and legal practice. Despite this, public perception of the role of the autopsy is clouded by misleading presentations in the media and by a degree of ignorance and indifference to the procedure communicated to them by some clinical medical practitioners. In order to understand the potential of the autopsy in human identification, it is important to consider what pathologists are attempting to achieve when they carry out the procedure.

The aims of the autopsy (forensic and clinical) include:

- confirmation or determination of the identity of the deceased;
- the identification of injuries and natural diseases;
- determination of the extent of injuries and natural diseases;
- determination of the effect of medical treatments;

- evaluation of the mode of death;
- determination of the cause of death;
- provision of an educational resource for the medical profession;
- provision of tissues for use in medical research and therapeutic procedures;
- retrieval of trace evidence and other samples for use as evidence in court;
- reconstruction of the circumstances surrounding the death.

In order meet these aims, all the stages of a death investigation must be carried out in a meticulous manner. In most cases, the identification of the deceased at autopsy is straightforward. However, where identification of the deceased is unknown, it is essential that the autopsy procedures used provide the best information possible on all the features that may be of use in determining identity. As discussed above, the autopsy serves many purposes, and in order for as many of these as possible to be accommodated, the pathologist must co-ordinate the activities of all forensic body examiners to ensure that they work as a team.

AUTOPSY PROCEDURES

The performance of an autopsy involves a series of medical tasks nearly all of which are similar to those performed in some aspects of clinical medical practice. Indeed the basic elements comprising all medical examinations are similar.

Preliminary matters

The first element of an autopsy is the identification of the goals or purpose of the examination. These goals may differ from case to case and depend upon the basis of the autopsy request. A coroner may have a different purpose in mind from the police, the family or a treating clinician. Each may separately be seeking answers to their own questions. It is up to the pathologist performing the autopsy to assure himself of the questions at issue in order to orientate the examination appropriately.

Where identification of the body is concerned, the pathologist must plan the autopsy in collaboration with the other investigators, including forensic odontologists, forensic anthropologists/osteologists and the police. This will ensure that the technical procedures carried out are complimentary and do not interfere adversely with each other. For example, in the case of procedures used in facial identification, it would be possible for some aspects of facial dissection to interfere with forensic radiology and photographic requirements. If the jaws are resected before skull or dental radiographs have been obtained, the relationship of the dental and facial structures cannot be used as a point of comparison with radiographs that may have been taken in life. The sequence of examination procedures is therefore of considerable importance and should never be left to chance.

Whether the autopsy is being performed for forensic or for medical reasons, some universal basic goals exist. These include identification of the deceased, discovery of significant disease processes and determination of the pathological states and injuries that have led, directly or indirectly, to the death. In the case of hospital autopsies, most of the disease processes and the cause of death will be known in advance. (Indeed, if the cause of death is unknown, the death *must* be referred to the coroner.) The main goal of the hospital autopsy is focused on determining the extent of the disease process and the effects of treatments provided in life. At the same time as investigating the death, the physical autopsy provides an opportunity for the collection of educational material for medical teaching and research. These autopsies require that consent for the procedure is given by those having legal control of the body, who must in turn ensure, in some jurisdictions, that relatives do not object. In practice, these requirements are met by obtaining the consent of the next-of-kin. In contrast to this, a medico-legal autopsy can be performed on the instructions of the coroner without consent having been obtained from the next-of-kin. This situation applies in the case of autopsies that are conducted principally to identify the deceased. There are instances in which the next-of-kin or other relatives can object to a coroner ordering an autopsy, but of course this cannot apply where the identity of the deceased is unknown.

Prior to examination of a body at a mortuary, the pathologist may already have carried out a superficial examination of the body in the place in which it was found. This is most likely to occur where the identity of the body is unknown and where the death appears to be suspicious. The scope of examination of a body at the scene of death depends on the circumstances but, in most cases, some initial information can be gathered from the position of the body, the presence or absence of rigor mortis or post mortem hypostatic lividity (discoloration of the skin) and the temperature of the body. A body that is fully clothed or otherwise wrapped and partly concealed may be difficult to examine adequately at the scene, and no definitive conclusions regarding the identity of the deceased or the nature of the death should be made until the body has been fully examined at autopsy and the necessary follow-up tests have been completed.

The next process involved in an autopsy is the retrieval and evaluation of information relating to the past medical and dental history of individuals who are missing and may be the deceased. The collection of ante mortem records is a specific phase in the processes involved in disaster victim identification, and most coroner and medical examiner jurisdictions will have protocols for this procedure. Mass disaster involving loss of life can be conveniently divided into two types: open disasters and closed disasters. Open disaster refers to the situation in which there is no record of the names of the individuals who may have been killed. Such a situation might be a major train crash: anyone in the community might be on a particular train, and it is not until friends and relatives report them missing that the investigators have an idea of who the deceased might be. In a closed disaster, there is a record of all people who might be involved. An example of a closed disaster is a plane crash where a list of passengers is immediately available from the airline. Clearly the task of identifying the individuals involved in a closed disaster is much simpler as the ante mortem investigation team know where to go for their information. This ante mortem information may include family and personal details, such as information regarding their last known activities, as well as background information on, for example, their work history, clothing and personal effects, and family background. Medical details, such as previous radiological examinations, drug history and previous surgical or dental procedures, are also important. While, in many cases, police investigators provide this information, it is often important for the pathologist and odontologist to be able to request particular information from or to speak to any dental or medical practitioners who have been involved with these suspected individuals prior to death. The ante mortem information collected should include actual medical and dental practitioners' files as well as photographs and radiographs of the suspected individuals taken in life.

Before the deceased's body is physically examined for identification purposes, it is necessary to carry out a number of preliminary investigations. This may involve the taking of specialist radiographs, blood tests for infectious diseases and/or photographs. Where the body is not too severely damaged, the deceased may have their fingerprints recorded or an attempt may be made to have them visually identified by a friend or a member of their family. These preliminary matters may take some time to complete before the physical autopsy can be commenced, and co-ordination of the whole process is essential at this time.

Post mortem radiology

Radiographic studies play an important part in the forensic autopsy and are particularly relevant in cases where the identity of the deceased is unknown. Comparison of post mortem radiographs with clinical radiographs taken in life can result in identity being established with a very high degree of certainty. The shapes of the frontal sinuses and dental structures are highly individual features and make post mortem radiography of the head almost mandatory in autopsies on unknown individuals. It is important to co-ordinate the radiological examination with the remainder of the autopsy procedures in order to minimize the risk that one process will interfere with another. For example, if the head is first opened with a saw, later radiographs of the frontal sinuses of the skull will be much more difficult to interpret. Similarly, the process of embalming a body may cause artefactual trauma and introduce air and fluids into body cavities, thus changing the radiological appearance (as well as interfering with the toxicological analysis of body fluids). Given its importance for craniofacial identification, some notes on the procedures for post mortem radiography of the head are covered here (see also Appendix VI).

While a variety of views of the head may be obtained, it is essential that the post mortem radiographs be comparable with clinical radiographs that may have been obtained in life. For this reason, standard views should be used at autopsy. In some cases in which clinical radiographs are already available, it may be necessary to take repeated post mortem radiographs with incremental repositioning of the deceased's head in order to obtain a post mortem radiographic view that is the same as the radiograph taken in life.

Anterior posterior skull

For this view, the body should be positioned supine with the film (24×30 cm) positioned lengthways immediately beneath (behind) the head. The head should be positioned so that there is no appreciable lateral rotation; a thin sponge placed behind the head can raise the head and make it stable on a flat surface. The skull base should be at 25 degrees from the perpendicular, and the head should be positioned so the central ray passes through the naison (the area just above the bridge of the nose).

Anterior posterior skull (angled 30 degrees down)

For this view, the body should be positioned supine in the anterior–posterior position so that the shoulders lie in the same transverse plane. The head should be positioned so that it lies in the mid-sagittal plane with the baseline perpendicular to the plane of the film (24×30 cm). The upper margin of the film cassette should be level with the uppermost part of the cranial vertex. With the head in this position, the X-ray tube should be orientated 30 degrees downward towards the feet so that the central ray passes through a point 6 cm above the eyebrows in the mid-sagittal plane.

Lateral skull

For this view, the body should be positioned supine in the anterior–posterior position, with the head slightly raised on a sponge. The shoulders should be positioned so that they lie on the same transverse plane, and the head positioned in the mid-sagittal plane without any lateral rotation. The film cassette, with grid, is placed in contact with the side of the head. The central ray is directed horizontally to the centre of the grid such that the central ray passes through the head 4 cm anterior to the external auditory meatus. Care must be taken to ensure that the field of view includes the entire skull.

Health and safety

Taking part in autopsy procedures necessarily involves some personal risk. This is particularly true when the identity and background of the deceased are unknown. Both physical injury and communication of infectious agents are potential hazards. Individuals infected with one of the types of infectious viral hepatitis, HIV or tuberculosis pose special risks. However, it should not be forgotten that commensal organisms can pose a threat to the operators if they are inoculated into their body tissues via a cutaneous injury. In deaths that have occurred as a result of major trauma, foreign materials present on or in the body may puncture protective clothing, including surgical gloves, and represent a significant hazard to the examiners. Any object, whether a part of the body or foreign material, that can cause a cutaneous injury needs to be identified in advance and counter measures instituted. Working with bodies that are very cold or frozen poses a particular risk as the operator's sense of touch and fine movement may become impaired. Control of the production of fluid splashes and aerosols during the autopsy should be given similar attention as these can also transmit infectious agents.

As well as physical injury being associated with the risk of transmitting infectious agents to the operator, other physical hazards can occur. The very act of moving heavy bodies and body parts can cause back and limb injuries, and these need to be avoided by the use of appropriate equipment and assistance. Chemical injuries to an operator can also occur if the body is contaminated, which can occur in a number of major disaster incidents and industrial deaths. Hydraulic fluids, caustic and corrosive chemicals, as well as gas and radiation hazards, must be anticipated and counter measures instituted at the appropriate time during the investigation. Deaths occurring in a setting of military action or terrorist activity may also involve complex highly toxic chemical contamination as well as explosive hazards from retained weapon projectiles and other explosive devices.

External examination

General aspects

The first stage of the physical examination of a body involves the removal of clothing, jewellery and any other wrappings from the body and is followed by inspection of the external surface of each region of the body. In doing this, great care must be taken not to lose any trace evidence that may be trapped in hair or adherent to the surface of the skin. For forensic and evidential purposes, all items removed from the body must be documented, including being described and photographed, before being collected in a controlled, safe and secure manner for later possible forensic examination. Amongst other procedures, this involves labelling and logging of specimens in such a way that a continuous chain of custody of the item is maintained from the time of its collection until its appearance in court as an exhibit.

Craniofacial region

The eyes, ears, mouth and nose are examined, together with the adjacent skin. Again, great care must be taken not to lose trace evidence that may be present in the external ears, the nose or the mouth. Such material may be foreign to the body or comprise body tissues such as fragments of bone or teeth. Where the body is grossly decomposed, there is a risk that easily detached structures may be lost from the body during handling and transportation. Teeth are a good example of such vulnerable structures, and every care must be taken to ensure that they are not lost during body recovery. In the case of badly burnt remains, the skeletal tissues themselves may become carbonized. In this state, the bony and dental hard tissue remains may be extremely friable and brittle, and, as a result, they may need to be stabilized with resins, glues and or waxes before the body remains are handled.

The initial stage of the external examination of the head is very similar to the general external medical examination performed on the living; indeed, similar medical and dental equipment can be used. For example, auroscopes may be of use in examining the nose and the mouth as well as the ears. The ordinary characteristics of faces with which we are all familiar should be noted. This includes features such as eye and hair colour, skin pigmentation, facial hair and the shape of the ears, nose and lips. In addition, the appearance of hairstyle and the distribution and type of cosmetics on the face should be described. Evidence of previous medical treatment and injuries, including scars as well as marks such as tattoos, must also be noted as these can assist with confirming identification as well as with corroborating other information from medical records or witness statements. In the case of a forensic autopsy, special attention is given to the classification and recording of injuries. Detailed injury descriptions are crucial if the pathologist is to assist with reconstructing the circumstances surrounding the death and effectively present such evidence in court. In this respect, the use of charts, diagrams and photographs to record the observations and findings is essential.

It is during the external examination of the head and neck that the pathologist and odontologist can plan the approach they will take in their internal examination of the head. Such discussions are essential to prevent any possibility that examination by one will impede examination by the other.

Post-cranial region

The external examination of a body in a forensic autopsy concentrates as much on the extraneous material as it does on human tissues. Such an examination therefore includes not only the surface of the body but also all of the clothing, jewellery and other foreign material that may be present. The identification of paint flakes, soil, grime and vegetable matter on the surface of the body may be of considerable importance in an investigation, and collection of that material for further forensic examination may be required. Similarly, the nature of jewellery, its type and its position on the body can be significant. In some cases, the presence of jewellery may contribute to particular injury patterns; in other cases, it may be a unique personal item that can help to confirm the identity of an individual.

A record of the basic morphometric features of the body is an essential element of all autopsies. In routine cases, this may simply take the form of measurements of height and weight. However, in the case of some autopsies, additional measurements will be needed. In the case of skeletal remains, morphometric assessment of key portions of the skeleton is relevant for anthropological assessment of race, sex, height and age.

The process of external examination at autopsy involves the largest organ of the body, namely the skin. The presence of old and recent injuries to the body surface is of particular interest to the forensic pathologist, but the recording of patterns of pigmentation, tattoos, hair distribution and the presence of dermatological diseases can be of considerable importance in determining the identity of an individual. The hands and feet may show anatomical features acquired as a result of a particular occupation, and the loss of digits is a useful identifying characteristic. Documentation of rigor mortis (stiffening of the muscles after death) and livor mortis (discoloration of the skin caused by settling of the blood in dependent blood vessels after death) is also important, but in bodies showing advanced decomposition, these features cannot usually be identified.

The description of wounds is critical to any forensic medical examination, whether the subject is deceased or living. Descriptions of all injuries should be recorded in detail in the autopsy notes, using terms that are objective rather than subjective. For example, an injury might be described objectively as 'a red zone of skin measuring 5 cm in diameter with areas of brown and yellow discoloration within it and having an indistinct border'. A subjective description of this same wound might be 'a 5 cm bruise showing signs of ageing'. The advantage of an objective description of a wound is that it does not presuppose the cause or nature of the injury. While cumbersome, such objective descriptions are of particular use to other medical experts who may be seeking alternative explanations for the injury.

Descriptions of identifying marks, wounds and injuries should always be given by reference to the patient in the standard anatomical position: the body standing erect and facing forwards, with the arms by the sides and the palms of the hands facing the front. This standard body position provides a constant reference point for terms such as superior, inferior, anterior and posterior, and provides consistency in the description of the location of marks on the body.

The position of marks and wounds on the body should also, whenever possible, be located by reference to fixed bony landmarks. This is preferable to using soft tissue landmarks such as the umbilicus or the nipples. The position of such characteristics can be measured in relation to bony prominences such as the tibial tuberosity, the iliac crest or the spinous process.

In describing a wound, the forensic medical examiner takes note of its site, its size, its shape and its surrounds. The colour, contour, course and contents of a wound should also be recorded. In addition to these general descriptive features, the forensic examiner should comment on other characteristics such as the depth of the wound and the nature of its borders.

The general principle for describing injuries in forensic autopsies is that the description in the notes made following an accurate forensic medical examination should assist in the identification of the individual and in the reconstruction of the events in which the injury occurred. As a result, it is vital that the recording of injuries and identifying features should be optimum. Charts, radiographs, photographs and videos should be used where appropriate.

While measurements of a body are difficult to obtain with a high degree of precision, it is important to record at least the weight and size of the body. Height, or crown–heel length, is only one of a variety of morphometric values that can be determined from a body. The use of multiple measurements as a technique for the identification of an individual is now only of historical importance, but isolated measurements can still be of value in distinguishing between a small number of different individuals. For example, shoe and hat sizes may be a good discriminator between some people.

Internal examination

On completion of the external examination, an internal examination is carried out. This part of the autopsy involves an examination of each of the body's main cavities and the organs within them. These cavities include the cranial, thoracic and abdominal cavities, but areas such as the head, face, neck, spine, limbs, pelvis and genitalia are also examined. The basic instruments used in these procedures are the same as those used in routine surgery. While the exposure of the body contents is more extensive during an autopsy, the way in which incisions are made and the organs dissected is again only a minor modification of routine surgical techniques.

The internal examination of the head and neck of a body may be performed in a variety of ways. In practice, the method chosen will depend on the identification issues that need to be addressed and the state of the human remains (burnt, decomposed, traumatized or skeletonized). Similarly, the procedures performed during the internal autopsy will depend on the particular comparison technique for identification that is to be employed. For example, if dental identification systems are to be used, one or all of such techniques as oral photography, jaw radiography, exposure of the oral cavity, dental impressions and excision of the jaws might be employed.

The conduct of the internal examination of the body at autopsy involves a systematic examination of the organs and tissues found within the body cavities and the solid tissues forming the musculoskeletal system. The recording of this process may be documented using an anatomical or body system approach. In either case, a high degree of importance is placed on the use of objective descriptive terms in the report that are later interpreted in relation to their significance regarding the presence of injury or disease. The cranial cavity, thorax, abdomen and pelvis comprise the regions of the body that receive the most attention during the internal examination. Not only are the major organs from these cavities examined but also the walls of the cavities themselves are assessed for characteristic features and signs of disease.

The visual inspection of body organs is only one part of the physical autopsy process. Some diseases involve alterations only to the microscopic appearances of body tissues. In other cases, a disease will first be visible as a microscopic change to the body tissues that precedes any changes to the 'naked eye' appearance of the relevant body organ. An example of the latter can be seen in the case of 'myocardial infarction', one of the pathological processes that can cause a heart attack. This pathology can occur when parts of the heart muscle are starved of blood and die. It may take several days of survival of the patient for the dead areas of heart muscle to become visible to the 'naked eye', and if the patient dies before this, the macroscopic autopsy may be unrevealing. However, the microscopic signs of damage are visible much earlier (in the case of electron microscopy, after a matter of hours), and it is therefore essential that the heart muscle is examined under the microscope. In practice, the only way to ensure that these issues are covered is to perform routine microscopy on all body tissues. Of course, it is logistically impossible to examine microscopically all of each tissue, but adequate sampling can be achieved so that an optimal pathology detection rate is established.

With some body organs, macroscopic examination at the time of the physical autopsy is particularly difficult. Organs such as the brain and the spinal cord are so soft and fragile that they may be damaged and distorted by the process of the dissection and tissue sampling. In these cases, it is often necessary to process the organs by 'fixing' them in a preservative solution in order that they can be made more rigid and capable of detailed dissection. In the case of brain diseases or trauma, this is generally advisable, although there are exceptional circumstances when dissection of the brain can be performed without fixation. These comments relating to the brain are also applicable to other body organs in particular circumstances of disease, so it may be necessary to retain such organs during the physical autopsy and 'fix' them for further examination. Unfortunately, the fixation process can take some time to render the organ suitable for specialist examination. In the case of solid organs such as the brain, it may take several weeks for fixation to be completed. This can result in difficulties with respect to the disposal of the body of the deceased. Families usually require that the funeral take place within a few days of the death and, as a result, the body may in some cases have to be buried or cremated without the organs that are undergoing fixation. For many families, this poses no significant problem. In many ways, the situation is no different from that when a person leaves hospital after surgery, a diseased part of their body having been removed and now being stored in a jar in the pathology department. What is important in both these situations is that, following the completion of the specialist pathology examinations, the tissues or organs are disposed of in a safe, secure and decent manner. For some families, however, the fact that a deceased person has been buried or cremated without all their organs is distressing and amounts to an incomplete disposal of their loved one. In these cases, it is often possible to arrange for a second, small, funeral-like process for the remaining tissues and organs after they have been examined.

As well as demonstrating the presence of disease or injury, the autopsy can reveal the extent of the disease and some of the effects of treatments that have been provided. However, many disorders are the result of functional disturbances of body systems that involve abnormalities of vital responses. Unless these abnormal responses have caused macroscopic or microscopic structural changes in the body tissues, they will not ordinarily be detected by the physical autopsy. The same is true in association with deaths due to some drugs and poisons. Although such chemicals can cause visible alterations to body organs, the changes are in many cases non-specific, and toxicological tests will have to be performed on tissues and fluids collected from the body during the physical autopsy in order to identify them. In both these cases, the physical autopsy may reveal no specific visible abnormalities. It is only by analysing the circumstances of the death, including the medical history, and by collecting samples from the body for testing that the death can be understood.

The physical autopsy is not complete until the body of the deceased person has been restored to a state in which the family, as part of their funeral tradition, can view it. The technical and scientific staff who are employed in assisting in this task are usually highly skilled and experienced. They are aware of the needs of the funeral industry, and a number will also be qualified embalmers. In all cases, the aim is to restore the outward appearance of the deceased to that visible before death. In deaths from severe trauma, specialized restorative techniques may be required to repair areas of the body damaged before the autopsy. Similarly, if large amounts of structurally significant tissue, such as the spinal column or the pelvis have been collected for investigation or transplantation, more extensive restorative work will be required. In most cases, relatively little restoration is required because the routine procedures employed in a standard autopsy are intrinsically non-disfiguring.

Post-autopsy procedures

Following completion of the restoration and reconstruction of the body, it is washed, wrapped and stored awaiting collection by the family's funeral director. However, even at this stage, various issues have to be kept in mind. The body must be stored in a safe and secure environment. Unless the body is being stored for several weeks, it should not be allowed to become frozen but must be kept cold enough to delay significant decomposition. This can be more difficult to achieve than is often realized since some deaths are associated with the rapid onset and progression of decomposition even in otherwise ideal environments.

When should a body be returned to the family for disposal? This question has been the subject of considerable debate amongst disaster victim investigators. For an event involving many deceased persons, the general principle is that no body should be released for disposal until all the victims have been identified. The alternate position is that, if a body has been identified by two or more independent criteria, it can be released. The major problem arises in closed disasters where identification uses a process of elimination to reconcile the lists of the presumed dead with the autopsy results. If a body is selected as being potentially two different individuals, more scientific and medical work will have to be performed to reconcile the ambiguity. If, however, one of these bodies has already been disposed of, it may be extremely difficult to resolve the problem.

In theory, a complex autopsy could take months to complete, but, in practice the physical autopsy takes in most cases a few hours. This means that the performance of an autopsy, be it for medical or medicolegal reasons, should not introduce any significant delay to a family's funeral arrangements.

Of course, even when the body of the deceased has been returned to the family, the autopsy process continues. There are chemical and toxicological tests to complete, histological specimens to be examined under the microscope and case conference discussions to be held. All of these processes take time, and it would be usual for it to take between 2 and 6 weeks for the final report on the death to be available. Despite this, limited information is usually available from the pathologist immediately following the autopsy and, in most circumstances, pathologists are happy to speak to family members or their personal medical practitioners about the interim findings.

The timely completion of an accurate and informative final autopsy report is an essential aspect of post-autopsy procedure. Such reports have to be clear and understandable to the various groups who require autopsy information. Unfortunately, the varied nature of the people who need the information makes it difficult to phrase an autopsy report in appropriate terms. For example, a family member may need information in non-medical language while the deceased's medical specialist may require more precise medical information. In the case of autopsies where people from different backgrounds all need access to the report, real communication problems can arise. In practice, the pathologist finds that he or she is working for several clients, each differing in their approach to the death investigation. Even though, strictly speaking, forensic pathologists are working solely for the coroner, they must keep in mind that their autopsy report may eventually make its way into the criminal or civil justice systems.

Recommended reading

Busuttil A, Jones JSP. 1990. *Deaths in major disasters: the pathologist's role*. London: Royal College of Pathologists.
Hill RB, Anderson RE. 1988. *The autopsy: medical practice and public policy*. Boston: Butterworths.
Knight B. 1991. *Forensic pathology*. London: Edward Arnold.
Selby, H. (ed.) 1992. *The aftermath of death: Coronials*. Leichhardt, NSW: Federation Press.

CHAPTER 4

Craniofacial anatomy

CA BRIGGS, M MARTAKIS

Introduction	37	Developmental and growth changes	42
General considerations	37	Factors of individualization	46
Normal anatomy	38		

Introduction

Craniofacial identification is based upon the premise that an individual's morphology is largely dependent upon his or her underlying bone structure. That is, facial details bear a reliable relationship to features of the skull. While other parts of the skeleton may provide important clues to the characteristics of an individual, it is the skull alone which conveys a personal portrait: the 'bony core of the fleshy head and face in life' (Krogman and Iscan, 1986, p. 417). However, before a likeness of the deceased can be produced, certain parameters need to be established. Principal amongst these are race, sex and age. Estimates of stature and weight may also be useful as facial soft tissue depth is said to bear a relationship to nutritional status and thus to body form (Rhine and Campbell, 1980; Caldwell, 1986). Although most of this information would be obtained from examination of a complete skeleton, the skull alone can provide valuable insights, especially with regard to racial features. It is not the purpose of this chapter, however, to describe the extensive anthropological characteristics of the skull, nor even detailed features of individual bones, but to indicate how the anatomical composition and salient features of the skull form a basis for craniofacial identification.

General considerations

The skull is broadly composed of two types of bone: cranial and facial. Cranial bones enclose a single cavity that surrounds the brain, while the facial bones form a number of smaller cavities (orbital, nasal and oral) around the sense organs. The cranial cavity is dome shaped with a smooth convex roof (cranial vault) and an uneven floor (cranial base). The latter is divided into three regions – anterior, middle and posterior cranial fossae – that lie at progressively lower levels from front to back. The ventral surface of the brain lies against this base, which consequently contains a number of foraminae for exiting cranial nerves and entering and exiting vascular structures. The facial skeleton is suspended below the anterior and middle cranial fossae, the upper end of the gut tube being attached to the back of the facial skeleton anteriorly and suspended from the middle fossa posteriorly, while below the posterior fossa lie the supporting vertebrae with their cavity – the vertebral canal – for the spinal cord. While the structure of the cervical spine is not discussed in this chapter, the degree of cervical lordosis influences the position of the head in relation to the cervical column and may therefore have a bearing on craniofacial morphology.

Normal anatomy

Study of the skull as a whole, and even of its individual bones, is best undertaken by viewing it from standard positions called 'norma' (Latin: a carpenter's square). These are the normae frontalis, lateralis, occipitalis, verticalis and basalis. The skull is placed in a standard reference position with a line connecting the inferior orbital margin to the upper aspect of the external auditory meatus set in the horizontal plane, the so-called 'Frankfort plane'. Of these views, the normae frontalis, lateralis and verticalis provide most of the salient information for craniofacial reconstruction; however, distinctive features of both the norma basalis and norma occipitalis may influence the final result.

NORMA FRONTALIS

This view illustrates aspects of all three cavities of the face as well as the larger facial bones. It is best to begin below with the lower jaw or mandible (Figs 4.1 and 4.2). This is a separate bone that articulates via its condylar head with the squamous temporal bone of the cranial base. Thus it may be studied alone and subsequently put aside to allow an unfettered view of the remainder of the skull.

The mandible consists of two rectangular plates on each side: a horizontal plate called the body and a vertical plate called the ramus. The body bears the teeth, within sockets in its alveolar process, while the ramus is for articulation and attachment of the muscles of mastication. On the body in the midline is the mental protuberance, with a median ridge above and an elevated triangular area below, representing the site of fusion of the two halves of the mandible and its modification by the process of remodelling. Anthropometrically, the lowest point of the mandible in the midline is referred to as the gnathion. Posterolaterally, the angle of the mandible – the gonion – represents a point on the ramus where the intersection of lines drawn along the inferior and posterior borders of the bone meet. It is often flared (gonial flare) or everted, particularly in males, by the attachment of the masseter muscle, and in these situations, the bigonial breadth is widened. The ramus diverges above into condylar (behind) and coronoid (in front) processes, with an intervening mandibular notch. Surmounted on the condyle is the expanded oval-shaped head, with its constricted neck just below bearing a pit (pterygoid fovea) anteriorly for the insertion of the lateral pterygoid muscle. The coronoid process receives the tendon of temporalis, a very large muscle of mastication, which, along with other masticatory muscles, may leave prominent

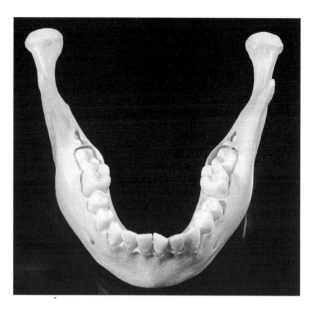

Fig. 4.1 Anterosuperior view of the human adult mandible

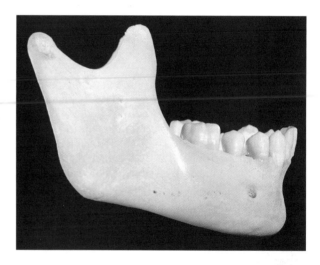

Fig. 4.2 Lateral view of the human adult mandible

characteristic markings on the bone. Since masticatory muscles give shape to the face and contribute to the contours of the cheek (Gerasimov, 1971), much useful craniofacial information can be gleaned from careful examination of these features.

The mandible is often used to sex skeletal remains, and several measures may be taken on the bone (Bass, 1987). For example, the bicondylar breadth, the direct transverse distance between the most lateral points on the two condyles, is usually greater in males. The mandible in the male is more robust, larger and thicker than in the female, with greater body height, especially at the protuberance, and a broader ascending ramus. The gonial angle is less obtuse (less than 125 degrees), the condyles are larger and the chin is square (Bass, 1987), in contrast to being V-shaped in females.

The remainder of the frontal view is dominated by the frontal bone, contributing to the cranial vault above the superior orbital margins (Fig. 4.3). The frontal tuber is a prominent swelling above each margin, the site of the primary centre of ossification of the bone (the two indicating its paired origin). The superciliary arches (brow ridges) are low, curved ridges immediately above the superior orbital margins. Their medial ends meet above the nose at another low prominence termed the glabella (Latin: 'glabrous' = smooth and bare), a smooth area of bone just above the frontonasal suture, the midpoint of which is termed the nasion. Lateral to the frontonasal suture, the frontal bone articulates with the frontal process of the maxilla, and further laterally it articulates with the lacrimal bone (within the orbit). At the superior margin of the orbit itself is the supraorbital notch, for passage of the supraorbital nerve and vessels. This is continued laterally by the zygomatic process of the frontal bone articulating with the zygomatic bone. The bony orbit is formed by contributions from adjacent bones: the frontal bone with part of the lesser wing of the sphenoid forms its roof;

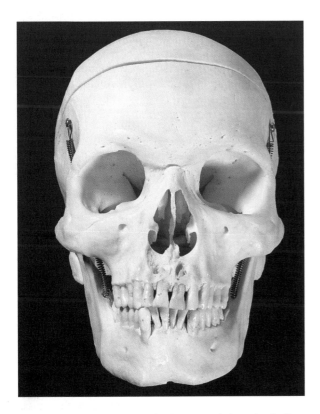

Fig. 4.3 Anterior view of the human adult male skull

the maxilla and zygomatic bones, with a small contribution from the palatine bone, comprising the floor; the lateral wall is formed by part of the zygomatic bone as well as by the orbital surface of the greater wing of the sphenoid; and the frontal process of the maxilla, lacrimal, ethmoid and a small part of the body of the sphenoid contribute to the medial wall.

The two nasal bones form the bony 'bridge' of the nose, their sinuous curve from above downwards, and convexity from side to side, providing important clues for identification. Inside the anterior nasal aperture can be seen the bony septum, comprising the perpendicular plate of the ethmoid and vomer, with the junction of the two parts of the maxilla in the midline forming the prominent anterior nasal spine (a uniquely human characteristic amongst the primates). Laterally, the bony conchae are visible, and on either side of the anterior nasal spine, the lower margin of the nasal aperture may be hollowed out to a variable depth in the form of the 'nasal gutter'.

The maxilla is characterized by a large alveolar process for the upper dentition (resorption of the alveolar processes occurs with ageing, particularly in edentulous skulls, and can be seen at the margins of the maxilla illustrated in Fig. 4.3) but has named bony processes, projecting to the frontal and zygomatic bones. Sutures develop at sites of articulation, that joining the maxilla to the zygoma being the most prominent. The zygomatic bone bridges the facial skeleton to the cranial bones from this articulation through its two processes to the frontal and temporal bones. The infraorbital foramen of the maxilla is visible below the lower margin of the orbit, lying in the approximate line of the supraorbital foramen. The canine eminence demarcates the root of the upper canine tooth, the longest of all the teeth. Medial to it is the incisive fossa and laterally the canine fossa (particularly prominent in Caucasian skulls).

A detailed tabulation of traits diagnostic of sex features in the skull may be found in Krogman (1955), but some are noted here. The bones comprising the frontal view are generally smaller in the female, with smoother and less pronounced landmarks. Features that distinguish the sexes include the contour of the forehead, which, due to a more prominent frontal tuber, is higher and more vertical in the female than in the male; the superciliary arches are much less strongly developed than in the male, the orbits are higher, more rounded and relatively larger compared with the upper facial skeleton (because of smaller maxillary antra), and the orbital margins sharper and less rounded than in the male. In the male, the nasal aperture is higher and narrower, and its margins are sharp rather than rounded. The male nasal bones are also larger and tend to meet in the midline at a sharper angle.

NORMA LATERALIS

Figure 4.4 clearly shows how the curvature of the cranial vault is influenced by three vault bones: frontal, parietal and occipital. It also illustrates the central role of the zygomatic bone, connecting the maxilla of the facial skeleton to the temporal bone (via the zygomatic arch) and to the frontal bone, forming part of the lateral margin of the orbit.

Above the temporal bone are the temporal lines that arch up and back before curving forwards again to form the supramastoid crest, continuous with the upper border of the zygomatic arch and enclosing the shallow temporal fossa, from where the temporalis muscle originates. Its depth may provide an indication of the thickness of the temporalis muscle and hence provide a clue to facial appearance, although the reliability of this feature is unproven (Keen, 1950). The zygomatic arch represents the widest part of the face and, because of its prominence, is commonly fractured, often with depression of the separated parts. The norma lateralis also shows the overall profile of the face, the degree of projection of the chin, protrusion of the teeth and prominence of the nasal bones and nasal spine. The body and ramus of the mandible are again clearly seen, with the temporomandibular joint, in front of the external auditory meatus, and the mastoid process projecting inferiorly behind this. Portions of the major vault sutures – coronal, squamous (squamoparietal) and lambdoidal – are all visible from the lateral view, as are lateral-anterior sites, for example sphenofrontal, sphenoparietal and sphenotemporal. Together with

the coronal and squamosal sutures, the anterolateral sutures form an intersecting pattern that demarcates the pterion, a region of bone deep to which branches of the middle meningeal artery groove the bone, these vessels being susceptible to laceration in skull fractures at this site.

NORMA OCCIPITALIS

The occipital view of the skull provides little information for craniofacial reconstruction that has not already been deciphered from the frontal and lateral aspects. Nevertheless, examination of the occipital region is worthwhile as it provides evidence of the robustness of the skeleton and hence a further clue to gender. For example, the external occipital protuberance is much larger in the male, as are the occipital condyles, and the transverse (nuchal) occipital lines are more evident. At the opisthocranion, a position just above the external occipital protuberance, the skull attains its greatest posterior extent. The distance from this landmark to the glabella provides an index of maximal cranial length. The occipital view may also be useful in determining race: in the Caucasian skull, the external occipital protuberance has a conical or hook-shaped appearance, while in the Australian aboriginal, the external occipital protuberance is absent but a pronounced transverse occipital torus often occurs. This view of the skull also shows convergence of the sagittal and lambdoidal sutures, which meet at the lambda. Sutural bones, small islands of bone lying within the suture, are common at this site and should not be confused with fractures of the skull.

NORMA VERTICALIS

This view shows the ellipsoid shape of the cranial contour, with the point of greatest maximal breadth of the vault at the parietal eminence (parietal tuber), a primary centre of ossification (Fig. 4.5).

This again illustrates the three vault sutures bordering the parietal bone: coronal, between the frontal and the two parietal bones; sagittal, between the two parietals themselves; and lambdoid, between the parietal bones and the occipital bone. The coronal and sagittal sutures meet at the bregma, and the sagittal and lambdoidal at the lambda, in the adult, but these are sites in the fetus of the anterior and posterior fontanelles. Sutural bones are most common at the borders of the parietal bone. While possessing few distinctive bony features, examination of the vertical view of the skull is important for craniofacial reconstruction as it may help to confirm the racial affiliation of the deceased. Because the zygomatic bones are large, prominent and angular in Mongoloid

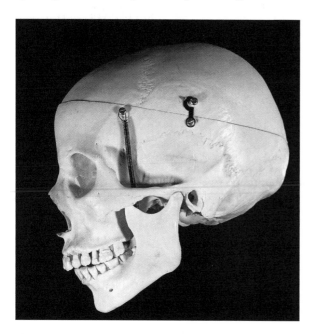

Fig. 4.4 Lateral view of the human adult skull

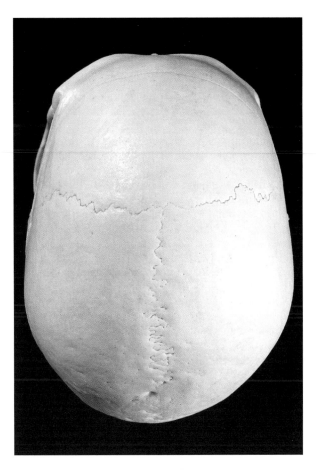

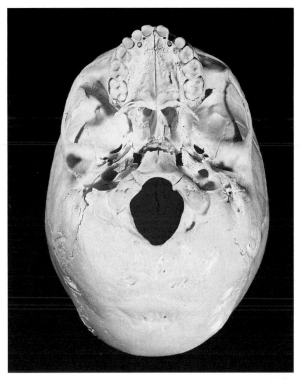

Fig. 4.6   View of the base of the human adult skull

Fig. 4.5   Vertical view of the human adult skull

skulls, they are usually visible lateral to the parietal bones, a feature not uncommon in the Australian aboriginal. In contrast, Caucasian skulls rarely reveal prominence of the zygomatic arches beyond the lateral margins of the parietals.

NORMA BASALIS

This inferior view of the skull is complex, displaying features both of frontal bones and of the cranial base, with its numerous foraminae for neurovascular structures. Therefore no attempt is made here to document its anatomy in detail. It is normally divided into three zones (Williams *et al.*, 1989) for descriptive purposes (Fig. 4.6).

The anterior zone comprises the hard palate and the upper dentition, i.e. the inferior view of the frontal bones as they attach to the cranial base. The posterior zone is located behind a transverse line drawn tangential to the anterior margin of the foramen magnum, that is, those features to which struc-

tures of the neck attach. The intermediate zone is occupied mainly by the base of the sphenoid, the petrous processes of the temporal bone and the basilar part of the occipital bone in between.

The width of the hard palate, as measured between the outside of the second molars, is quite variable, although it tends to be broader and shallower in males than females (El Najaar and McWilliams, 1978). The hard palate is often dome shaped and, in the Mongoloid skull, short and wide. A palatine torus, a bony exostosis alongside the intermaxillary suture, and mandibular tori are often present. The site of the spheno-occipital synchondrosis (basilar 'suture') and its status is of considerable importance. Redfield (1970) indicated that this 'suture' is united between the ages of 20 and 29, while Krogman and Iscan (1986) suggested a mean age of 23 and a range of 20 to 25 years. Suchey (1993), basing her observations on documented skulls of teenagers, indicates that the 'suture' can close as early as 14 in females and 16 in males. Thus, if the basilar 'suture' is closed in a skeleton of unknown sex, its age can be determined to be 14 or older. If the 'suture' is open, the individual is likely to be 18 or younger. Suchey (1993) further points out that skulls with an open 'suture' are generally too young to determine sex accurately.

Developmental and growth changes

The skull is a composite of individual bones. As a general rule, those of the cranial base develop by endochondral ossification while those of the cranial vault and facial skeleton develop in membrane. Regardless of the process of ossification, however, bone first appears as a model made up of a condensation of mesenchyme. The terms 'endochondral' and 'intramembranous' refer only to the process by which the bones are formed; histologically, they are identical. However, this distinction is important since it determines not only the process of ossification occurring at the different growth sites but also the type of articulation between individual bones. Some bones are found exclusively in the vault, for example the parietal (therefore a membrane bone), or in the cranial base, for example the ethmoid (an endochondral bone). Others (the occipital, temporal and sphenoid) have parts in each and are therefore formed by both processes. This has sequelae should these parts later fail to fuse.

PATTERN OF OSSIFICATION

Where and at what time ossification commences within the model (be it of cartilage or membrane), how it spreads to form the bone and the manner by which that bone grows describe the pattern of ossification. While it is not the purpose of this chapter to review the processes of ossification, it is pertinent to note that bone formation in membrane, as well as in a cartilage model, is preceded by the appearance of a 'primary' centre of ossification. Subsequent sites or centres are referred to as secondary centres of ossification. At a typical endochondral site, a primary centre appears in early intra-uterine life, normally between the sixth and eighth weeks, in which primary mesenchyme condenses at the surface of the model to form a membrane called the periosteum. Here, osteoblasts lay down compact or periosteal bone so that the bone grows by apposition to its surfaces. Interestingly, some dermal bones of the facial skeleton also develop cartilaginous growth plates, for example the condylar and coronoid cartilages of the mandible and the malar cartilage of the maxilla. The most important of these is the condylar cartilage because of its significant contribution to the growth of the mandible and therefore the lower facial skeleton. These cartilages are secondary cartilages and, although ossifying by endochondral ossification, do so by a process different from that seen with primary cartilage (Johnson and Moore, 1989).

CRANIAL BASE

The bones of the cranial base are 'cartilage' bones. The cartilage model thus replaced is called the chondrocranium. It develops between the overlying brain and underlying foregut by the condensation and segmentation of intervening mesenchyme, which thus produces head somitomeres and occipital somites. Their sclerotomes subsequently undergo chondrification to form the discrete hyaline cartilages of the chondrocranium. The first cartilages appear as early as the fifth to seventh week of intrauterine life, and while some develop adjacent to the midline, others develop laterally. Foramina form in the cranial base for exiting cranial nerves and entering vascular structures, some where adjacent lateral cartilages join with paramedian ones and some between cartilages. They occur between lateral and paramedian cartilages or between lateral cartilages themselves. The internal acoustic meatus and cribriform plate of the ethmoid form in conjunction with the two sensory capsules (otic and nasal), while the hypoglossal canal develops between occipital sclerotomes. With ossification of the chondrocranium, the bones of the cranial base meet each other at primary cartilaginous (synchondrotic) joints, which represent remnants of the original cartilage model.

CRANIAL VAULT

The bones of the cranial vault are 'membrane' bones. The membrane model is formed from the mesenchyme of the head somitomeres and occipital somites. As is typical of intramembranous ossification, centres of ossification appear directly in the mesenchymal membrane surrounding the developing brain. Vault bones meet each other at sutural joints that represent remnants of the original mesenchyme. It is worth noting that those parts of the greater wing of the sphenoid and squamous occipital bones contributing to the vault are dermal bones. They unite with the base (endochondral) parts of their respective bones. In fact, the temporal bone is a composite of four bones: the petrous develops by endochondral ossification in the cartilage of the otic capsule; the squamous and tympanic develop from intramembranous ossification; and the styloid forms by endochondral ossification of the dorsal end of Reichert's cartilage (the cartilage of the second branchial arch).

FACIAL SKELETON

These bones develop mainly by the intramembranous ossification of membrane derived from neural crest

cells, there being a small contribution from the endochondral ossification of the cartilages of the nasal
capsule and those of the first and second pharyngeal
arches. In the development of the head and neck,
mesoderm of the first pharyngeal arch forms the
maxillary and mandibular processes of the face.
Intramembranous ossification of this mesoderm subsequently forms the dermal bones of the facial skeleton. The maxillary process gives rise to the
development of an arc of four dermal bones: from
front to back, premaxilla, maxilla, zygoma and squamous temporal. (Other dermal bones to develop in
this mesoderm are the palatine, vomer, lacrimal and
nasal.) The mandibular process gives rise to only one
dermal bone, the mandible. There is a single ossification centre in each of these dermal bones. In the
mandible, the primary centre of ossification appears
near the centre of its membrane model, adjacent to
Meckels' cartilage at the terminal division of the
inferior alveolar nerve. Ossification proceeds below
the nerve, forms a cradle for it and finally entraps it.
Secondary cartilage subsequently develops on the
condylar and coronoid processes of the ramus,
which, by endochondral ossification, become growth
sites. The condylar process is an important site for
lower facial growth postnatally. The pattern for the
maxilla is similar, its primary centre appearing in the
membrane of the maxillary process. The bony capsule of the nose is preformed in cartilage (of the
chondrocranium) and it too ossifies endochondrally.
Part of the cartilage of the septum remains unossified
and is believed to be an important primary growth
site for the face.

PATTERNS OF SKULL GROWTH

The extent to which the skull increases in size and
thickness with age is arguable. Israel (1973, 1977)
examined the degree of craniofacial expansion
occurring during ageing and reported symmetrical
enlargement in all areas, with the exception of the
skull tables, sella turcica and frontal sinus, enlargement in these being considerably greater than in
other skull components. Johnson and Moore (1989)
reviewed the postnatal growth of the skull and indicated that the bones of the neurocranium follow,
as does the developing brain they house, a 'neural
growth curve', while the bones of the viscerocranium
follow a 'somatic curve'. It is therefore not surprising to observe in the fetal skull a ratio of neurocranium to viscerocranium in the order of 8:1 (Fig. 4.7).

The face subsequently grows predominantly postnatally, particularly under the influence of the teeth
and jaws, which are responsible for significant facial
growth (Berkovitz and Moxham, 1988). Johnson and
Moore (1989) also consider the dimensions of the

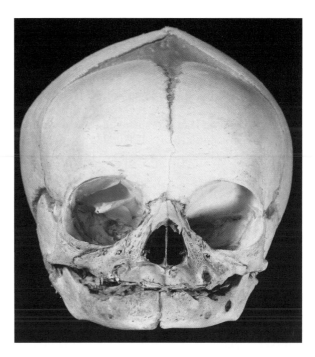

Fig. 4.7   Anterior view of the human fetal skull

vault to increase along all three axes so that the contained cranial cavity expands equally. Following
maturity, the vault bones become thicker, muscle
markings become more prominent and there is
enlargement of the superciliary arches. Parameters
have also been defined which allow a measure of the
growth of the cranial base (Johnson and Moore,
1989). These include the 'basicranial axis', from the
anterior margin of the foramen magnum to the pituitary fossa, the 'anterior extension' from the pituitary
fossa to the nasion, and the 'sphenoethmoidal angle',
which represents the angle between the two. The basicranial axis and anterior extension both follow a
somatic growth curve. However, that of the anterior
extension has been shown to follow a neural curve if
measured to the anterior edge of the cribriform plate
of the ethmoid (the adolescent growth spurt being
attributable to an increase in thickness of the frontal
bone). The sphenoethmoidal angle increases prena-
tally from 130 to 150 degrees but after birth decreases once more. Parameters used to determine growth
of the facial skeleton are its height, anteroposterior
length and width. All follow a somatic growth curve,
but the increase in height is relatively greater than
that in length, which is in turn greater than the
increase in width.

It is important to note that, while the orbits functionally house and protect the eyeball, they make a
major contribution to the facial skeleton. Because the
eyeball is an outgrowth of the developing brain, the
bones of the orbit, like the eye itself, follow a neural

growth curve. By adolescence, they are fully developed, and the increase in height of the facial skeleton seen at that time occurs suborbitally (Figs 4.8 and 4.9). The enlargement of the maxillary air sinuses is a major contributory factor to this change. The increase in anteroposterior length of the facial skeleton is again least in the orbits, greater below the orbits in the upper face and greatest in the lower jaw. This mandibular growth is attributable to growth at the condylar cartilage.

GROWTH SITES IN THE SKULL

Bone grows and remodels on all its surfaces. Nevertheless, that site where the rate of bone deposition is greatest forms the major growth site for the bone. The dermal bones of the cranial vault follow a neural growth curve, allowing the enclosed cranial cavity to expand equally, with growth occurring at the major sutures. Growth at the sagittal suture leads to enlarged width of the cranial cavity, growth in a transverse suture, such as the coronal and lambdoid sutures, gives rise to increased length, while growth

at a horizontal suture such as the squamoparietal leads to an increase in height. Concomitantly, remodelling occurs at the surfaces of the bones, accommodating the change in curvature necessitated by the increase in all three diameters of the cavity. Various types of skull deformity may result from premature closure of cranial sutures. If there is early closure of the sagittal suture, the skull becomes elongated (dolichocranic), whereas if the coronal suture closes prematurely, the skull becomes round (brachycranic). Reichs (1989) documents a case of dolichocrania in which early closure of the sagittal suture complicated determination of sex. Skeletal remains consisted of a long narrow skull with predominantly male features but with a mandible that had distinctly female characteristics. Because changes in the width of the skull were affected by closure of the sagittal suture, most growth had occurred in an anteroposterior direction, affecting the shape not only of the cranium but also of the mandible. The 'lop-sided' appearance of the skull (plagiocephaly) illustrated in Fig. 4.10 is taken from the osteological collection of the Department of Anatomy and Cell Biology at the University of Melbourne, Australia. The malformation illustrated was probably induced in this case not by premature suture closure of a longitudinal suture but by artificial deformation. The skull is from the south-western part of America, and the deformation may be due to the use during development of cradleboards. Other types of cranial deformation, due both to congenital and artificially induced mechanisms, are well documented in Brothwell (1981) and El Najaar and McWilliams (1978).

Some sutures may remain open well beyond closure of the remainder. The mediofrontal or metopic suture is one such example (Limson, 1924; Brothwell, 1981). The frontal bone ossifies in fibrous mesenchyme from two primary centres that appear *in utero* during week eight (these are the sites of the frontal tubers in the adult). At birth, the bone is in two halves, the metopic suture intervening. This suture usually disappears within the first or second year after birth but may in some persist into late adult life (Brothwell, 1981). There may be racial differences regarding its appearance, Woo (1949) suggesting an incidence as high as 10% in Mongoloids, although probably less than 1% in other racial groups.

In general, closure of sutures is associated with a loss of elasticity of the skull, especially from that seen in the young. Todd and Tracy (1930) and Cobb (1942) both noted changes in the 'texture' of the skull, from being smooth in the young adult to increasingly granular and roughened in appearance with age. After maturity, vault sutures begin to ossify from inside out (starting with the coronal at approximately 30 years of age). Krogman and Iscan (1986)

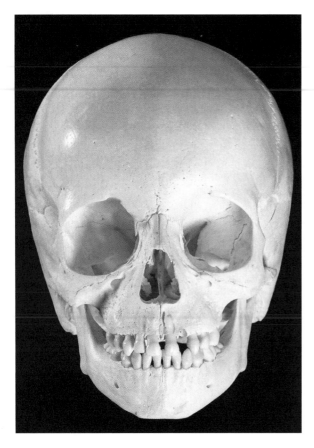

Fig. 4.8 Anterior view of the human infant skull (aged 6 years)

indicate that an age range of 17 to 50 years is not unreasonable for vault suture closure, while the circummeatal sutures may not fuse until the eighth or ninth decade. Meindl and Lovejoy (1985) examined specific sites for suture closure and correlated their findings with the known chronological age of their sample. They found the strongest correlations between age and anterolateral sites, including those demarcating the pterion as well as the sphenofrontal, midlambdoid and lambdoid sutures. They also found that closure of some sutures seemed to give a better indication of specific age; for example, the pterion was the best monitor of ages between 40 and 50 years.

The bones of the cranial base are endochondral bones that ossify in the cartilage model known as the chondrocranium and articulate with one another at primary cartilaginous (synchondrotic) joints. Growth at the spheno-occipital synchondrosis, between basiocciput and basisphenoid, leads to an increase in the basicranial axis. As described earlier, this 'suture' may close as early as 14 years. Cartilage at the sphenoethmoidal synchondrosis, between sphenoid and mesoethmoid ossification sites is replaced by fibrous tissue and forms a 'suture' after birth. Growth here increases the anterior extension. It should be noted that growth at the midsphenoidal synchondrosis, between presphenoid and basisphenoid ossification

sites, ceases when these fuse to form the body of the sphenoid by the time of birth. As with the vault, remodelling of the cranial base occurs at the same time as growth at the above growth sites.

The bones of the facial skeleton follow a somatic growth curve, increasing height, length and width (in that order) of the face. Growth sites exist at the fibrous or sutural joints of the facial bones. The craniofacial and circummaxillary sutures are arranged obliquely so that growth results in an increase in all parameters of the facial skeleton. The sagittal sutures (internasal, intermaxillary and palatal) increase the width of the face. Paradoxically, despite the facial bones being dermal in origin, a major contribution to the growth of the suborbital part of the facial skeleton occurs by the process of endochondral ossification. This takes place in the upper face in the cartilage of the nasal septum and in the lower facial skeleton in the secondary condylar cartilage of the mandible. Both result in the forward and downward movement of the facial skeleton relative to the cranial base. As in the cranial vault and base, there is concomitant remodelling occurring on the surfaces of the bones. The process is a balance between bone deposition and resorption, and proceeds throughout life. During the growth phase, the external periosteal surface of the facial skeleton is resorbed over a wide Y-shaped area, which has its stem just below the cen-

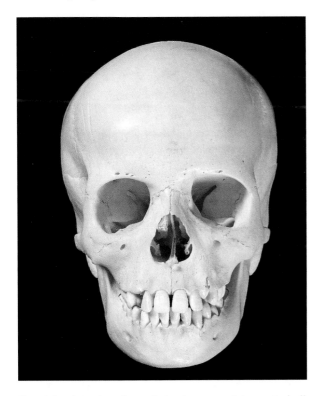

Fig. 4.9 Anterior view of the human adolescent skull (aged 14 years)

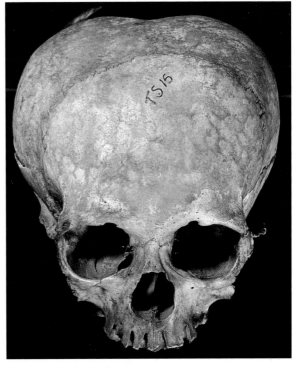

Fig. 4.10 Anterior view of an anomalous (plagiocephalic) human adult skull

tral incisors of the mandible, involves the premaxilla above and extends laterally across the body of the maxilla, the zygoma and its frontal process (Johnson and Moore, 1989). Remodelling involves the bones of the upper and lower jaws that need to change to accommodate the erupting dentition.

Factors of individualization

Several reports (Gerasimov, 1971; Angel, 1978; Gatliff and Snow, 1979; Caldwell, 1986) have documented the relationship between fixed bony landmarks and the location of facial features. Caldwell (1986) suggests that the three most significant features for facial recognition are 'the eyes', 'the nose' and 'the mouth'. In a study of skulls and accompanying death masks derived from the Terry Collection, she located the position of the eyebrows approximately 3–5 mm above the superior orbital margin following the supraorbital arches, confirming the observations of Angel (1978). Although unable to comment on the placement and projection of the eyeball, Caldwell provided some interesting observations of how body build may affect eyelid closure: 'the thinner the face, the shorter the distance between the two inner canthi and vice versa' (Caldwell, 1986; p. 244). Gerasimov (1971) points out that the size of the orbit correlates well with the size of the eyes but, paradoxically, that Mongolians, presumably with Mongoloid racial characteristics, although possessing a relatively large orbit (in comparison to Europeans and Negros), have the smallest eyes. It is therefore very important that racial affiliation is carefully documented.

Caldwell (1986) suggests that the nasal bridge formed by the paired nasal bones gives the profile slope for septal and lateral nasal cartilages. She also indicates that the nasal bridge is usually straight in Caucasoids, although it may be concavo-convex (Caldwell, 1986). The orientation of the nasal spine – up, horizontal or downward – pointing may have a bearing on the orientation of the nasal tip. Furthermore, a high vertical orientation of the nasal spine may indicate a vertical slant of alar cartilages and more lateral visibility of the nares.

A parasagittal line joining the infraorbital and mental foraminae may provide a reference point for the position of the 'corners of the mouth', as does the interval between the canine and first premolar. Evidence of markings for the levator and depressor anguli may indicate the relative strengths of these muscles and therefore a further guide to facial appearance (Angel, 1978, in Caldwell, 1986).

These studies illustrate the importance of detailed anatomical analysis of the skull in obtaining information on identity from human skeletal remains. Such analysis need not be limited to matters of race, gender and age but can contribute substantially to the assessment of the possible soft tissue structures of the face, with all that this means for facial identification.

Acknowledgements

The authors would like to thank Mrs Michelle Gough and Mr Stuart Thyer, Department of Anatomy and Cell Biology, University of Melbourne, for the preparation of all photographic material.

References

Angel JL. 1978: Restoration of head and face for identification. Paper presented at the 30th Annual Meeting of the American Academy of Forensic Sciences, 20–25 February, St Louis, Missouri.

Bass WM. 1987: *Human osteology. A laboratory and field manual* (3rd edn). Columbia, MO: Archeological Society.

Berkovitz BKB, Moxham BJ. 1988: *A textbook of head and neck anatomy*. London: Wolfe.

Brothwell DR. 1981: *Digging up bones: the excavation, treatment and study of human skeletal remains* (3rd edn). British Museum: Oxford University Press.

Caldwell PC. 1986: New questions (and some answers) on the facial reproduction techniques. In Reichs KJ (ed.) *Forensic osteology. Advances in the identification of human remains*. Springfield, IL: Charles C. Thomas, 229–55.

Cobb WM. 1942: Physical anthropology of the American Negro. *American Journal of Physical Anthropology* **29**, 113–23.

El Najaar MY, McWilliams KR. 1978: *Forensic anthropology. The structure, morphology and variation of human bone and dentition*. Springfield, IL: Charles C. Thomas.

Gatliff BP, Snow CC. 1979: From skull to visage. *Journal of Biocommunications* **6**(2), 27–30.

Gerasimov MM. 1971: *The face finder*. New York: Lippincott.

Israel H. 1973: Age factor and pattern of change in craniofacial structures. *American Journal of Physical Anthropology* **39**(1), 111–28.

Israel H. 1977: The dichotomous pattern of craniofacial expansion during aging. *American Journal of Physical Anthropology* **47**(1), 47–51.

Johnson DR, Moore WJ. 1989: *Anatomy for dental students* (2nd edn). Oxford: Oxford University Press.

Keen JA. 1950: Sex differences in skulls. *American Journal of Physical Anthropology* **8**, 65–79.

Krogman WM. 1955: The skeleton in forensic medicine. *Postgraduate Medicine* **17**(2): A48–A62.

Krogman WM, Iscan MY. 1986: *The human skeleton in forensic medicine*. Springfield, IL: Charles C. Thomas.

Limson M. 1924: Metopism as found in Philipino skulls. *American Journal of Physical Anthropology* **7**(3), 317–27.

Meindl RS, Lovejoy CO. 1985: Ectocranial suture closure: a revised method for the determination of skeletal age at death based on the lateral-anterior sutures. *American Journal of Physical Anthropology* **68**, 57–66.

Redfield A. 1970: A new aid to aging immature skeletons: development of the occipital bone. *American Journal of Physical Anthropology* **33**, 207–20.

Reichs KR. 1989: Cranial suture eccentricities: a case in which precocious closure complicated determination of sex and commingling. *Journal of Forensic Sciences* **34**(1), 263–73.

Rhine JS, Campbell HR. 1980: Thickness of facial tissues in American blacks. *Journal of Forensic Sciences* **25**(4), 847–58.

Suchey J. 1993: Lecture notes, Sixth Annual Forensic Anthropology Course, University of New Mexico, June 21–25.

Todd TW, Tracy B. 1930: Racial features in the American Negro cranium. *American Journal of Physical Anthropology* **15**, 53–110.

Williams PL, Warwick R, Dyson M, Bannister LH. 1989: *Gray's Anatomy*. Melbourne: Churchill Livingstone.

Woo J. 1949: Racial and sexual differences in the frontal curvature end and its relation to metopism. *American Journal of Physical Anthropology* **7**, 215–26.

CHAPTER 5

 Anthropological assessment

CA BRIGGS

Introduction	49	Racial characteristics of the postcranial skeleton	53
Determination of racial affiliation	49	Cultural indicators of race in the skeleton	53
Racial identification in juvenile bones	50	Determination of sex	53
Racial identification in adults	50	Determination of age	55

Introduction

In life, individuals may be distinguished one from another on the basis of their appearance: their facial features, their hair and eye colour, how they dress, their mannerisms and so on. After death, and particularly following skeletonization, when these superficial characteristics have disappeared, determination of identity is more difficult. Fortunately, the skeleton retains some evidence that helps in identifying the person who, in life, clothed the bones. Clues that leave their mark on the skeleton relate in particular to an individual's race, sex and age. These may be deduced on the basis of a number of features: variability in shape and size of bones and bony features between the sexes and traits distinguishing different racial groups as well as morphological changes evident with ageing. The traditional approach to eliciting these clues has been through documenting their presence or absence using the naked eye. The accuracy of such assessment is, however, only as good as the expertise of the examiner. Because of its less subjective nature, metrical analysis (particularly of the skull) as well as discriminant function analysis, in which the discriminatory power of selected measurements is also used to determine a function, have been used successfully to provide objective data, particularly of race and gender traits.

Determination of racial affiliation

While the notion that humans may be categorized into clear-cut subdivisions of racial groups is rejected by many anthropologists (Sauer, 1992), forensic anthropologists, osteologists and anatomists, when presented with a set of skeletal remains by the police, are regularly asked to nominate the racial grouping to which the remains belong. In helping to establish identity, there are some traits or features that allow one clearly to distinguish a high proportion of individuals of one major racial group from another. However, in all racial groups, there are those who exhibit extreme variance from what is normally expected. According to Brothwell (1981, p. 107), 'there are skulls which display, say, the Negroid character of strong alveolar prognathism, or the flat, broad cheeks of a Mongoloid, yet do not belong to either group'. One reason for this apparent anomaly may be, in part, the intermingling of races that has occurred in the latter part of the twentieth century, owing to a breakdown of traditional barriers to migration. Australia has, since the middle of the 1940s, seen the inward migration of peoples from Europe, and in the past 20 years people from China and South East Asia, as well as from India and Melanesia. This movement of different racial groups has also been a factor in determining the current community racial mix in the USA and the UK. What influence this genetic admixture is having and will continue to have on the traits by means of which race is assessed is uncertain, although some 'blurring' at the margins of traditional groupings may be expected. Perhaps some racial traits will in future be retained while others will be masked or may even disappear. Undoubtedly, the mixing that results will only confound racial identification.

In establishing racial affiliation, five major groups or populations tend to be considered:

1. Caucasian/Caucasoid
2. Mongoloid
3. Negroid
4. Australian Aboriginal
5. Polynesian.

In forensic anthropology, only the three 'major' groups are normally encountered (at least outside the Pacific rim and Australia): Caucasian (including Europeans, Asians from the Indian subcontinent, Mediterraneans and Americans with similar ancestry); Mongoloid (Asiatics and Native Americans); and Negroid (Africans and African Americans). Populations of American Indians (Native Americans) have received considerable anthropological investigation in the USA, particularly in the south west. This unique population is generally considered to be derived from Mongoloid stock, which separated from its 'Asiatic' ancestors approximately 10 000 to 15 000 years ago (Boyd, 1950; Dunn, 1967).

Distinction between the racial subgroups is best made from features of the skull and, secondarily, from the postcranial skeleton. If a skull is in good condition, it may also provide information helpful in the determination of sex and, within a general range, age at death. Both morphological and metrical methods may be used to assess race. As mentioned in the introduction to this chapter, morphological assessment requires the identification of selected traits or features of the cranium and mandible, with associated documentation of their absence, presence or degree of development. Traits useful in the assessment of racial affiliation include the overall morphology of the skull – its length, breadth and height – the shape of the face, the width of the zygomatic arches, the shape of the orbits, the interorbital breadth, and the size, shape and degree of guttering of the nasal aperture. In the hands of an experienced observer, morphological methods are relatively fast and accurate (up to 90% correct). Because of the subjective nature of such assessment, attempts have been made to determine the probability of correct observation using discriminant function analysis or other objective measures. Accuracy of metrical analysis is reported to range between 77% and 95% correct assessment, depending on the measurements used (Giles and Elliot, 1962; Birkby, 1966; Howells, 1970; Rhine, 1990).

Racial identification in juvenile bones

Many racial traits do not appear fully until puberty and, even in adolescence, they may not be completely formed. As the adult dentition augments and replaces the deciduous, the midfacial region undergoes dramatic growth and modification, with increases in all midfacial projections (Gill *et al.*, 1988; Brues, 1990). In conjunction with these changes, there is enlargement of the frontal sinuses, the brow ridges change in shape and size, and the nasal root is modified. However, these alterations occur at varied stages of development in different populations, with considerable individual variation. It is therefore often a difficult proposition to identify race in juvenile material (St Hoyme and Iscan, 1989).

Racial identification in adults

MORPHOLOGICAL FEATURES

As the juvenile face changes into its adult form, certain traits become pronounced, whereas others may be masked to a greater or lesser degree. The major racial traits of the flesh-covered face that are preserved in the skull are those relating to head shape, face shape, nose shape and chin shape (Brues, 1990). None of these is unique to any one racial group, although some seem to appear more frequently in certain groups, while others are not always found, owing perhaps to genetic mixing. For example, European Caucasoid populations show differences in skull length and breadth. On the basis of this variability, they may be separated into three subgroups: Northern European (Nordic), Central European (Alpine) and Southern European (Mediterranean). Table 5.1 illustrates these differences as well as the traits commonly found in typical Caucasoid, Negroid and Mongoloid skulls.

Caucasoids show vault characteristics that range from long, narrow and low, to short, broad and high; in anterior relief, the vault is rounded, there is mild-to-moderate development of the brow (supraorbital) ridges and a conical or hook-shaped external occipital protuberance. Mastoid (and styloid) processes are large, while the cranial sutures are tortuous. The lat-

Table 5.1 Cranial traits common in the three major racial groups

Trait	Caucasoid	Mongoloid	Negroid
Skull length			
Long	*		*
Short	*	*	
Skull breadth			
Narrow	*		*
Broad	*	*	
Skull height			
High	Medium to high	Medium	
Low			*
Cranial sutures	Tortuous	Simple	
Parietal bossing	Small to medium	Large	Small
Zygomatic projection	Absent	Prominent	Slight
Mastoid process	Large		Small
Sagittal contour	Rounded	Rounded	Flat
Face breadth	Narrow to wide	Very wide	Narrow
Face height	Short to high	High	Low
Facial morphology	Long, narrow	Flat, rounded	Prognathic
Orbital opening	Angular	Rounded	Rectangular
Interorbital distance	Narrow	Narrow	Wide
Brow ridges	Moderate	Absent	Moderate
Nasal opening	Narrow – medium	Narrow – medium	Wide
Nasal root	High – depressed	Medium	Low
Nasal root contour	'Steepled'	'Tented'	'Quonset hut'
Nasal spine	Prominent – sharp	Short – dull	Small – troughed
Prognathism	None	Moderate	Marked
Incisal shovelling	Absent	Present	Absent
Carabelli's cusps	Present		Absent
Shape of dental arcade	Narrow – parabolic	Wide – U-shaped	Wide – rectangular
Profile of chin	Prominent	Vertical	Vertical
Lower border mandible	Undulating	Straight	Undulating

* Trait present.
Data from: Krogman and Iscan (1986), Brues (1990) and Rhine (1990). For a more comprehensive compilation of racial characteristics associated with selected populations, the reader is referred to Howells (1970), Rhine (1990) and Brues (1990).

eral margin of the orbit is sharp and the interorbital distance narrow. The nasal spine is prominent, and the lower margin of the nasal opening is sharp. There is a deep canine fossa. Prognathism is not marked, and the dental arcade is parabolic. Features of the mandible are a prominent chin and an undulating lower mandibular border.

The Mongoloid cranium is relatively short, broad and high, the vault is rounded and brow ridges are absent or show only slight development. Cranial sutures are simple. There is prominence of the zygomatic bones giving a rounded appearance to the face. The root of the nose is broad and flat, the nasal spine is short and there is absence of canine fossae. A classic feature is 'shovelling' of the upper incisor teeth.

The typical Negroid skull, as seen in African and American blacks, has a long narrow vault, which is rounded in anterior relief and has sharp upper orbital margins, a wide interorbital distance and wide and rounded nasal apertures. A distinctive feature of most Negroid skulls is the presence of marked alveolar (subnasal) prognathism.

A more recent distinction between the racial groups is based on the contour of the nasal root. Brues (1990) has identified three types of root appearance: a high nasal root, narrowed below, with a break in contour at the nasomaxillary suture (a 'steepled' appearance) is said to be characteristic of Caucasoids; a nasal root of low-to-moderate height with straight sides angled at the midline (a 'tented' appearance) is characteristic of Mongoloids; while a nasal root which is low and rounded in contour ('Quonset hut'-like in appearance) is characteristic of Negroids. Brues (1990) indicates that these features are also clear in the living.

While most readers outside the Antipodes will be

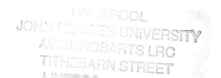

unfamiliar with Aboriginal crania, their unique features warrant some comment. Larnach (1978) lists traits, in hierarchical order, that discriminate Australian Aboriginals from other racial groups, and Pounder (1984) describes their relevance in a forensic setting. The sagittal contour of the vault in Australian Aboriginals is flattened or 'keeled'. The nasal aperture is broad, with low nasal bones. There is no external occipital protuberance, but a distinct occipital torus (transverse bony prominence) is instead found. This occipital torus can show considerable variation in size, shape and lateral extension. The supraorbital arches are moderate to large, as is the glabella. The zygomatic bones are also medium to large and are visible from above (phaenozygy), while the skull tends to be long (dolichocephalic). The cephalic index – ratio of skull length to width – may be less than 75, particularly in males, making dolichocephaly a characteristic trait of Aboriginals. There is a good chance of marked subnasal prognathism, although tribal differences may magnify or reduce some of these features, particularly when comparing Aboriginal cranial remains from the north with those from the south of Australia (Pietrusewsky, 1990).

The Polynesian cranium, as evident in the New Zealand Maori, shows a high vault profile with prominent parietal bossing and keeling. Nasal bones may be absent or markedly reduced in size. The zygomatic arches are visible from above. The facial profile tends to be vertical (orthoganism), while the upper facial height is large, with minimal subnasal prognathism. The chin is prominent, the ramus of the mandible high and broad, and the inferior border of the mandible curved, producing a 'rocker jaw' (when the jaw is placed on a flat surface and the condyle is tapped, the jaw 'rocks' to and fro). This feature is reported to be present in 69% of males and 78% of females in the South Pacific (New Zealand), and 71% of males and 88% of females from the Hawaiian islands (Snow, 1974; Houghton, 1977, 1978).

CRANIOMETRY

Because of the subjective and experiential nature of visual inspection, attempts have been made to standardize evaluation procedures. Giles and Elliot (1962) were the first to use a discriminant function technique for the determination of race from the skull. They utilized eight cranial indices (Table 5.2) to discriminate whites (Caucasians) from Negroes and American Indians, and claimed an accuracy of 82–89%. Their technique requires two separate tests, one to distinguish between blacks and whites and another for American Indians and whites. In both tests, race is indicated by the scores falling above or below a predetermined sectioning point value.

Birkby (1966) also used eight measurements, while Howells (1970) performed discriminant function analysis on 72 observations. One limitation of these techniques is, in general, their inability to discriminate between more than two racial groups. Furthermore, many formulae are suitable only for the population under study and do not compare well with other racial groups (Birkby 1966).

Johnson *et al.* (1989) computed discriminant function analysis of skulls of modern racial groups, including Australoid material, using 25 craniometric points covering the entire cranial vault, facial skeleton and mandible. They were able correctly to classify 70–95% of their sample and suggested that the use of a large number of craniometric measurements may not be necessary for the determination of race.

Table 5.2 Discriminant function weights for distinguishing American whites from American blacks on the basis of cranial measurements

Measurement	Male weights	Female weights
Basion–prosthion	+3.06	+1.74
Glabello-occipital length	+1.60	+1.28
Maximum width	−1.90	−1.18
Basion–bregma height	−1.79	−0.14
Basion–nasion	−4.41	−2.34
Maximum bizygomatic diameter	−0.10	+0.38
Prosthion–nasion height	+2.59	−0.01
Nasal breadth	+10.56	+2.45

Race is assessed by determining each measurement on a specimen and adding the constant for each function. Male sectioning point: above 89.27 = black; below 89.27 = white. Female sectioning point: above 9.22 = black; below 9.22 = white. The test sample included 108 white males, 79 white females, 113 black males and 108 black females from the Terry and Todd collections. Age, sex and ethnic group were known.

Reproduced from Giles and Elliot (1962) with permission.

Racial characteristics of the postcranial skeleton

The postcranial skeleton has not been found to provide information as useful as that from the cranium and mandible in racial assessment. However, selected morphological features attributable to specific postural traits or tribal rites have been documented. It is claimed (Brothwell, 1981) that where there is a lack or scarcity of household furniture, particularly in more primitive groups, these populations tend to spend more time in a squatting posture. Amongst several features associated with squatting are facets on the tibia and foot bones, and on the anterior neck of the femur. Additional features are anterior femoral bowing and tibial flattening (St Hoyme and Iscan, 1989). Body and limb proportions, such as tibial retroversion, have also been documented (Lovejoy *et al.*, 1976; Brothwell, 1981; Pounder, 1984). However, St Hoyme and Iscan (1989) caution against overreliance on such features to distinguish 'primitive' from 'civilized' populations, pointing out that 'intraseries variability in all races seems so great that the anthropologist should not depend too heavily on body proportions for his decisions' (p. 85). This view is reinforced in the same authors' comments on the presence of squatting facets (p. 80): 'their occurrence in non-squatting populations is frequent enough to make them, alone, of dubious value for diagnosing race, nationality, or sitting habits'.

St Hoyme and Iscan (1989) documented the accuracy of race determination from selected bones of the postcranial skeleton (Table 5.3) and compared them with the face or with features of the face and vault in combination.

As may be seen, adding measurements of long bones (for example, the femur and tibia) to pelvic formulae increases the accuracy of race determination to over 90%, while use of the transverse breadth of the pelvic inlet alone provides an accuracy of only 75–88%.

Cultural indicators of race in the skeleton

Skeletal remains may show evidence of the cultural beliefs and habits of a racial group and the environment in which they lived. Brothwell (1981) documents intentional cranial deformation, seen particularly in the Central and South Americas, and the distortion of feet seen amongst past generations of Chinese women. Evulsion of the front teeth, usually the upper central incisors, is a common initiation procedure amongst Australian Aboriginals but is also performed amongst the Masai tribe of Kenya. Healed fractures of the ulnae are common among Aboriginal skeletons and probably represent 'parry' fractures associated with warding off a direct blow (Pounder, 1984). The presence of associated grave goods or the use of colouring agents and dyes on skeletal remains may also provide helpful clues to racial affiliation.

Determination of sex

Once ethnicity has been attributed, perhaps the most important of parameters to determine from a skeleton is the sex of an individual. If a bone is successfully sexed, approximately 50% of the population are immediately eliminated from the process of identification. Sex-distinguishing characteristics of the

Table 5.3 Accuracy rate of race determination in various bones using the discriminant function formulae

Bone or structure	Variables	Race	Percent accuracy	Source
Face	1	C, I	M = 80–95/F = 91–95	Gill *et al.* (1988)
Face and neurocranium	7	N, C, I	M = 80–85/F = 88–93	Giles and Elliot (1962)
Pelvic inlet	1	N, C	M = 75–77/F = 79–88	Iscan (1983)
Innominate and femur	15	N, C	M = 94–97/F = 88–92	DiBennardo and Taylor (1983)
Innominate and femur	3	N, C	M = 82/F = 78	Schulter-Ellis and Hayek (1984)
			M = 84/F = 77	
Pelvis, tibia and femur	10	N, C	M = 95/F = 91	Krogman and Iscan (1986)
Femur	4	N	M = 77	Krogman and Iscan (1986)
	4	C	F = 67	
Tibia	4	N	M = 83	Krogman and Iscan (1986)
	4	C	F = 71	

C = Caucasoid, I = American Indian, N = Negroid.

Reproduced from St Hoyme and Iscan (1989) with permission.

skeleton are based on the differences that arise in males and females as a consequence of sexual maturation. Sex determination may be made from the cranium or from bones of the postcranial skeleton, although, in general, evaluation of the pelvis and the modifications that occur to permit childbirth provides a more reliable estimate of sex than do cranial measurements. While sexual differences begin to develop in the skeleton before birth (Fazekas and Kosa, 1978), it is not until the individual approaches the age of about 16–18 years that decisions on sex differences can be made with any confidence. Because sex differences are unique to a given race, if it is possible to establish racial affinity, this should be done first before attempting to document sex (Brothwell, 1981; Johnson *et al.*, 1989).

SEX DETERMINATION BY MORPHOLOGICAL CHARACTERISTICS OF THE CRANIUM

Sex determination from the cranium and mandible relates to their relative size and robustness, so it is necessary to take into account the specific sexual dimorphism of the racial group to which the skull belongs. For example, sex determination for Caucasoids and Mongoloids may require the use of a different, unique set of discriminant functions (Table 5.4; Johnson *et al.*, 1989, p. 52).

As the majority of sex-distinguishing features do not become pronounced until puberty, they are most appropriate for sex determination within the age range 20–55 years (Krogman and Iscan, 1986), before the onset of senile changes. Male and female skulls may be distinguished by a number of characteristics (Table 5.5).

In general, the female skull shows a rounded appearance, 'tending to retain more the adolescent form' (Brothwell, 1981, p. 61). The male skull tends to be larger and heavier (up to 200 cm^3 more cranial capacity) than the female, and it is more rugged, with prominent landmarks for muscular and ligamentous attachments. The male supraorbital ridges are better defined and the frontal sinuses larger. The mastoid and styloid processes, and external occipital protuberance, are well developed in the male, whereas parietal and frontal eminences are not prominent. The upper margin of the orbit in the male is more rounded (in the female, it is sharper), and the cheekbones are heavier. The male palate is large and broad, and the posterior root of the zygomatic process extends beyond the external auditory meatus for some distance as a clearly defined ridge. The male mandible is more robust, with a U-shaped chin, broad ramus and flared gonial regions. When an entire skeleton is available for inspection, sex determination is usually immediately possible with 95–100% accuracy. Accuracy of prediction decreases to approximately 95% with the pelvis alone, 90% with the skull alone and 80–90% with bones of the postcranial skeleton.

SEX DETERMINATION BY METRICAL CHARACTERISTICS OF THE CRANIUM

Where they are available, quantitative methods should be used to support the visual assessment of sex characteristics. Several attempts have been made to determine gender from cranial measurements, comparing weighted measures of the skull with known sectioning points. The reliability of metrical analysis depends on the bony features used but usually lies somewhere between 70% and 95%. Keen (1950) documented an accuracy of 85% based on selected cranial traits and the dimensions of 'Cape Coloured' skulls from South Africa, while Hanihara (1959) reported an 83–89% accuracy in sexing Japanese skulls. Giles and Elliot (1962) and Giles (1970) used discriminant function analysis to sex the crania of American blacks and whites, and also

Table 5.4 Best variables for classification by sex

Caucasoids	Mongoloids
1. Bizygomatic breadth	1. Angle opisthion–basion–nasion
2. Maximum length glabella–opisthocranion	2. Maximum length glabella–opisthocranion
3. Nasal breadth	3. Foraminal length
4. Subnasal height	4. Foraminal breadth
5. Palatal length	5. Subnasal height
6. Angle opisthion–nasion	6. Nasal breadth
	7. Angle lambda–opisthion–basion
	8. Basi-prosthion length

Reproduced from Johnson *et al.* (1989) with permission.

Table 5.5 Sex differences in the appearance of the skull

Trait	Male	Female
General size	Large	Small
Architecture	Rugged	Rugged
Supraorbital ridges	Smooth	Small to medium
Mastoid processes	Medium to large	Small to medium
Occipital region	Marked muscle lines and attachments	Not marked muscle lines and attachments
Frontal eminences	Small	Large
Parietal eminences	Small	Large
Orbits	Square with round margins	Round with sharp margins
Forehead	Sloping – less rounded	Vertical
Cheekbones	Heavier, laterally arched	Light, compressed
Palate	Large, broad, U-shaped	Small, parabolic
Occipital condyles	Large	Small
Mandible	Large, high symphysis, broad ramus	Small, lower symphysis and smaller ramus
Chin shape	U-shaped	V-shaped
Gonial angle	Angled	Vertical
Gonial flare	Pronounced	Slight

Data from Krogman and Iscan (1986).

reported an accuracy of between 83% and 89%. As with racial determination, Birkby (1966) warns that discriminant function measures should only be used on bones for which the function has been developed.

SEX DETERMINATION FROM THE POSTCRANIAL SKELETON

Sex determination from the postcranial skeleton is often based merely on observed differences in size and ruggedness of the bones. Because there is considerable overlap between males and females, both in the same population and between populations, this approach to sexing is, however, prone to error. Specific postcranial landmarks appropriate for sexing include the overall breadth of the pelvis, the width of the sciatic notch and subpubic angles, the presence of a ventral arc on the anterior surface of the pubis and the contour of the medial part of the ischiopubic ramus. Sutherland and Suchey (1991) report that the ventral arc alone has an accuracy of 96% for determining sex. A 'precursor' arc, represented by a faint line on the ventral surface of the pubis, may be present as early as 14 years, while the well-developed form may not appear until the mid-20s. The preauricular sulcus, a groove between the auricular area and the sciatic notch, is suggested to be indicative of parturition, although a shallow groove has been reported in some males, making its use as a predictive index less reliable. Discriminant functions for sex determination from the sacrum in American

whites, blacks and Japanese were developed by Kimura (1982), utilizing the transverse width of the sacral base and the transverse width of the ala of the sacrum. The functions resulted in the correct sexing in 75% of Japanese, 80% of whites and 83% of blacks.

While metrical sexing of bones of the postcranial skeleton has generally concentrated on the pelvis and sacrum, attempts have been made to show sex differences among many other bones. Washburn (1948) used the ischiopubic index (length of the pubis divided by length of the ilium multiplied by 100), in conjunction with the width of the sciatic notch, correctly to allocate sex in over 90% of cases. Other variations on this index have been developed by St Hoyme (1982, 1984) and Schulter-Ellis *et al.* (1983). Amongst other bones to have received attention are the scapula (Bainbridge and Genoves, 1956) and the sternum and ribs (Jit *et al.*, 1980). Maximum diameters of the heads of the femur, humerus and radius are also good indicators of gender when their values fall outside the zone of overlap (Stewart, 1979).

Determination of age

The human skeleton passes through several major stages of development and growth:

1. At birth, rapid fetal growth is represented in the commencement of ossification and the presence, with few exceptions, of primary (diaphyseal) cen-

tres of ossification. The exceptions are secondary, or epiphyseal, centres in the distal condyle of the femur, in the proximal condyle of the tibia and possibly in the head of the humerus. Numerous primary centres, for example at the wrist, do not form until a number of years after birth.

2. The increasing mechanical stresses on the skeleton in the first 2 years of life serve to stimulate skeletal growth, ossification and remodelling. During this time, new primary centres of ossification develop, and secondary centres begin to make an appearance, especially at the ends of long bones, to facilitate continued longitudinal growth.

3. Between puberty and adolescence, secondary centres start to fuse, and the skeleton increasingly approaches maturity.

4. From late adolescence, when secondary centres of ossification fuse, into middle and later life, the skeleton passes through stages of active remodelling, which may result in characteristic marking in bones. This is followed by a period of quiescence, and degenerative processes ultimately replace restorative ones. Bones may thin and become osteoporotic, and parts of the skeleton, such as vertebrae and the weight-bearing surfaces of lower limb bones, reveal some of the stresses and strains to which they have been exposed over a lifetime of use.

AGE ESTIMATION IN IMMATURE SKELETONS

In general, immature remains are those of individuals who are less than 20 years of age. Age at death in immature skeletons is usually assessed by determining the maturation stages of several bones, determining the presence or state of closure of secondary epiphyseal centres, and then formulating a 'mean' age. This 'bone' or 'skeletal' age represents an equivalent level of skeletal development rather than a true chronological age. The relationship between chronological age and skeletal age was first established in the 1950s by assessing the age at which radiological ossification centres appear in the wrist, hand, knee and foot, and the sequence of closure of secondary epiphyses in the adolescent (Gruelich and Pyle, 1959).

In an immature skeleton, where longitudinal growth is not yet complete, epiphyses separate from the diaphysis once the supporting soft tissue is removed (as with skeletonization). Once growth is complete and the epiphyses fuse with the diaphysis, a bony scar is left as evidence of the union. The degree of 'openness' of this scar provides an indication of how recently fusion took place.

In the case of fetal and prepubescent material, age

estimation is best determined from diaphyseal lengths and the appearance of ossification centres (Fazekas and Kosa, 1978). In individuals from prenatal to about 6–7 years of age, the length of the long bone diaphysis can be used to estimate age, although growth rates vary greatly between different racial groups and between the sexes, and are strongly influenced by dietary intake. Age estimation based on epiphyseal union is most commonly used in the teenage (10–20) years, and standards are available for the humerus, clavicle, scapula, hip, elbow, hand, wrist, foot, ankle and knee.

If an entire skeleton is present, it is best to provide an 'average' age based on the state of union of all epiphyseal centres. Stewart (1979, p. 156) illustrates the approximate sequence of closure: from elbow to hip, to ankle, to knee, to wrist and finally to shoulder. It must be appreciated, however, that epiphyseal union is an ongoing process rather than a single event. Indeed, a range of up to 4 years may be seen between the onset of fusion in early-maturing and the completion of fusion in late-maturing individuals. As a result, the above pattern of fusion is useful only as a guide. Because skeletal maturation occurs earlier in girls, usually by anything up to 3–4 years, it is important first to determine gender. Furthermore, individual differences make it difficult to indicate with absolute confidence when closure of epiphyses is likely to take place. Where radiographs are used to estimate epiphyseal closure (Flecker, 1932/33), earlier age estimates commonly result.

NON-DENTAL AGE ESTIMATION FROM THE CRANIUM

For the determination of age in children, development of the teeth is by far the most important factor. However, in the absence of jaws and teeth, age may be determined, in the first years of life, from closure of the fontanelles, completion of ossification of the sphenoid and occipital bones, fusion of the two halves of the frontal bone (the site of an unfused metopic suture) and ossification of the upper cervical vertebrae (Table 5.6).

Cranial suture closure was historically the first aspect of the skeleton to undergo systematic investigation for estimation of age at death in adults, and many studies were conducted at the turn of the century and into the 1920s. However, limitations of the technique were also reported (Montagu, 1938; Singer, 1953). While most sutures commence closure between the mid-20s and mid-40s, the order and timing of closure shows great variability, leading to wide age estimates (Table 5.7).

This is further compounded by the fact that sutures tend to close endocranially before they do so ectocra-

Table 5.6 Approximate times of union of primary centres of ossification from birth to about 6 years of age

Centre	Approximate time of union
Fontanelles	
Sphenoid and mastoid	Soon after birth
Occipital	During first year
Frontal	During second year
Mandible	
Symphysis	Complete by second year
Frontal	
Metopic suture	Begins closure in second year
Atlas	
Posteriorly	Closed by third year
Anteriorly	Closed by about the sixth year
Axis	
Dens, body and two sides	During third or fourth year
Occipital	
Squamous with lateral parts	Closed in fifth year
Lateral parts with basilar parts	Before seventh year

Reproduced from Terry RJ. 1942: Osteology and articulations. In Parson J (ed.) *Morris's human anatomy*, 10th edn, Blakiston, Philadelphia. Reprinted in Bennett (1987).

Table 5.7 A simplified presentation of stages of vault suture closure to show its variability: vault sutures (in %)

Age	N	0	1	2, 3	4	0	1	2, 3	4	0	1	2, 3	4
17–18	55	75	4	12	9	92		5	3	99			1
19	52	66	4	10	19	83	5	5	7	84	7	5	4
20	45	54	10	13	23	82	11	3	4	77	17	2	4
21	37	56	9	10	25	72	10	10	8	86	7	2	5
22	24	54	17	5	24	75	17	4	4	72	20	4	4
23	26	42	11	15	32	65	6	23	6	49	34	11	6
24–25	27	34	7	11	48	53	11	18	18	67	12	14	7
26–27	25	12	8	40	40	32	28	16	24	28	16	24	32
28–30	29	18	12	19	51	27	17	35	21	26	25	25	24
31–40	45	10	4	14	72	24	17	20	39	20	20	35	25
41–50	6	2	16	66	16	1	66		33	50	33		16

Suture stage: 0 = no closure anywhere; 1 = suture is closed, but clearly visible as a continuous zigzagging line; 2 = suture line becomes thinner, has fewer zigzags and may be interrupted by complete closure; 3 = only pits indicate where the suture is located; 4 = suture completely obliterated: even its location cannot be recognized.

Reproduced from McKern (1970) with permission.

nially. Because of the difficulty of opening the vault to allow comparison of the two sides, and owing to variation in the amount of obliteration at any age level, documentation of suture closure appears at the moment to be useful only for the corroboration of other ageing techniques or for a general classification into child, adolescent or young, through middle age, to old adult. Nevertheless, papers by Meindl and Lovejoy (1985) have provided the impetus to re-examine the entire technique of age estimation from cranial suture closure. More recently, Mann *et al.* (1987) documented the amount and pattern of closure of the maxillary suture (between the two palatine bones) occurring at different ages. They found that males typically exhibit more suture obliteration at all ages than do females but that race has only a minor influence on this parameter.

The spheno-occipital (basilar 'suture') synchondrosis is reported not to close until the early 20s (Williams *et al.*, 1995). However, McKern's (1970) data on American males killed during the Korean War (Table 5.8) indicate that closure is complete before the age of 20 years, while Suchey (1991) has reported closure as early as age 14 in females and age 16 in males. Thus, in the case of its closure in a skeleton of unknown sex, age may be determined as 14 years or older. Similarly, if the 'suture' is open, age may be estimated as 18 years or younger.

Table 5.8 Age distribution of stages in closure in the spheno-occipital synchondrosis (%) (*N* = 213)

Age	Number	0	1	2	3	4
17–18	55	3	2	7	10	78
19	52				3	97
20	45				2	98
21	37					100
22	24					100

Epiphyseal union is recorded on a scale of 0–4, where: 0 = non-union, $1 = \frac{1}{4}$ united, $2 = \frac{1}{2}$ united, $3 = \frac{3}{4}$ united, 4 = complete union. Sample consisted of 375 American males, predominantly white, killed during the Korean War. Age range 17–50, the younger ages being most frequent.

Reproduced from McKern (1970) with permission.

AGE ESTIMATION FROM THE POSTCRANIAL SKELETON

The regions of the adult skeleton (with the exception of sutures of the vault and cranial base) that are most commonly used in determining age are the pubic symphysis, the sternal ends of ribs, the auricular surfaces of the ilium and sacrum, the anterior iliac crest and the medial end of the clavicle. Unlike in the developmental stages of growth, when the epiphyses of long bones close and teeth form and erupt, ageing in the adult tends to be associated initially with remodelling of the skeleton and ultimately, in middle to old age, with degenerative changes. Because there is no regular age-related sequence of growth and development on which to rely, the techniques used in ageing adult bones are generally less precise than those in the juvenile and adolescent population. They involve observation and analysis at both the morphological and microscopic levels, but as age changes often vary between the sexes, as well as amongst different populations, the task of age assessment from adult material is considerably more difficult. Parts of the skeleton where the ageing process is most evident are the articular ends of the bones at synovial, cartilaginous and fibrous joints. Ageing at each of these sites is, however, quite different. At synovial joints, it is predominantly one of wear and tear, with erosion of articular cartilage and the appearance of osteo-

phytes at the joint margins. At the rib ends and the pubic symphysis, both cartilaginous joints, there is mineralization of cartilage and characteristic erosion and metamorphosis of articular surfaces.

PUBIC SYMPHYSIS

Age-related changes at the pubic symphysis have been recognized for many years (Todd, 1920, 1921; McKern and Stewart, 1957; Gilbert and McKern, 1973; Suchey *et al.*, 1984; Suchey and Brooks, 1988). Ageing here is associated with the disappearance of a 'billowing' pattern to the bone, represented by a distinct complex of ridges and grooves on the articular surface. The articular margins become 'built up', and ultimately, beyond the age of 50, there is erosion of the symphyseal surface. It becomes smooth and 'grainy' in appearance; marginal osteophytes develop and are associated with separation of the pubic tubercle from the remainder of the face. Suchey and Brooks (1988) developed an age-determination system of symphyseal changes for both males and females, based on a modern sample of known age. Their technique correlates closely with matched age samples of both males and females in the age range 15–25 years; however, the confidence of prediction declines markedly with older samples. Furthermore, using the same sample, Katz and Suchey (1987) revealed significant race differences in the mean age at death among white, black and Mexican Americans, suggesting that there may be racial variation in the degree of age changes. Therefore, when dealing with skeletal remains that fall into older age categories, it is apparent that a multiple age indicator, which relies on additional subjective criteria, such as the sternal end of the rib, vertebral lipping and scapular changes, may be more appropriate than is examination of the pubic symphysis alone.

STERNAL RIB

The sternal end of the rib also shows an age-related 'metamorphosis' throughout life, involving change in pit shape, increased pit depth and scalloping of the rim as well as a decline in overall condition of the bone. Nine phases of progression spanning the age period from the teens through to the 70s have been identified (Iscan *et al.*, 1984). Reported benefits of using the sternal rib in comparison with other ageing sites relates to the fact that the rib is not subject to weight-bearing forces or to changes associated with pregnancy and parturition, as are the joints of the pelvis. One of the limitations of the technique is that the standards devised by Iscan *et al.* (1984) were derived from the fourth right rib, and it is not known how much the other ribs differ in their ageing response. In addition, preservation of the rib ends may not always occur, especially where skeletal remains are scattered. The progression of age changes in the sternal rib, furthermore, appears to be both sex and population specific, with variation in time of onset, rate and pattern in females compared with males. As with the pubic symphysis, the age range of the various phases is most reliable for those between 16 and 25 years (Iscan *et al.*, 1984, 1985).

AURICULAR SURFACE

The ear-shaped 'auricular' surface of the iliac component of the sacroiliac joint has also been examined for age-related modifications (Lovejoy *et al.*, 1985). Changes are similar to those occurring at the pubic symphysis. There is loss of billowing and increasing fine granularity, the process passing through eight arbitrarily attributed stages of increasing irregularity in appearance of the articular surface, porosity and destruction of the subcortical bone. While there are a number of components to this technique, making it more difficult to learn than that for the pubic symphysis, the major advantages are that it provides age estimation beyond the age of 50 years. In addition, because of its relative robustness, the auricular surface of the hip bone is, if the skeletal remains are scattered, often likely to survive carnivore activity wheras smaller and more delicate bones may be susceptible to damage or removal.

GENERAL AGE CHANGES

Osteoarthritic changes, particularly those involving 'lipping' at the margins of lumbar vertebrae, degeneration of articular surfaces at facet joints and migration of osteophytes into the vertebral canal and intervertebral foraminae of the vertebral column, are common features of ageing. As well as indicating age, osteophytes also develop as a result of occupational stress. Lipping at the margins of lumbar vertebral bodies is rarely present until the mid- to late-40s, therefore, without consideration of the level of physical activity, there is a danger that a young adult skeleton may be 'over-aged' (Iscan and Loth, 1989, p. 27).

OTHER AGE INDICATORS

The most accurate technique for ageing adult skeletal material is to count Haversian units (osteons) per unit area in a thin section of cortical bone (Kerley and Ubelaker, 1978; Stout, 1989). This is a laboratory-based histomorphological technique, and while involving an objective assessment of bone, the method requires both specialist equipment and specialized training. Furthermore, the technique is destructive of bone. Nevertheless, it does have advantages as it involves the application of quantitative techniques over more subjective traditional approaches.

The degree and progression of ossification of the thyroid cartilage may also be used to assess age. Cerny (1983) documented nine stages through which the thyroid ossifies, from ages 15 to 68 years. Information on the early stages of ossification is relevant for both males and females, while the later stages are valid for males only.

Radiographic estimation of thinning of the cortex of long bones has also been used. Age-related changes in both the humerus and femur, as a result of endosteal resorption, as well as regression of trabecular bone from the shaft with associated enlargement of the medullary cavity, have been documented (Schranz, 1959; Acsádi and Nemeskéri, 1970). Schranz (1959) indicated that during the age period from 31 to 40 years cancellous bone almost reaches the surgical neck, by 41–50 the upper level of the surgical neck, and not until between 61 and 74 years of age the epiphyseal line. Acsádi and Neméskeri (1970) documented six phases of structural change between the ages of 41 and 62 years, with the appearance of increasingly fragile and porous bone over this period. It might be anticipated that these changes will be more apparent in females who show an early onset of osteoporosis. Other bones have been examined, but the changes are highly variable and tend to be 'site specific'.

The anthropological approach to human identification involves the anatomical examination of a variety of body regions. The examination of skeletal remains represents one of the most useful medical investigative procedures to assist in the determination of identity. This is primarily because assessment of race, sex and age provides the foundation upon which other identification techniques, involving human individualization, are based.

References and recommended reading

Acsádi G, Nemeskéri J. 1970: *History of human life span and mortality*. Budapest: Akademiai Kiado.

Bainbridge D, Genoves ST. 1956: A study of sex differences in the scapula. *Journal of the Royal Anthropological Institute* **86**(2), 109–34.

Bennett KA. 1987: *A field guide for human skeletal identification*. Springfield, IL: Charles C. Thomas.

Birkby WH. 1966: An evaluation of race and sex identification from cranial measurements. *American Journal of Physical Anthropology* **24**, 21–7.

Boyd WC. 1950: *Genetics and the races of man: an introduction to modern physical anthropology*. Boston: Little, Brown.

Brothwell DR. 1981: *Digging up bones*. British Museum: Oxford University Press.

Brues AM. 1990: The once and future diagnosis of race. In Gill GW, Rhine S (eds) *Skeletal attribution of race. Methods for forensic anthropology*. Maxwell Museum of Anthropology: University of New Mexico, 1–9.

Cerny M. 1983: Our experience with estimation of an individual's age from skeletal remains of the degree of thyroid cartilage ossification. *Acta Universitatis Olomucensis*, **3**, 121–44. In Krogman MW, Iscan MY. 1986: *The human skeleton in forensic medicine*. Springfield, IL: Charles C Thomas, 127–9.

DiBennardo R, Taylor JV. 1983: Multiple discriminant function analysis of sex and race in the postcranial skeleton. *American Journal of Physical Anthropology* **61**, 305–14.

Dunn LC. 1967: Race and biology. In Korn N, Thompson F (eds) *Human evolution. Readings in physical anthropology*. New York: Holt, Rinehart & Winston.

Fazekas I, Kosa F. 1978: *Forensic fetal osteology*. Budapest: Akademiai Kiado.

Flecker H. 1932/33: Roentgenographic observations of the times of appearance of the epiphyses and their fusion with the diaphyses. *Journal of Anatomy* **67**, 118–64.

Gilbert BM, McKern TW. 1973: A method for aging the female os pubis. *American Journal of Physical Anthropology* **38**, 31–8.

Giles E. 1970: Discriminant function sexing of the human skeleton. In Stewart TD (ed.) *Personal identification in mass disaster*. Washington, DC: National Museum of Natural History.

Giles E, Elliot, O. 1962: Race identification from cranial measurements. *Journal of Forensic Sciences* **7**, 147–57.

Gill GW, Hughes SS, Bennett SM, Gilbert BM. 1988: Racial identification from the midfacial skeleton with special reference to the American Indians and whites. *Journal of Forensic Sciences* **33**, 92–9.

Greulich WW, Pyle SI. 1959: *Radiographic atlas of skeletal development of the hand and wrist*. Stanford: Stanford University Press.

Hanihara K. 1959: Sex diagnosis of Japanese skulls and scapulae by means of discriminant functions. *Journal of the Anthropological Society of Nippon* **67**, 21–7.

Houghton P. 1977: Rocker jaws. *American Journal of Physical Anthropology* **47**, 365–9.

Houghton P. 1978: Polynesian mandibles. *Journal of Anatomy* **127**, 251–60.

Howells WW. 1970: Multivariate analysis for the identification of race from crania. In Stewart T (ed.) *Personal identification in mass disasters*. Washington: National Museum of Natural History, 111–21.

Iscan MY. 1983: Assessment of race from the pelvis. *American Journal of Physical Anthropology* **62**, 205–8.

Iscan MY, Loth SR. 1989: Osteological manifestations of age in the adult. In Iscan MY, Kennedy KAR (eds) *Reconstruction of life from the skeleton*. New York: Alan R Liss.

Iscan MY, Loth SR, Wright RK. 1984: Age estimation from the rib by phase analysis: white males. *Journal of Forensic Sciences* **29**(4), 1094–104.

Iscan MY, Loth SR, Wright RK. 1985: Age estimation from the rib by phase analysis: white females. *Journal of Forensic Sciences* **30**(3), 853–63.

Jit I, Jhingan V, Kulkarni M. 1980: Sexing the human sternum. *American Journal of Physical Anthropology* **53**, 217–24.

Johnson DR, O'Higgins P, Moore WJ, McAndrew TJ. 1989: Determination of race and sex of the human skull by discriminant function analysis of linear and angular dimensions. *Forensic Science International* **41**, 41–53.

Katz D, Suchey JM. 1987: *Determination of age in the male os pubis: consideration of the race variable*. American Academy of Forensic Sciences, Program 1987, p. 122 (abstract).

Keen JA. 1950: A study of the differences between male and female skulls. *American Journal of Physical Anthropology* **8**, 65–79.

Kerley ER, Ubelaker DH. 1978: Revisions in the microscopic method of estimating age at death in human cortical bone. *American Journal of Physical Anthropology* **49**, 545–6.

Kimura K. 1982: A base-wing index for sexing the sacrum. *Journal of the Anthropological Society, Nippon* **90** (suppl.), 153–62.

Krogman MW, Iscan MY. 1986: *The human skeleton in forensic medicine*. Springfield, IL: Charles C. Thomas.

Larnach SL. 1978: Australian aboriginal craniology. *Oceania Monographs*, **21**, 1.

Lovejoy CO, Burstein AH, Heiple KG. 1976: The biomechanical analysis of bone strength: a method and its application to platycnemia. *American Journal of Physical Anthropology* **44**, 489–506.

Lovejoy CO, Meindl RS, Pryzbeck TR, Mensforth RP. 1985: Chronological metamorphosis of the auricular surface of the ilium: a new method for the determination of age at death. *American Journal of Physical Anthropology* **68**, 1–14.

McKern TW. 1970: Estimation of skeletal age: from puberty to about 30 years of age. In Stewart TD (ed.) *Personal identification in mass disasters*. Washington, DC: National Museum of Natural History.

McKern TW, Stewart JH. 1957: *Skeletal age changes in young American males*. Analysed from the standpoint of age identification. Environmental Protection Research Division Technical Report No. EP-45. Natick, MA: Quartermaster Research and Development Center, US Army.

Mann RW, Symes SA, Bass WM. 1987: Maxillary suture obliteration: aging the human skeleton based on intact or fragmentary maxilla. *Journal of Forensic Sciences* **32**(1), 148–57.

Meindl RS, Lovejoy CO. 1985: Ectocranial suture closure: a revised method for the determination of skeletal age at death and blind tests of its accuracy. *American Journal of Physical Anthropology* **68**, 57–66.

Montagu MFA. 1938: Aging of the skull. *American Journal of Physical Anthropology* **23**, 355–75.

Pietrusewsky M. 1990: Craniofacial variation in Australian and Pacific populations. *American Journal of Physical Anthropology* **82**(3), 319–40.

Pounder DJ. 1984: Forensic aspects of Aboriginal skeletal remains in Australia. *American Journal of Forensic Medicine and Pathology* **5**(1), 41–52.

Rhine S. 1990: Non-metric skull racing. In Gill GW, Rhine S (eds) *Skeletal attribution of race. Methods for forensic anthropology*. Maxwell Museum of Anthropology, University of New Mexico, Albuquerque, 9–21.

St Hoyme LE. 1982: A simple statistical method for estimating sex distribution and dimensions in dissociated long bone series. *Ossa* **7**, 119–27.

St Hoyme LE. 1984: Sex differences in the posterior pelvis. *Collegium Anthropology* **8**, 139–54.

St Hoyme LE, Iscan MY. 1989: Determination of sex and race: accuracy and assumptions. In Iscan MY, Kennedy KAR (eds), *Reconstruction of life from the skeleton*. New York: Alan R Liss, 5.

Sauer NJ. 1992: Forensic anthropology and the concept of race: if races don't exist, why are forensic anthropologists so good at identifying them? *Social Science and Medicine* **34**(2), 107–11.

Schranz D. 1959: Age determination from the internal structure of the humerus. *American Journal of Physical Anthropology* **17**, 273–8.

Schulter-Ellis FP, Hayek LC. 1984: Predicting race and sex with an acetabulum–pubis index. *Collegium Anthropology* **8**:155–62.

Schulter-Ellis FP, Schmidt OJ, Hayek L-A, Craig J. 1983: Determination of sex with a discriminant analysis of new pelvic bone measurements. Part 1. *Journal of Forensic Sciences* **28**, 169–80.

Singer R. 1953: Estimation of age from cranial suture closure. A report on its reliability. *Journal of Forensic Medicine* **1**(1), 52–9.

Snow CE. 1974: *Early Hawaiians*. Lexington: University of Kentucky Press.

Stewart TD. 1979: *Essentials of forensic anthropology, especially as developed in the United States*. Springfield, IL: Charles C. Thomas.

Stout SD. 1989: Histomorphometric analysis of human skeletal remains. In Iscan MY, Kennedy KAR (eds), *Reconstruction of life from the skeleton*. New York: Alan R. Liss, 4.

Suchey JM. 1991: *Instructional materials accompanying female pubic symphyseal models of the Suchey-Brooks*. Distributed by France Casting (available from Diane France, 20102 Buckhorn Road, Bellvue, Colorado 80512).

Suchey JM, Brooks ST. 1988: *Skeletal age determination on the male os pubis*. Twelfth International Congress of Anthropological and Ethnological Sciences, Zagreb, Yugoslavia, July 24–31.

Suchey JM, Owings PA, Wiseley DV, Noguchi TT. 1984: Skeletal aging of unidentified persons. In Rathbun TA, Buikstra JE (eds), *Human identification: case studies in forensic anthropology*. Springfield IL: Charles C. Thomas, 278–97.

Sutherland LD, Suchey JM. 1991: Use of the ventral arc in pubic sex determination. *Journal of Forensic Sciences* **36**, 501–11.

Todd TW. 1920: Age changes in the pubic bone. Part 1: The male white pubis. *American Journal of Physical Anthropology* **3**, 285–334.

Todd TW. 1921: Age changes in the pubic bone. Part 6: The interpretation of variations in the symphysial area. *American Journal of Physical Anthropology* **4**, 407–24.

Washburn SL. 1948: Sex differences in the pubic bone. *American Journal of Physical Anthropology* **6**, 199–208.

Williams PL, Bannister LM, Berry MM *et al.* 1995: *Gray's anatomy*. Edinburgh: Churchill Livingstone.

CHAPTER 6

Dental identification

JG CLEMENT

History and introduction	63	Unwritten records	71
The need for expert opinion	65	General pattern agreement versus specific feature	
Establishment of identity is a comparative process	66	recognition	73
Problems with ante mortem records	67	Age at death	75

History and introduction

Forensic odontology is one of the fastest emerging subdisciplines within the broader subject of dental science. Implicit in its title is the conjunction of the law and dentistry in all its manifestations. In essence, the forensic odontologist has to be an experienced practitioner of clinical dentistry who is also able to observe, record, gather, preserve and interpret dental evidence in order to make it meaningful in a legal context, often a court of law.

While forensic odontology therefore rightly encompasses ethical issues and events relating to claims of negligence and malpractice by dentists and paradental professionals, the main thrust of day-to-day casework still remains primarily that of the corroboration of the identity of deceased persons.

There are numerous historical accounts of famous persons being identified post mortem by the recognition of certain peculiarities within their dentitions. Many of these cases have been collated by Hill (1984). However, it is not merely enough for various combinations of teeth, dental restorations and prostheses to be highly individual in order for them to find application in the post mortem identification of the dead. Durability in life and especially after death, often in extremely adverse conditions, is also an essential attribute.

The natural teeth are the most durable organs in the bodies of vertebrates, and humankind's understanding of their own past and evolution relies heavily upon remnant dental evidence found as fossils (Tobias, 1990). Teeth can persist long after other skeletal structures have succumbed to organic decay or destruction by some other agency, such as fire (Fig. 6.1). It may be argued that dental enamel, the hardest skeletal tissue, is not a tissue at all in the strictest sense but virtually a fossilized secretion from the time of its formation upon the teeth, which are then still entombed in bony crypts within the jaws prior to their emergence into the mouth.

Teeth and bone can be heated to temperatures approaching the melting point of skeletal mineral ($\geqslant 1600°C$) without appreciable loss of microstructure or tertiary architecture (Clement *et al.*, 1992; Holden *et al.*, 1995a, b, c) (Fig. 6.2). Such permanence of structure has spawned the emergence of yet another subspecialty preoccupied with the interpretation of dental evidence. Dental anthropology can draw its study material from the living (e.g. studies of variation of tooth morphology within a population), when it may be considered to be part of the wider discipline of anthropology. However, dental anthropology is often concerned with issues akin to those of the forensic odontologist, such as the proper recovery of remains and their identification, cleaning, storage, tabulation and interpretation.

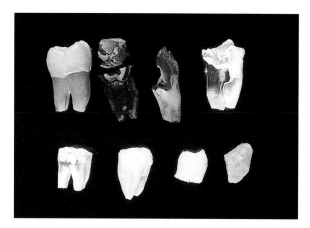

Fig. 6.1 A series of teeth, each incinerated in air at increasing increments of 200°C for 2 hours. Top left to top right: 200, 400, 600 and 800°C. Bottom left to bottom right: 1000, 1200, 1400 and 1600°C. The early colour changes (charcoal gray) are attributable to the combustion of organic constituents, the later ones (pale pink) to crystallographic changes. The specimen at 1600°C shows some evidence of slight melting and resolidification on cooling. At all other temperatures, the tertiary architecture of the tissues is retained despite thermal shock damage shattering parts of the organ. (Courtesy of Dr Olsson–Jacques)

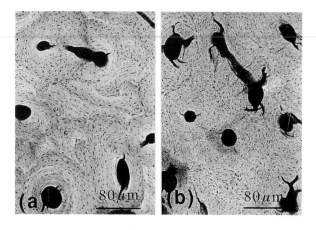

Fig. 6.2 Microradiographs of two transverse sections taken from the mid-shaft of the femur of a person aged 12 years. (a) Heated at 1000°C for 2 hours. (b) Heated at 1400°C for 2 hours. Note the retention of the bone microstructure. Haversian systems and osteocyte lacunae are still clearly visible. (Courtesy of Dr J Holden)

It is therefore obvious that many of the interests, skills and techniques of dental anthropology are shared with forensic dentistry. The principal difference between the specialties lies in the context within which their respective studies are undertaken rather than in the nature of their investigations *per se*. An excellent review of non-forensic dental anthropology is provided by Hillson (1996), which represents an ideal companion volume to this text.

The final requirement for the utility of dental findings for identification purposes is based in the almost universal need for people to attend a dentist for an examination of their oral health status. The 'byproducts' of such visits are the dental records of the person in life.

Such records need not only be in the form of written clinical notes. Plaster casts of the patient's mouth, clinical photographs and in particular radiographs ('dental X-rays') are invaluable for the forensic odontologist's comparison between ante mortem status and post mortem findings. It is commonly surmised that if no treatment has been provided, dental records will be of little use. This is a serious misconception. With improvements to diet, oral hygiene and the adjustment of the fluoride content of the drinking water supply to optimize its anticaries effects, many young people in first-world countries do not now experience significant dental decay. While such people obviously do not have dental restorations and repairs to their teeth that might have been used for identification purposes, they nevertheless still have radiographic examinations of their teeth to check for the signs of dental decay beginning at the regions of contact between adjacent teeth in the dental arches.

A decline in dental decay in modern populations is also accompanied by an increasing attention on the part of the public to aspects of their oral status that were once generally considered less important or a luxury. The growth in orthodontic practice in 'Western' societies is a good example of this change in attitude and sophistication (Kingman, 1997).

When advice has been sought concerning either functional or aesthetic malocclusion of the teeth in adolescence, cranial radiographs are taken as part of the orthodontic examination (Fig. 6.3). Plaster casts of the patients' mouths are invariably made as part of the assessment, diagnosis and treatment planning for orthodontic cases. These 'study models' record tooth number, size, crown form and tooth position very accurately (Fig 6.4). Wax wafers or some other temporarily deformable substance is used permanently to record how the patient's jaws and teeth fit together when the mouth is closed. These records of the occlusal relationships can also be important for identification purposes, particularly if reconstruction of facial features upon remnant skull evidence or the use of superimposition techniques is proposed.

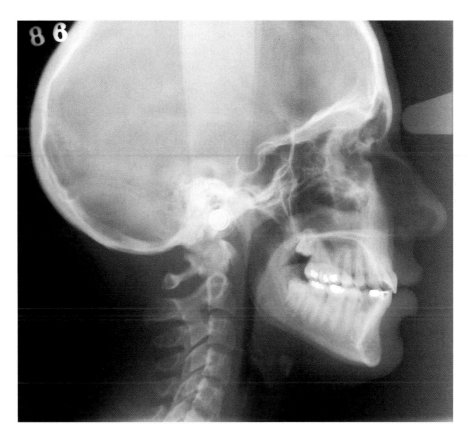

Fig. 6.3 Lateral cephalometric radiograph taken as part of the initial examination and assessment of patients seeking orthodontic treatment. Further radiographs of the same type are taken either throughout treatment to monitor progress, or at the end of treatment to record changes to the size of patient's jaws and the positions of their teeth. The incorporation of an aluminium step wedge over the soft tissues of the face attenuates the X-ray beam and reveals the soft tissue profile

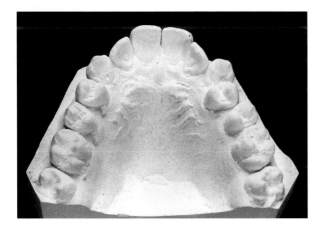

Fig. 6.4 Typical dental study model or cast made from an inexpensive alginate impression. Note the enormous amount of individualizing detail displayed in the combination of the number and positions of teeth, and their crown micromorphology. Casts made from rubber-based silicone impressions show even more detail, but such models are less plentiful for forensic application

The need for expert opinion

The dental examination of a corpse is quite different from the dental examination of a living person, whether he or she is awake and co-operative, or anaesthetized and unresponding. These skills are not taught as part of the undergraduate dental curriculum.

The corpse may be rigid or semirigid due to rigor mortis or refrigeration. The musculature may have been fixed by heat, so it may be impossible to open the jaws without a dissection or resection (see Chapter 8). The body may have multiple injuries, which, in addition to disfigurement, may give rise to the presence of sharp-edged skeletal fractures, presenting a health risk to the examiner.

Since the main thrust of forensic odontology is the identification of the deceased, it follows that many of the bodies that need to be examined are unidentifiable by other means. Many are therefore partially decayed or even completely skeletalized.

Each of these different sets of circumstances presents the examiner with a particular challenge, and dealing with these challenges and risks should not be the responsibility of the general dental practitioner who has not had any graduate training in forensic odontology. When such people have been pressed into service, many have performed well at the time, only privately to carry the emotional legacy of their ordeal for years to come. This is an unwise practice. Similarly, when the legally naive are later asked to present evidence or be cross-examined as an expert witness, when they are often not fully expert in all aspects of the task they have been asked to undertake, it is likely to give rise to problems for the courts. This can be to no-one's benefit.

Another source of stress can arise from the enthusiasm of police investigators to avail themselves of autopsy findings at the earliest opportunity. It is often the case that a period of quiet reflection to consider all aspects of the evidence is needed before the expert is in a position to give a truly expert opinion. If the tempo of the investigation or the immediate public interest in the case subverts this requirement, mistakes can happen, and it is usually the least experienced practitioner who feels the most coercive pressures. The conjunction of a high-profile case and inexperienced practitioners is a potentially dangerous combination. In Australia, one prominent murder investigation – 'the pyjama girl case' – was thwarted for years because the initial dental examination of the victim resulted in a mischarting of some of the teeth of the deceased (Coleman, 1978).

It is therefore important that dentists who wish to become practitioners of forensic dentistry undergo an appropriate course of graduate training and instruction before undertaking any obligations and casework in their own right. The cultivation of a mentor is to be encouraged. Regular case presentations and audit before one's peers are invaluable as a source of help and advice for one's own professional development. It is isolated practitioners who are most at risk of becoming out of date with their thinking, with the accompanying risk of eccentricity of opinion. The stressful nature of the work needs to be recognized and steps taken to make provision for rest and recuperation. This is very important in mass disaster investigations where the temptation to overcommit one's personal resources is very high.

The contribution that a truly expert, professionally detached and non-aligned forensic odontologist can make to an investigation is considerable. In cases of homicide, the establishment of the identity of the deceased is obviously of paramount importance. Problems can arise if one is working in a legal system in which different courts have different requirements or standards of proof. In the British system of justice and its various offshoots and derivatives, the coroner only requires that persons be identified 'on the balance of probability'. Conversely, higher courts require proof 'beyond reasonable doubt'. It is therefore likely that a body will sometimes be discovered and identified to the satisfaction of the coroner before the criminal circumstances surrounding the case come to light. If, in the meantime, the body has been interred or, even worse, cremated, this may well preclude any later opportunity for a more rigorous examination of the remains to establish identity 'beyond reasonable doubt'. The forensic odontologist should be alert to this from the outset and take the necessary preventive steps if possible.

In the wake of catastrophe, family members are often asked to help with the identification of their relatives. This will sometimes be the first occasion that many will ever have had to look at a dead person. This is obviously an additional burden for people who are already suffering great distress.

In the immediate aftermath of the *Herald of Free Enterprise* shipwreck in Belgian waters at Zeebrugge in March 1987, families of the deceased were required to inspect many corpses already casketted in order to identify their next of kin. At the time, many bodies still had to be recovered, so it was likely that, for some families, the ordeal would be in vain. In one instance, all the relatives failed to recognise the remains of their family member, who fortunately had a constellation of dental treatment and whose dentist had supplied very comprehensive dental records. The forensic dental evidence to corroborate identity was irrefutable and was accepted by both investigators and family.

In other investigations, families have disputed the identity of the deceased, resulting in two different families laying claim to the same body. Again, the role of an expert investigator, emotionally detached and unconnected by strong social, cultural or religious affiliations to the victims, paired with a legal system in which all parties have implicit trust, is essential for a satisfactory outcome.

Visual identification is so vulnerable to genuine mistakes, fraud or other attempts to 'pervert the course of justice' that its use without further corroboration of identity by other means is unwise.

Establishment of identity is a comparative process

The definite establishment of identity for a body essentially comes from a detailed comparison and matching of tangible ante mortem records and post mortem findings. It is rarely the case that the two match in all respects, so some judgement is required.

This often requires the application of logic, and unless the person dies on the day of their last dental appointment, it always requires the investigator to grasp the temporal framework in which the ante mortem records were amassed relative to the time at which the corpse was examined.

It is commonly the case for more than one set of dental records to exist for the same person. Such records may be sequential, perhaps reflecting a shift of abode or workplace on the part of the deceased. However, this is not always the case. Patients may attend both a general dental practitioner and a dental specialist over the same period of time. Unless the first set of dental records collected by the police are scrutinized by the forensic odontologist at the outset, the existence of other records relating to the same person but housed elsewhere, perhaps by a specialist, may go overlooked until it is too late to recover them.

However, whatever complexities exist in the ante mortem pattern of treatment, it is the responsibility of the forensic odontologist to compile a single master ante mortem record summarizing all the available dental evidence (Fig. 6.5). This is then compared with the single post mortem record to identify features that are common to both records and also to look for any incompatible inconsistencies that may exclude a positive identification.

This is in essence a simple procedure, but in reality, it is often quite a complex task. Why should this be so?

Problems with ante mortem records

NOTATION

In common with many other groups whose workload is heavy and somewhat repetitive, dentists have evolved shorthand methods for recording what they see and what they do. All dentists are trained in at least one of these methods, but in a lifetime of practice many will extend, embellish or even further prune the particular shorthand so that it efficiently reflects their own choice of restorative materials and the nature of their practice. These metamorphoses may be opaque to an outsider. This often necessitates a conference between the forensic odontologist who has performed the post mortem examination and the treating dentist from whom the ante mortem records of the presumed deceased have been obtained.

This problem is exacerbated by the fact that there exist at least four major shorthand languages within dentistry (see Appendix III). Fortunately, many have

a predominant geographical location, usually related to what has been taught in the local university dental schools. This means that most practitioners within a particular country share at least a common notation for ascribed tooth-numbering systems on dental charts.

Historically, the Haderup system has been restricted to Scandinavia, where it was invented. It is declining in usage with the increasing move to the Fédération Dentaire Internationale (FDI) system, which is gaining adoption.

The Palmer/Zygmondy system was invented almost simultaneously in two different places. It was the most widespread system in use in the UK and many countries that were once in its sphere of influence. The system is simple, intuitive but not really compatible with keyboard data entry. It is now a system in declining use. All dental schools in Australia now use the FDI system. Consequently, most dental practitioners in Australia today are 'bilingual', understanding both Palmer and FDI notation.

The Universal system is not universally used. Its use is almost entirely restricted to the USA where it can be anticipated to continue. Like the FDI system, it is a two-digit code, so it is possible to completely misidentify a tooth and any associated treatment unless the type of notation being used is explicitly specified. This is particularly true in mass disaster situations in which US nationals and people from other parts of the world may have died together.

INCOMPLETENESS

Incompleteness is the most commonly encountered shortcoming in dental records. This may extend from the omission of patients' personal details such as date of birth, through to a failure to record treatment provided. In the latter case, a search of the bills sent to the patient can help to augment otherwise incomplete records.

One common, widespread but unfortunate practice is the custom for many practitioners to chart only the work necessary to restore oral health rather than sound restorations that may have been done elsewhere on previous occasions by another practitioner (Fig. 6.5). The use of panoramic radiography is becoming more popular as a screening procedure. These radiographs often conveniently summarize much of the patient's previous treatment experience and can be used to augment otherwise deficient notes. They can also be used for direct comparison with similar post mortem radiographs, but this is quite a challenging procedure to attempt owing to complexities in the geometry of the system needed to generate identical projections between the two views. It is sometimes necessary to use exactly the

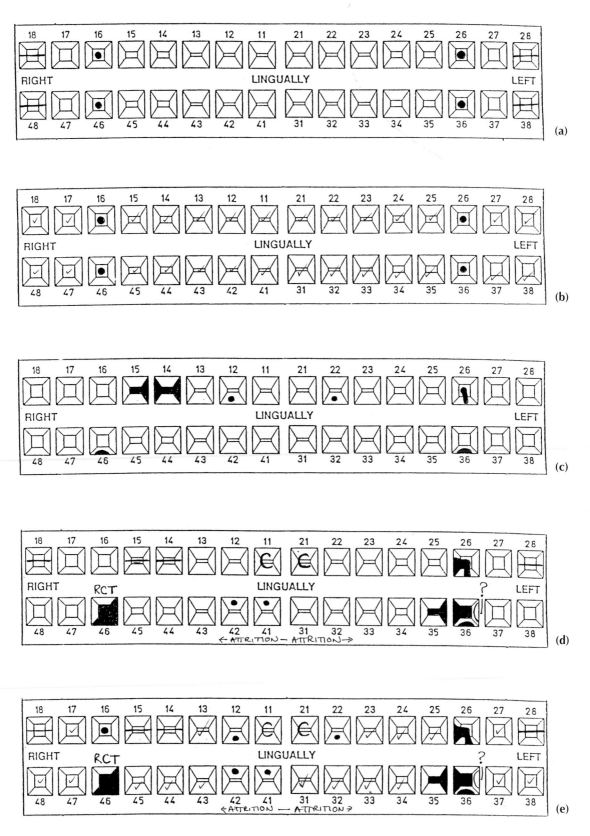

Fig. 6.5

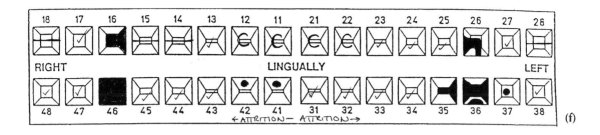

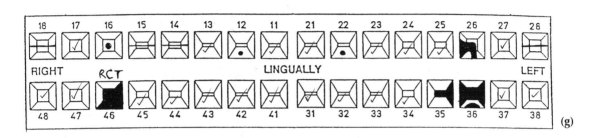

Fig. 6.5 A series of dental charts from the same individual throughout life compared with post mortem records. (a) Dentist 1 only charts four simple restorations and notes the absence of all four wisdom teeth. The status of all other teeth is unrecorded. The patient is in the late teens. It may be reasonable to presume that all teeth unrecorded are nevertheless still present. (b) Dentist 2 corroborates the presence of a full dentition, including wisdom teeth, which have now appeared in the oral cavity. Patient aged in the early 20s. (c) Dentist 3 records additional restorations in teeth 15, 14, 12, 22, 46 and 36. Restoration in tooth 26 has now been replaced and extended. Patient aged in the mid-30s. (d) Dentist 4 records some but not all of the existing restorations. Crowns are fitted to teeth 11 and 12. Teeth 15 and 14 (previously heavily restored) are now missing, presumed extracted. Tooth 46 is now extensively repaired, including root canal therapy (RCT). Lower anterior teeth 42, 41, 31 and 32 are now heavily worn, 42 and 41 have lingual restorations and tooth 35 has been restored. Tooth 36 has had the existing restoration extended, and the presence of the older restoration is noted. The patient is now aged 55. (e) Odontologist's composite ante mortem chart compiled from (a)–(d). (f) Odontologist's chart made from a post mortem examination of an unidentified body. This chart is compatible with the composite ante mortem chart (e). Further treatment has obviously taken place since the patient was seen by Dentist 4. Additional crowns have been fitted to teeth 12 and 22. Restorations to teeth 16, 36, 46 have been extended. Identity would have to be corroborated by an X-ray examination and the comparison of specific, stable features, for example the restoration in tooth 26. (g) Odontologist's chart made from a post mortem examination of an unidentified body. This odontogram has some incompatible inconsistencies when compared with the composite ante mortem chart (e). Most notable is the apparent disappearance of the artificial crowns from teeth 12 and 11, which have been charted as present and sound. Similarly, teeth 42 and 41 have 'self-repaired'. Tooth 36 has a more extensive restoration than previously recorded, but this is not incompatible. Should a chart like this arise in the context of a busy investigation, for example a mass disaster situation, it would be prudent to re-examine the remains to double-check for the presence of crowns on teeth 11 and 12, and restorations in teeth 42 and 41, which may have been so good as to have been overlooked

same type of panoramic X-ray machine in order exactly to reproduce the original set of circumstances in which ante mortem radiographs were generated.

INACCURACY AND MISINTERPRETATION

In the forensic dental autopsy, two practitioners examine the remains. One should ideally act as the examiner while the other records the information that is dictated. The scribe can also act as an interrogator, thereby prompting the examiner to pay particular attention to any features of interest or special importance. This protocol also ensures that any written notes, which have to be taken out of the mortuary, remain free from contamination with blood or any other body fluids. At the end of the first examination, the forensic odontologists reglove and swap roles, repeating the examination process. This is an essential step to ensure the fidelity of any post mortem records. It also provides the opportunity for discussion on any issues that may be unclear.

A commonly encountered problem is the disparity between the description of posterior teeth by the treating dentist and that found in the later dental autopsy report. The explanation is often quite simple. People often have third molar (wisdom) teeth that remain unerupted. These are frequently removed because of lack of space in the mouth for them to fit properly in the dental arches. Only two molars remain, and they are then correctly named as first and second molars. However, there are numerous instances in which people have had their first molars extracted early in life, usually because of severe decay. The second and third molars emerge and drift anteriorly so that no gaps remain where the first molars have been lost. These teeth are then commonly misnamed as first and second molars when they are in fact second and third molars in slightly unusual positions. This is more likely if the teeth have been heavily restored, thereby hiding their original differences in morphology. The forensic odontologist has to be alert to these and other similar charting discrepancies, take them into account and be prepared to explain them to a lay jury (Fig. 6.6).

FRAUD

Much dentistry is funded on a fee for item of service basis. As a sound means of providing health care, this approach has come in for much discussion, particularly by those who see the prevention of illness and disease as more important than the repair of damage that has been sustained by the same arguably preventable diseases (Pine, 1997). It is beyond the scope of this chapter to join this important philosophical debate. The results of a successful prevention strategy are easy to recognize. However, cause and effect cannot always be identified. As a health care fund manager, it is much more difficult to monitor and police provision of care using purely preventive programmes.

Conversely, a fee for item of treatment system is easier to police. The results of clinical work done and for which payment is claimed can easily be verified. This may to some extent, encourage overprescribing

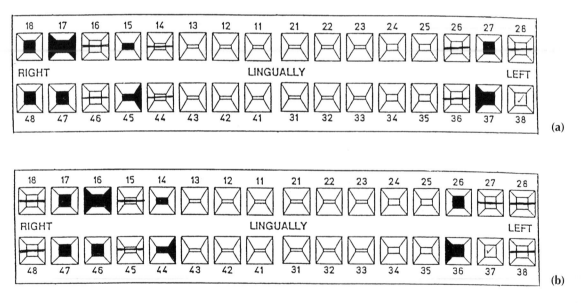

Fig. 6.6 Common charting discrepancies due to misidentification of teeth within a particular series. Odontogram (a) records the absence of the first molar teeth 16, 26, 36, 46 and premolars 14 and 44, together with wisdom tooth 28. (b) Another odontogram of the same patient made by a second dentist. The missing first molars have not been noted. This can easily occur if the first molars are extracted early in life, whereupon teeth distal to the extraction sites drift mesially to obliterate the gap. In this case, it has been erroneously assumed that it is the third molars which are missing. A similar situation can arise when there is only one remaining premolar in any quadrant of the mouth. Note the discrepancies with respect to teeth 15, 14, and 45, and 44 between charts (a) and (b). A sound knowledge of tooth morphology minimizes such errors. This knowledge can still be thwarted by the presence of large dental restorations that obliterate natural tooth form

but it does not encourage spurious claims. Deliberate falsification of dental records is virtually unknown.

Unwritten records

RADIOGRAPHS

Ante mortem X-ray photographs of the head and oro-dental region are excellent evidence for identification purposes. The size, shape and dimensions of many structures are very stable in the skeleton of the head. The paranasal sinuses are small early in life, but the pneumatization of the bones of the face and base of skull with growth to adulthood gives rise to a series of large air-filled cavities that are complex in form and unique in outline.

The frontal sinuses housed in the ridge of bone just above the eye sockets have numerous chambers, with lobes separated by walls or septae. These sinuses are ideal for comparison between ante mortem records and corresponding post mortem views (Fig. 6.7). The simplest way to make a comparison is by overlaying the ante mortem and post mortem films either directly or in an electronic environment (Andersen and Wenzel, 1995; Clement *et al.,* 1995; Ranta and

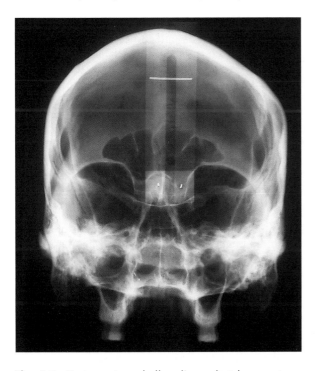

Fig. 6.7 Post mortem skull radiograph taken postero-anteriorly. The outline of the frontal sinuses above the eyes and within the substance of the forehead can be clearly seen. These structures are stable in adulthood

Kerosuo, 1995). The biggest impediment to the more widespread use of this technique is attributable to the relative rarity of ante mortem posteroanterior plane film radiographs of the skull. (This is the situation with many types of medical treatment: the records are excellent when they exist; unfortunately, for an identification requirement, they are rare.)

The maxillary sinuses are equally complex. Their images are frequently recorded on dental radiographs. It is only on panoramic views such as orthopantomographs that they are seen in their entirety (Fig. 6.8). Their images are often poorly recorded because the bones surrounding them are in places little thicker than an eggshell. The original films are usually taken to record the status of the teeth and their associated alveolar processes that are much more radio-opaque. Consequently, the air-filled sinuses are frequently overexposed in ante mortem films. When their shape and form is clearly depicted, they are excellent for comparison purposes.

Lateral skull radiographs are often taken under rigorously reproducible conditions because they are used to monitor growth and the results of orthodontic tooth movements in adolescents. Serial views are often taken at intervals. While some parts of the craniofacial complex can change appreciably through the teenage years, other parts of the skull can achieve adult size and shape much earlier in life. The inner aspect of the anterior cranial fossa is a good example of early dimensional stability, which is readily seen in all lateral cephalometric radiographs, as is the sella tursica more posteriorly (see Fig. 6.3 above). If an aluminium step wedge was used during the initial exposure to attenuate the X-ray beam over the face, the soft tissue profile, including the lip positions, may be clearly visible. If, in addition, the position of the anterior teeth is clearly visible, the radiograph may be suitable for a superimposition on a near life-sized photograph of the deceased. The images of the teeth can be used as fine scaling factors since lateral skull radiographs taken in a cephalostat produce an enlarged image of the skull, which is approximately 12% larger than life size in the midline. Unfortunately, very few people (except criminals) have true lateral photos taken of their face, so the technique, despite having great potential, rarely finds an application for identification purposes.

Post mortem radiographs of skulls can, however, be taken under conditions identical to those which were employed during life, allowing superimposition comparisons to be made. This technique finds much more widespread application because of the more plentiful availability of lateral skull radiographs over facial photographs taken from the side view (see Chapter 12).

The most common type of dental radiograph is the intra-oral bitewing film (Fig. 6.9). These views are

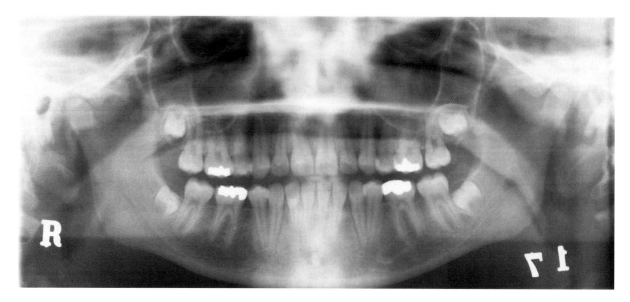

Fig. 6.8 Orthopantomograph (OPG) of the lower face. These panoramic X-ray views conveniently summarize the dental status of the patient. In this case, the person is a late teenager. These are four restorations, one in each first molar. The third molar crowns are complete within their crypts. The outline of the floor of the maxillary sinus can be seen above the roots of the maxillary teeth

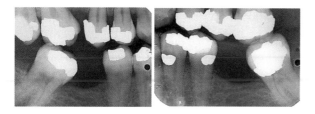

Fig. 6.9 Bitewing radiographs. This pair of intra-oral films images the cheek teeth in both upper and lower jaws for each side of the mouth. This patient has many radio-opaque silver amalgam dental restorations, each of which may be individualizing

taken to examine the crowns and part of the roots of the teeth in the buccal segments of the dental arches. Each film images teeth from both the maxilla and the mandible, and potentially contains myriads of 'points of concordance' with corresponding post mortem views of the same subject when taken under the same geometric conditions.

The longstanding acceptance by courts of law of fingerprint evidence has led to serious conceptual misunderstandings when the same criteria for judging closeness of fit or concordance are applied to comparisons of radiographs. It is fallacious to label an arbitrary number of features that concur between two radiographs that are being compared. It can lead to pointless argument and obfuscation about how many points have to concur before a statistically valid measure of uniqueness is satisfied.

The difference between the techniques of comparison in fingerprints and radiographs has to be understood. With fingerprints, the initial print is examined and enhanced until certain *discrete* features can be recognized subjectively. Complex matrices are then constructed by a computer to relate these features spatially to each another. In such an analysis, the number of points of concordance is therefore an important parameter. It is not the direct comparison of one image with another which is being undertaken but a comparison between transforms.

With radiographs, one set of raw data is being compared with another *in its entirety*. Consequently, it does not matter which feature is selected as a match because *all features have to match simultaneously* (Fig. 6.10). When asked 'How many points of concordance are there?' between matching radiographs, the answer should therefore be 'Either one or an infinite number, depending on the resolution at which the images are to be compared'. Counsel who are more accustomed to dealing with fingerprint evidence may find it difficult to grasp these concepts.

Even in the absence of any ante mortem radiographs, it is often useful to make a post mortem radiographic survey of the remains. Root canal therapy can be detected (Fig. 6.11). Recently healed extraction sockets can be seen, and tooth-coloured restorations that so closely resemble the real tooth substance that they have eluded detection during the routine forensic dental examination may be revealed (Fig. 6.12). This occurs because the restorative materials have a different radio-opacity from the rest of the tooth.

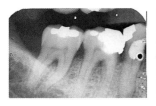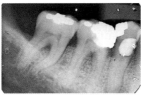

Fig. 6.10 Two intra-oral periapical radiographs, one taken ante mortem (left), the other post mortem (right). The two images match closely in many ways: root morphology, bone trabecular patterns and the number and shape of amalgam restorations

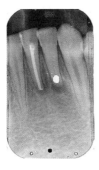

Fig. 6.11 Post mortem intra-oral periapical radiograph. This reveals two examples of root canal therapy that were undetected by the oral examination alone. The conjunction of these two root-filled teeth and the manner in which they have been filled is good evidence to corroborate identity

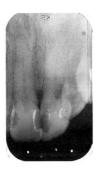

Fig. 6.12 Intra-oral radiograph of the maxillary anterior teeth. The presence of tooth-coloured restorations can be seen as crescentic, radiolucent outlines at the contact areas of adjacent teeth. The restorations were very difficult to detect clinically, matching very closely the colour and form of the natural teeth. On X-ray, their presence is obvious

General pattern agreement versus specific feature recognition

One of the most important skills for the forensic odontologist to develop is the sense of what is truly individualizing. Attempts have been made to calculate the probability of two persons having the same pattern of dental restorations on all of their 160 tooth surfaces. The various combinations theoretically provide 2.5 billion possibilities of uniqueness. The analysis employed to generate such statistics was not particularly sophisticated, and the real situation is likely to be somewhat different, particularly with respect to the diminishing rates of tooth decay amongst the young.

Put simply, the more restorative work that anyone has had done to their teeth, the more individual that person's dentition is likely to become *when depicted in the form of a dental chart*. Earlier analyses paid no attention to the relative frequencies with which specific tooth surfaces were restored. In treating all surfaces as equally susceptible to decay (and hence repair), it is likely that the individual nature of a person's dentition was overemphasized when seen only as dental chart.

Anyone who has any experience of forensic dental casework will recall numerous instances where the remains of young people are found to have very few restorations. Such restorations are not randomly distributed throughout the mouth but are frequently found in the pits and fissures of those permanent teeth which have been present in the mouth for the longest time. Put crudely, four single-surface amalgam restorations, each placed in one of the first permanent molars, is commonplace. What is individualizing is their specific shape, which may have been recorded on clinical photographs or dental radiographs (Fig. 6.13).

Conversely, the situation can arise where there is such an unusual juxtaposition of unusual treatment or the detection of an uncommon developmental anomaly that the finding is instantly recognized as individualizing (Fig. 6.14).

If no restorations are present, the patient may still have had impressions taken of the mouth, perhaps for the construction of a mouthguard for use during sport or as part of an orthodontic examination. The resulting plaster casts, which are often retained by the patient, faithfully record not only the number, position and alignment of teeth present in the mouth but also huge amounts of information in the record of ridges, furrows, cusps, tubercles and other fine surface detail, much of which has a high level of heritability, somewhat akin to fingerprints (Zubov, 1977;

Zubov and Nikityuk, 1978). While the inheritability of fissure patterns is still deserving of wider study for identification purposes, many of the more easily recognized and quantified anatomical variations of tooth form can be interpreted for forensic benefit.

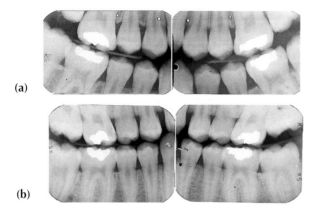

(a)

(b)

Fig. 6.13 Two sets of bitewing radiographs, each from a different person. If odontograms only were compared, these two people would have the same, simple dental charts. However, a comparison of radiographs (a) and (b) clearly reveals differences in the silhouettes of the restorations

Broadly speaking, dental anatomists and anthropologists study the human dentition and the dentitions of our nearest relatives in an evolutionary sense in two ways. There have been a multitude of studies in which the sizes of tooth crowns have been measured. Foremost amongst the exponents of this 'metric' methodology are Moorees (1957), Moorees *et al.* (1957), Moorees and Chandha (1962), Goose (1963, 1971), Moorees and Reed (1964), Garn *et al.* (1965, 1968), Townsend and Brown (1978), Townsend (1980) and Kieser (1990).

The subjects studied usually represent geographically or culturally separate populations who may be assumed to share some common genetic features. Large numbers of measurements are made on large numbers of teeth from large numbers of individuals. Such studies are very useful for identifying evolutionary change within the dentition and investigating patterns of inheritance of tooth sizes and proportions or the relation of tooth size to overall body size, but these studies find very little application in the examination of a specific individual, which so often characterizes the forensic situation.

The second way in which tooth form has been studied is in recognizing the presence, absence or degree of expression of features that vary in their

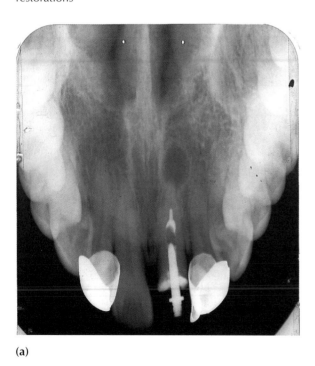

(a)

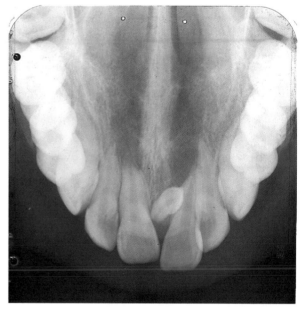

(b)

Fig. 6.14 Anterior occlusal radiograph views of the maxillae of two people. Both have highly significant individualizing features. (a) Reveals two metal crowns, a post in the root of a central incisor, some cementing material in the same root canal and some apical rarefaction of bone. (b) Reveals the presence of a small supernumary tooth in the midline of the maxilla. This developmental anomaly has adversely affected the alignment of the adjacent central incisor teeth. The presence of the mesiodens is unusual, but when viewed in conjunction with all the other anatomical information contained in this radiograph, its presence is as individualizing as a fingerprint

prevalence between individuals. Scoring systems have been developed to make such 'non-metric' studies interpretable by others, and identical sets of dental casts have been manufactured from type specimens and distributed in an attempt to standardize scoring ascribed to any particular feature that is being examined. Dahlberg (1945, 1949, 1963) pioneered the best-known and most widely used set of plaques depicting variants of tooth form. These have recently been augmented by others from Arizona State University, USA (Turner *et al.*, 1991; Buikstra and Ubelaker, 1994). It is non-metric variations of tooth form that find application in a forensic context.

The best known example of morphological variation of crown form is Carabelli's trait. In its most overt form, this is expressed as an additional cusp found on the mesiopalatal aspect of the large mesiopalatal cusp of human maxillary first permanent molars and second deciduous molars (which have a very similar morphology and are closely related in their development) (Fig. 6.15). In less florid forms, Carabelli's trait may manifest itself as a shallow groove or a dimple in the enamel (Hanihara, 1963). It is found in approximately four-fifths of those with European origins but in less than half of Pacific Islanders. In conjunction with other skeletal ethnic traits, this can find obvious forensic application in a country such as New Zealand, where both groups collectively represent the bulk of the population.

Another important variant is shovelling of the maxillary incisors. It can also occur in mandibular teeth, but this is much less common. In extreme forms, shovelling can be accentuated by fluting on the labial aspect of the teeth, leading to a 'double shovelling' effect. It is most common amongst Mongoloid peoples (Asians and American Indians), in whom its presence is almost ubiquitous. Conversely, it is very rare in persons of European origin (Fig. 6.16).

Many other non-metric traits, such as deflecting wrinkle, variations in the numbers of cusps in mandibular premolars and fissure pattern variation in molars, have been described. A good review of these is provided by Hillson (1996).

In the edentulous, it is still possible to find palatal rugae, which can be compared with the fitting surface of an unworn denture. Rugal patterns, in common with the product of many other epithelial/mesenchymal interactions, have a high heritability. In societies where different ethnic groups have for some reason been segregated, it is possible to utilize rugal patterns to help establish ethnicity (Thomas and Kotze, 1983) (Fig. 6.17).

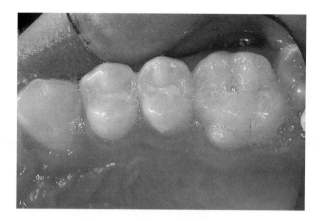

Fig. 6.15 Carabelli's trait. In this person, it appears as an extra cusp on the palatal aspect of the larger mesiopalatal cusp of the first permanent molar. It can also appear as a groove or an indentation, but it is always in the same position irrespective of its degree of expression

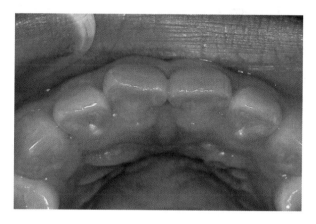

Fig. 6.16 Shovelled anterior teeth. Almost all mongoloid people exhibit this trait to some extent

Age at death

One of the most common situations in which the forensic odontologist's opinion is sought follows the discovery of skeletalized or badly decomposed human remains. One of the most essential things to ascertain, after assigning race and gender to the remains, is an estimate of the age at death. The teeth and jaws are very helpful in this regard.

LIFE AND DEATH BEFORE BIRTH

One of the single, most comprehensive accounts of the development and growth of the skeleton through-

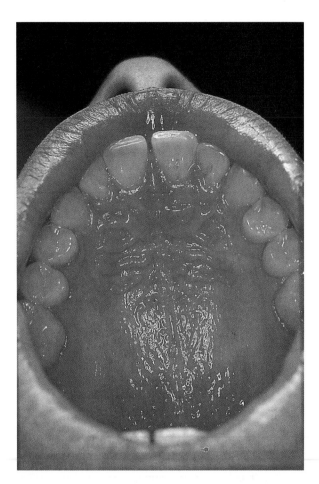

Fig. 6.17 Photograph of the maxilla in life. Immediately posterior to the anterior teeth in the hard palate, a series of transverse, branching, raised soft tissue elevations are seen. These are palatal rugae. Their number and shape can indicate family or racial relationships

out the period of gestation can be found in Fasekas and Kosa (1978). Shorter, more dentally oriented accounts can be found in Clement and Kosa (1992) and Clement (1993), so the topic will not be covered in any detail here. The principles for age estimation from the skeleton in the fetal period are:

1. the recognition and assignment of *all* bones found to confirm that they are indeed human and that one and only one set of remains needs thereafter to be considered;
2. the measurement of all bones in accordance with established guidelines for comparison with published values;
3. the recognition and dating of the processes of fusion between component parts of what would be considered single bones in later life post parturition.

In common with most methods of ageing remains, the more information to hand, the better the estimate. Ribs are difficult to identify if not all are recovered. Bones from the upper and lower limbs can similarly be misidentified. This seems surprising until it is discovered that it is really only the various mid-shafts (diaphyses) that are mineralized and hence available for study. It is the ends of bones (metaphyses) that really assist in their unequivocal identification. Calvarial vault bones are friable and subject to distortion, which often invalidates measurements.

The human mandible is very easily recognized, and its full length from articular condyle to midline symphysis can be measured reliably, this dimension bearing a surprisingly constant proportional relationship with respect to the rest of the fetal dimensions. The length of the half mandible is almost exactly an order of magnitude less than the total crown–heel length of the fetus at all times. Since the crown–heel length relates well to gestational age (Hasse's rule), so too does that of the mandible.

Fetal age estimation from a full consideration of all the above points is as good as any other method of inference and better than most. In the experience of the author, the method is accurate to ±2 weeks throughout the latter 5 lunar months of pregnancy, which is when most legislation relating to the unborn finds application.

TEETH BEFORE BIRTH

It is less common for the antenatal remains of the dentition to be found than the rest of the fetal skeleton. The crypts or 'alveoli' of the jaws are not completely formed even at birth. For this reason, when soft tissues decay, the calcifying and calcified parts of the teeth become lost from the incomplete crypts, in which they are no longer retained by the soft tissue components of the tooth germs. Sometimes, however, a child or fetus is buried or hidden wrapped in a plastic bag. If, after recovery, the remains are then carefully enzymatically digested, leaving just the calcified remains to be gathered by careful sieving or collection on black filter paper, they can be studied to great benefit (Clement, 1992) (Fig. 6.18).

Others have dissected entire tooth germs from aborted fetuses and stained the calcified parts with a calcium-seeking dye such as Alizarin Red S (Kraus and Jordan, 1965). While this has been invaluable for the visualization of dental development, it is difficult to apply such an approach in a forensic context. Essentially, the principles for age estimation are similar to those used for the fetal skeleton. The teeth have to be cleaned, dried and identified to check that commingling of remains has not occurred. The developmental stages of the teeth can

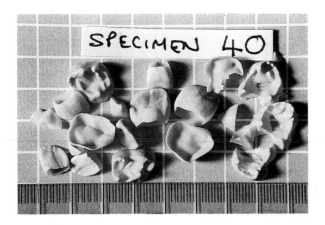

Fig. 6.18 Calcified parts of the human dentition just before birth. Unfortunately, these small structures are hardly ever recovered from the site of the burial

be compared with published standards. A further step employed by Stack (1964, 1967, 1971; Luke *et al.*, 1978) was to dry teeth of different ages to constant weight for comparison and to establish good correlations with gestational age. Liversage *et al.* (1993) found similarly good correlations between crown heights and age. The biggest impediment to the more widespread application of this knowledge is attributable to poor recovery of remains at the scene.

CALCIFICATION PATTERNS/EMERGENCE DATES FOR THE TEETH

Postnatally, the human is at first edentulous, this being followed by a period during which deciduous dentition emerges. This initial deciduous dentition is later augmented by the emergence of some permanent teeth before a progressive replacement of the deciduous dentition takes place. Eventually, more permanent teeth are added to the jaws as they enlarge until towards the end of the second decade of life, the full adult dentition has been established.

Two features of this progression are used to age postnatal remains until the beginning of the third decade of life. The first is the pattern of crown and root formation of the teeth, which was alluded to in the previous section. The second phenomenon having a predictable sequence is the emergence of the teeth through the gingivae into the oral cavity. This process is sometimes called 'eruption', but the term incorrectly implies that the process is brief and temporary when it is, in reality, often slowly continuous throughout life, the teeth constantly adjusting their position to adjust for wear on their external surfaces. Most studies of the chronology of tooth emergence

are combined with the patterns and timing of dental growth because the two events are to some extent synchronized and functionally interrelated.

Early forensic application of this knowledge was widespread during the years of the industrial revolution in Britain. Wholesale dental examinations of the juvenile workforce were conducted by factory inspectors who used Saunder's method (1837), which chronicled molar emergence, to corroborate a child's age and hence fitness to work.

The most famous tooth formation and 'eruption' chart is still that of Schour and Massler (1941). It is well known that it is inaccurate but not so inaccurate that its use has been discontinued. Rather, it remains a convenient chart to memorize for the visualization of what may be found within the jaws corresponding to what can be observed in the oral cavity. The chart owes a great deal to the work of Logan and Kronfeld (1933) and may have been derived from this source or some of Kronfeld's later work in the late 1930s. This early work used terminally ill children as the subjects from whom the data set was derived. If one considers this, and the effects that secular trends may have exerted in the past 65 years, it is hardly surprising that the information is now somewhat inaccurate.

It is advisable to construct local modifications of the values depicted in the Schour and Massler chart to take account of different ethnic mixes in different societies. This practice is widespread and often incompletely reported. Conversely, a well-researched and well-reported example is that of Ubelaker (1987). There are many others, some using various combinations of teeth within the dentition rather than the entire data set. Foremost amongst these are the works of Demirjian and Goldstein (1976) and Moorees *et al.* (1963), the method of the former now often being used as a template for comparative studies on other populations (Knott and Clement, 1995). One study notable for the helpful manner in which the data are depicted for ease of use in the field situation is that of Ciapparelli (1992).

The final event in the establishment of the permanent dentition is the formation of the roots of the third molars. Studies of third molar root development are therefore an attempt to extend age determination from a consideration of normal developmental events to the final events of tooth formation. Unfortunately, third molar emergence is very variable. This is probably due to problems of impaction and crowding as these are the last teeth to be accommodated within the dental arches. This has led to widespread belief that third molars are unreliable landmarks for temporal events. Although their emergence may be unreliable, Anderson *et al.* (1976) found that root formation showed less variation than crown formation.

Forensic investigators (Dalitz, 1963; Johanson, 1971; Harris and Nortje, 1984) have found staging of root formation and its correlation with age to be useful.

AGE CHANGES

Changes in the teeth and supporting tissues after their formative period are highly dependent upon diet, oral hygiene and many lifestyle factors (Fig. 6.19). Gustafson (1966) consolidated many of the age-related changes of the teeth into a unifying series of age-predictive regression equations. Factors taken into account were infilling of the dental pulp chambers by secondary dentine, attrition, migration of gingival attachments, increasing cementum deposition and increasing translucency of dentine due to increased peritubular (intratubular) dentine deposition. Many others have critically reconsidered and revisited all or part of Gustafson's method, introducing minor modifications from time to time (Bang and Ramm, 1970; Johanson, 1971; Nkhumeleni *et al.*, 1989).

In essence, Gustafson's method was probably successful because of the homogeneity of his Swedish sample at that time in terms of genes, social factors and diet. The methods are of much less use in countries where there is recent, large-scale immigration from many different places.

Of all the factors considered by Gustafson and his emulators, the increasing translucency of dentine with age is probably the most physiologically related and hence the least affected by environmental influence. The quantification of translucency is currently measured from planoparallel ground sections. The mapping of sclerosis in dentine could now be extended to volumetric analyses, thereby freeing the technique from sampling errors attributable to selection of the plane of section. An excellent recent study of age-related changes to tooth structure has been made by Kvall (1995). This includes a comprehensive review of the literature.

A great deal of study has been devoted over a long period to tooth wear patterns for the estimation of age at death (Hojo, 1954; Murphy, 1959; Heithersay, 1960; Miles, 1963; Kambe *et al.*, 1991). These studies are generally focused on burial site populations that may not represent the contemporaneous population at large. The applications are therefore usually archaeological rather than forensic.

Cement accretion and annulation are used very effectively to age wild animals such as deer, moose and elk (Low and Cowen, 1966). These animals experience large fluctuations in climate and food supply, and some fast during the mating season. Consequently, growth increments are easily seen in their hard tissues. Their cementum is thick, so the spacing between seasonal increments is large enough for them to be resolved. This is not the case in human

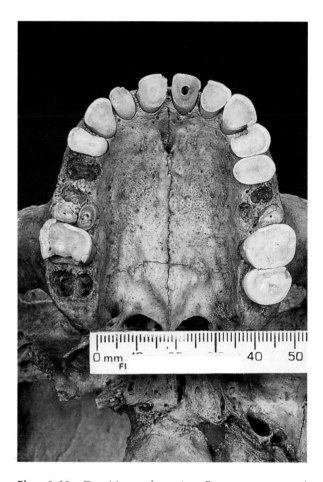

Fig. 6.19 Dentition of a 'pre-European contact' Australian aboriginal. Note the degree of tooth wear. The degree of attrition has been so great as to expose the pulp chambers of several teeth, which have subsequently died. In the case of the first molars, the crowns have been completely destroyed, and the remaining roots have been loosened by bone destruction caused by dental abscesses. Such remains are rarely of interest in a coronial context but have to be treated with due regard and sensitivity to the customs and practices of indigenous peoples

teeth, and attempts to image and use incremental lines in human cementum to age individuals have not lived up to their early promise (Romaniuk and McGrory, 1990).

In addition to these essentially morphological means of determining age at death, in the last two decades there have been moves to utilize time-dependent changes to the structural constituents of the skeleton in order to estimate the age of the deceased.

Changes to the inorganic matrices of the skeleton, in environments which permit their continuing existence, take place at the rate of solid state diffusion in crystals and are therefore orders of magnitude too slow for application in a forensic context. Changes to the organic matrices are much more rapid and therefore potentially much more useful.

Foremost amongst these is the slowly progressive and predictable conversion of aspartic acid from its *levo*, or left-handed form to its *dextro*, or right-handed enantiomer. This conversion begins from the time of the initial deposition of the tissue. Knowledge of the chronology of changes to the D/L radio allows good correlations with age at death to be established. This is particularly true for tissues in which there is practically no turnover of constituents following their original formation e.g. dentine (Ogino *et al*., 1985; Ogino and Ogino, 1988; Ritz *et al*., 1990).

Later work has striven to extend the technique to other tissues for application in cases where teeth may not be found or are not available. Pfeiffer *et al*. (1995a) obtained very good correlations between changes to the D/L aspartic acid ratio in rib cartilage and chronological age at death. Somewhat poorer, but still useful correlations were obtained when femoral bone was studied (Pfeifer *et al,*, 1995b).

These results are what might have been anticipated given the dynamic nature of bone, for in bone organs there is a continuous process of turnover of bone tissue throughout life. At death therefore some bone within the bones of an elderly person will still be very young.

The validity of attempting to extend this technique to studies of root cementum, which is slowly deposited throughout life, yet experiences little resorption, must be viewed with some scepticism.

At the conclusion of this brief chapter devoted to the principles rather than the practice of identification from a study of dental evidence, it is worth reiterating that forensic odontology is not for the inexperienced dental practitioner. Not only does additional specialist knowledge have to be acquired but also a sound and broad experience of all aspects of dentistry has to be ever present as a reference against which observations can be compared. These are two of the essential basic requirements for a competent forensic dental practitioner. The other needs are to develop a sound working knowledge of the legal framework in which one operates, to develop a systematic and analytical approach to all of one's tasks and to be circumspect in opinion.

References

Andersen L, Wenzel A. 1995: Digital subtraction radiography applied to bitewing radiographs. In Jacob B, Bonte W. (eds) *Advances in forensic sciences*, Vol. 7 *Forensic odontology and anthropology.* Berlin: Verlag Dr Köster, 193–5.

Anderson DL, Thompson GW, Popovitch F. 1976: Age of attainment of mineralisation stages of the permanent dentition. *Journal of Forensic Sciences* **21**, 191–200.

Bang G, Ramm E. 1970: Determination of age in humans from root dentine transparency. *Acta Odontologica Scandinavia* **28**, 3–35.

Buikstra JE, Ubelaker DH. (eds) 1994: *Standards for data collection from human skeletal remains.* Arkansas Archeological Survey Research Series No. 44. Fayetteville: Arkansas Archeological Survey.

Ciapparelli L. 1992: The chronology of dental development and age assessment. In Clark DH. (ed.) *Practical forensic odontology.* London: Wright, 22–42.

Clement JG. 1993: Forensic dentistry. In Freckelton I, Selby H. (eds) *Expert evidence – practice and advocacy*, Vol. 1. Australia: Law Book Company.

Clement JG, Kosa F. 1992: The fetal skeleton. In Clark DH (ed.), *Practical forensic odontology.* London: Wright, 43–52.

Clement JG, Olsson C, Phakey PP. 1992: Heat induced changes in human skeletal tissues. In York LK, Hicks JW. (eds) *Proceedings of an international symposium on the forensic aspects of mass disasters and crime scene reconstruction*, FBI Academy Quantico 1990, Laboratory division of the FBI, Washington DC: US Government Printing Office.

Clement JG, Officer RA, Sutherland RD. 1995: The use of digital image processing in forensic odontology: when does 'image enhancement' become 'tampering with evidence'? In Jacob B, Bonte W. (eds) *Advances in forensic sciences*, Vol. 7, *Forensic odontology and anthropology.* Berlin: Verlag Dr Köster, 149–53.

Coleman R. 1978: *The pyjama girl.* Melbourne: Hawthorn Press.

Dahlberg AA. 1945: Paramolar tubercle (Bolk). *American Journal of Physical Anthropology* **3**, 97–103.

Dahlberg AA. 1949: The dentition of the American Indian. In Laughlin, WS (ed.), *The physical anthropology of the American Indian.* New York: Viking Fund, 138–76.

Dahlberg AA. 1963: Analysis of the American Indian dentition. In Brothwell DR (ed.) *Dental anthropology*, London: Pergamon Press, 149–78.

Dalitz GD. 1963: The root development of third molar teeth. *Journal of Forensic Medicine* **10**(1), 30–5.

Demirjian A, Goldstein H. 1976: New systems for dental maturity based on seven and four teeth. *Annals of Human Biology* **3**, 411–21.

Fasekas I, Kosa F. 1978: *Forensic foetal osteology.* Budapest: Akadémiai Kiadó.

Garn SM, Lewis AB, Kerewsky RS. 1965: Size interrelationships of the mesial and distal teeth. *Journal of Dental Research* **44**, 350–4.

Garn SM, Lewis AB, Kerewesky RS. 1968: Relationship between buccolingual and mesiodistal crown diameters. *Journal of Dental Research* **47**, 495.

Goose DH. 1963: Dental measurement: an assessment of its value in anthropological studies. In Brothwell DR (ed.) *Dental anthropology.* London: Pergamon Press, 125–48.

Goose DH. 1971: The inheritance of tooth size in British families. In Dahlberg AA (ed.) *Dental morphology and evolution.* Chicago: University of Chicago Press, 263–70.

Gustafson G. 1966: *Forensic odontology.* London: Staples Press.

Hanihara K. 1963: Crown characteristics of the deciduous dentition of the Japanese–American hybrids. In Brothwell DR (ed.) *Dental anthropology.* London: Pergamon Press, 105–24.

Harris MPJ, Nortje CJ. 1984: The mesial root of the third mandibular molar. *Journal of Forensic Odontostomatology* **2**, 39–43.

Heithersay GS. 1960: Attritional values for Australian aborigines. Haast's Bluff. *Australian Dental Journal* **5**, 84–8.

Hill IR. 1984: *Forensic odontology: its scope and history.* In Hill IR (ed.) Solihull, UK: Alan Clift Associates.

Hillson S. 1996: *Dental anthropology,* Cambridge: Cambridge University Press.

Hojo M. 1954: On the pattern of dental abrasion. *Okajimas Folia Anatomica Japonica* **26**, 11–30.

Holden JL, Clement JG, Phakey PP. 1995a: Age and temperature related changes to the structure and chemistry of human bone mineral. *Journal of Bone and Mineral Research* **10**(9), 1400–9.

Holden JL, Phakey PP, Clement JG. 1995b: Scanning electron microscope observations of incinerated human femoral bone: a case study. *Forensic Science International* **7**(4), 17–28.

Holden JL, Phakey PP, Clement JG. 1995c: Scanning electron microscope observations of heat-treated human bone. *Forensic Science International* **74**, 29–45.

Johanson G. 1971: Age determination from human teeth. A critical evaluation with special consideration of changes after fourteen years of age. *Odontologisk Revy,* **22**, 1–126.

Kambe T, Yonemitsu K, Kibayashi K, Tsunenari S. 1991: Application of a computer assisted image analyser to the assessment of area and number of sites of dental attrition and its use for age estimation. *Forensic Science International* **50**, 97–109.

Keiser JA. 1990: *Human adult odontometrics.* Cambridge Studies in Biological Anthropology 4. Cambridge: Cambridge University Press.

Kingman A. 1997: Statistics in community oral health. In Pine CM (ed.) *Community Oral Health.* Oxford: Wright.

Knott SC, Clement JG. 1995: Dental maturity of children in Perth, Western Australia-based on four teeth employing the method described by Demirjian and Goldstein 1976. In Jacob B, Bonte W (eds), *Advances in forensic sciences,* Vol. 7, *Forensic odontology and anthropology.* Berlin: Verlag Dr Köster, 225–34.

Kraus BS, Jordan RE. 1965: *The human dentition before birth.* Philadelphia: Lea & Febiger.

Kvall SI. 1995: Age related changes in teeth. A microscopic and radiographic investigation of the human permanent dentition. PhD thesis, University of Oslo, Norway.

Liversage HM, Dean MC, Molleson TI. 1993: Increasing human tooth length between birth and 5.4 years. *American Journal of Physical Anthropology* **90**, 307–13.

Logan WHG, Kronfeld R. 1933: Development of the human jaws and surrounding structures from birth until the age of fifteen years. *Journal of the American Dental Association* **20**, 379–427.

Low WA, Cowen McTI. 1966: Age determination of deer by annular structure of dental cementum. *Journal of Wildlife Management* **27**, 466–71.

Luke DA, Stack MV, Hey EN. 1978: A comparison of morphological and gravimetric methods of estimation of human foetal age from the dentition. In Butler PM, Joysey, KA. (eds) *Development, function and evolution of teeth.* London: Academic Press, 511–18.

Miles AEW. 1963: Dentition in the assessment of individual age in skeletal material. In Brothwell DR (ed.) *Dental anthropology.* London: Pergamon Press, 191–209.

Moorees CFA. 1957: *The Aleut dentition.* Cambridge, MA: Harvard University Press.

Moorees CFA, Chandha JM. 1962: Crown diameters, of corresponding tooth groups in the deciduous and permanent dentition. *Journal of Dental Research* **41**, 466–70.

Moorees CFA, Reed RB. 1964: Correlations among crown diameters of human teeth. *Archives of Oral Biology* **9**, 685–97.

Moorees CFA, Thomsen SO, Jensen E, Yen PKJ. 1957: Mesiodistal crown diameters of deciduous and permanent teeth. *Journal of Dental Research* **36**, 39–47.

Moorees CFA, Fanning EA, Hunt EE. 1963: Age variation of formation stages for ten permanent teeth. *Journal of Dental Research* **42**, 1490–502.

Murphy T. 1959: The change in pattern of dentine exposure in human tooth attrition. *American Journal of Physical Anthropology* **17**, 167–78.

Nkhumeleni FS, Raubenheimer EJ, Monteith BD. 1989: Gustafson's method for age determination, revisited. *Journal of Forensic Odontostomatology* **7**, 13–16.

Ogino T, Ogino H. 1988: Application to forensic odontology of aspartic acid racemization in unerupted and supernumerary teeth. *Journal of Dental Research* **67**(10), 1319–22.

Ogino T, Ogino N, Nagy B. 1985: Application of aspartic acid racemisation to forensic odontology: postmortem designation of age at death. *Forensic Science International* **29**, 259–67.

Pine CM, 1997: Introduction and principles and practice of public health. In Pine CM (ed.) *Community oral health,* Oxford: Wright.

Pfeiffer H, Mornstad H, Teivens A. 1995a: Estimation of chronologic age using the aspartic acid racemization method. I. On human rib cartilage. *International Journal of Legal Medicine* **108**(1), 19–23.

Pfeiffer H, Mornstad H, Teivens A. 1995b: Estimation of chronologic age using the aspartic acid racemization method. II. On human cortical bone. *International Journal of Legal Medicine* **108**(1), 24-6.

Ranta H, Kerosuo E. 1995: Computerized image analysis of panoramic tomograms. In Jacob B, Bonte W (eds) *Advances in forensic sciences,* Vol. 7, *Forensic odontology and anthropology.* Berlin: Verlag Dr Köster, 178–80.

Ritz S, Schultz HW, Schwarzer B. 1990: The extent of aspartic acid racemization in dentin: a possible method for a more accurate determination of age at death? *Zeitschrift fur Rechtsmedizin – Journal of Legal Medicine* **103**(6), 457–62.

Romanuik K, McGrory MA. 1990: Age determination by cementum annulation counts in human teeth. Paper presented to the International meeting of the International Association of Forensic Science, Adelaide, Australia, October 1990.

Saunders E. 1837: *The teeth as a test of age, considered with reference to the factory children: addressed to the members of both Houses of Parliament.* London: H. Renshaw.

Schour I, Massler M. 1941: The development of the human dentition. *Journal of the American Dental Association* **28**, 1153–60.

Stack MV. 1964: A gravimetric study of crown growth rate of the human deciduous dentition. *Biology of the Neonate* **6**, 197–224.

Stack MV. 1967: Vertical growth rates of the deciduous teeth. *Journal of Dental Research* **46**, 879–82.

Stack MV. 1971: Relative rates of weight gain in human deciduous teeth. In Dahlberg AA (ed.) *Dental morphology and evolution.* Chicago: University of Chicago Press, 59–62.

Thomas CJ, Kotze TJVW. 1983: The palatal rugae in forensic odonto-stomatology. *Journal of Odontostomatology* **1**(1), 11.

Tobias PV. 1990: *Olduvai Gorge*, Vol. 4, *The Skulls, endocasts and teeth of* Homo habilis. New York: Cambridge University Press.

Townsend GC. 1980: Heritability of deciduous tooth size in Australian aboriginals. *American Journal of Physical Anthropology* **53**, 297–300.

Townsend GC, Brown T. 1978: Heritability of permanent tooth size. *American Journal of Physical Anthropology* **49**, 497–505.

Turner CG II, Nichol CR, Scott GR, 1991: Scoring procedures for key morphological traits of the permanent dentition: the Arizona State University Dental Anthropology System. In Kelly MA, Larsen CS (eds) *Advances in dental anthropology.* New York: Wiley–Liss, 13–31.

Ubelaker DH. 1987: Estimating age at death from immature human skeletons: an overview. *Journal of Forensic Sciences* **32**, 1254–63.

Zubov AA. 1977: Odontoglyphics: the laws of variation of the human molar crown microrelief. In Dahlberg AA, Graber TM (eds) *Orofacial growth and development.* Hague: Mouton, 269–82.

Zubov AA, Nikityuk BA. 1978: Prospects for the application of dental morphology in twin type analysis. *Journal of Human Evolution* **7**, 519–24.

PART 2

Techniques

CHAPTER 7

Preservation, restoration and duplication of remains

PJG CRAIG, JL LEDITSCHKE, RG TAYLOR

Introduction	85	Freezing	88
Bodily changes after death	85	Plastination	88
Natural means of preservation	86	Restoration of appearance	89
Artificial preservation	86	Conditions of viewing	89
Embalming for forensic purposes	87	Duplication of remains	90
Public health considerations	87	Traditional methods of replication	90
Modern embalming techniques	87	Method for fabrication of a replica of a skull	91
Embalming after autopsy	88	Computer-assisted methods	93
Refrigeration	88		

Introduction

All material of a biological nature proceeds to undergo change and decay immediately following death. The rate of change depends upon a complex interaction between biochemical breakdown reactions and extrinsic factors such as ambient temperature, the availability of oxygen and the bacterial and insectival flora that happen to be in the vicinity. Under favourable conditions, natural tissue breakdown can be extremely rapid (Iserson, 1994). Consequently, forensic investigation may depend on the artificial preservation of the remains so that investigation may proceed.

Remains may be preserved by chemical means (embalming or plastination), refrigeration, desiccation or freezing. Facets of forensic interest may be preserved by reproduction in model form. When the object in question is a cadaver, the method employed will take into consideration whether or not a visual identification of the remains is to be attempted. This chapter will be restricted to the preservation, restoration and duplication of remains or parts thereof which may be of interest to the forensic investigator.

Bodily changes after death

There are two ways in which death can be described: somatic death and cellular death. Clinical death proceeds to brain death, biological death and cellular death. Whereas cells in the brain and nervous tissues die within 5 minutes of cessation of the circulation, cells that have a reserve of oxygen, such as blood, will survive for up to 6 hours. Immediately prior to somatic death is a period of agonal algor, a cooling of bodily temperature, or in the case of an individual suffering from an infection, agonal fever. Hypostasis, i.e. cessation of blood flow and loss of blood pressure during this period, will cause the blood to settle in dependent areas and coagulate. Capillary expansion and increased permeability can cause oedema.

Post mortem changes are both physical and chemical. The physical changes are a continuation of those changes seen peri mortem, or immediately prior to death. An example of this is body cooling, in which the body temperature lowers further until it is equivalent to the surrounding environment. Other examples include the pooling of blood and other bodily fluids to the dependent areas. Chemical changes are responsible for the onset of rigor mortis, post mortem skin staining (from the haemolysis of blood constituents) and decomposition. The rate at which these changes occur is dependent on the physical condition of the individual and the environment in which he or she dies. These variables are of importance when attempting to establish time of death. For example, in a warm humid environment, the cooling of bodily organs occurs more slowly and bacterial decomposition more quickly. A corpulent body cools more slowly than that of a small thin person (Mann *et al.*, 1990).

Natural means of preservation

Bodies may be naturally preserved for centuries if the surroundings are unfavourable for decomposition. Extremely hot, cold or dry, or certain chemical, conditions will enable preservation to occur to varying degrees. A body may be frozen in a glacier or under snow and ice on a mountaintop, as was the case with the 'ice man' recently discovered in the Alps in Europe. Peruvian mummies have been found at high altitudes where the cold, combined with the dry climate, produced desiccation before decomposition could take place. Exposure to extremes of dry, cold air will produce a freeze-dried mummy. This process was used in a mortuary on a mountaintop in Switzerland, where the construction of the building allowed a freezing cold, dry current of air to pass over the corpses. Dry heat will also produce mummification by natural desiccation. The mummification of bodies in ancient Egypt was performed by burying the bodies in the dry sand of the desert, a procedure that was also used by cultures in other hot, dry countries such as south-western America. Certain types of soil are conducive to preservation. The peat bogs of northern Europe have a wet acid environment, which can preserve bodies for hundreds of years. The high natural tannin content and lack of oxygen in the bog halts decomposition to such an extent that parts such as skin, hair and nails are still evident. A similar situation can occur when a body is buried in soil highly impregnated with salts of aluminium or copper.

The surface features of a body can be preserved for years by the formation of adipocere. This lipid substance (formerly called grave wax) can be formed naturally by hydrogenation of the fatty tissues of the body under moist, warm conditions. Once adipocere begins to form, decomposition is retarded, and a form of mummification begins (Aidan and Cockburn, 1982).

Artificial preservation

Controlled drying by slow heat will produce desiccation, thus removing the moisture that aids decomposition. Setting a body in the sun to dry out has been used as a means of preservation throughout history. In more recent times, indirect heat, such as that from a slow oven, has been used. This is the means employed by monks in the Capuchin monastery near Palermo, Italy. The bodies are dried in an oven heated by slaked lime until they are quite shrunken and desiccated, before being placed in the catacombs beneath the monastery. Early experiments by anatomists, seeking to preserve bodies for dissection, resulted in a technique by which the hot air was driven through the large blood vessels of the body, thus speeding the desiccation process.

Application of preserving powders such as a mixture of potassium nitrate and sodium chloride, carbonate, sulphate and nitrate (Natron) was used by the ancient Egyptians during the complex preparations for mummification as practised during the period from 3200 BC until about AD 650. Common salt has been used by various cultures to pack the cavities of eviscerated bodies, often prior to drying in an oven or in the sun. A nineteenth-century French physician, Dr Falonry, preserved bodies for anatomical purposes by placing them on a bed of sawdust to which powdered zinc sulphate was added.

Immersing bodies in preserving liquids has also been used to preserve them. After his death, Alexander the Great was said to have been carried from Babylon to Egypt sealed in a jar of honey. This practice was a feature of funeral practice of the ancient Persians. Alcohol and brine have been used to preserve bodies for hundreds of years: the body of Lord Nelson was shipped back to England in a barrel of brandy. In fact, many dead sailors were carried across the world in sailing ships sealed in a barrel of brine or alcoholic spirit so that they could be buried in their home country. In some cases, the body was first eviscerated, the organs being treated separately. This allowed better penetration of the preservative and thus better preservation of the body, particularly in a hot climate.

The practice of *arterial injection* for preservation arose from the increased knowledge of anatomy that was amassed throughout the sixteenth and seventeenth centuries. Alcohol, turpentine and arsenic were purported to have been used for embalming purposes by the Dutchman Frederick Ruysch (1638–1731). Although he never published his methods, a collection of his preparations still exists today in the St Petersburg museum. William Hunter, the British surgeon, injected the femoral artery of his specimens with a mixture of essential oils to which was added vermilion dye, the latter being used to impart a more lifelike colour to the embalmed body. Desiccation of the treated body was aided by placing it on a bed of plaster of Paris and gypsum.

The use of pressure is necessary to drive preserving fluid through the vascular system of a corpse. A more efficient system than brute force was devised by John Morgan, Professor of anatomy in Dublin in about 1863. He injected the fluid through the left ventricle of the heart, having made an opening in the right auricle to allow the blood to escape. By positioning the injecting fluid container 12 ft above the body, sufficient perfusion pressure was obtained.

Embalming for forensic purposes

The first account of embalming being used for forensic purposes appeared in a newspaper article in Paris in 1840. It described the murder of a young boy whose identity was unknown. Because decomposition was imminent, the Magistrate ordered that his body be embalmed pending further investigation of his identity. M. Jean N. Gannal, a French chemist, was mentioned as the embalmer. He had devised a simple yet effective method of arterial infusion, using as a fluid a mixture of acids to which arsenic was added. However, because arsenical poisoning was a common crime at the time, the use of arsenic in embalming fluids was soon prohibited by law on the grounds that it would mask any traces of poison in a suspect body.

Public health considerations

In many parts of the world, embalming, or at least disinfection and decontamination of human remains, is a legal requirement for the protection of those handling the body. In an unembalmed state, human remains constitute an ideal environment for the growth of pathogenic bacteria. It has been found that endogenous invasion of the cerebrospinal fluid by colonic bacteria will occur within 4–6 hours of death. Peak densities of organisms occur within 24–30

hours after death and consist of $3.0–3.5 \times 10^6$/g body tissue. Leakage from bodily orifices will contaminate all adjacent surfaces and thus create a significant potential health hazard (Mann *et al.*, 1990). All too frequently, little knowledge is available after death as to whether the deceased was previously infected or carrying a communicable disease. Varying forms of hepatitis, systemic mycoses, respiratory infections and human immunodeficiency virus infections constitute a considerable health risk for the pathologist or other examiner of the body. Public health guidelines have been established to prevent transmission of pathogens from human remains to those handling them or coming in to close contact with them. In many jurisdictions, disinfection and decontamination of the body, the handler and the mortuary are mandatory.

Modern embalming techniques

Embalming is performed for a variety of reasons. It may be required to render the body fit for viewing by the relatives of the deceased, or a religious belief in the resurrection of the body may encourage relatives to ensure that the body is preserved from decomposition. A body may also need to be preserved for transportation or for forensic investigation purposes, particularly in times of war or other mass disaster. Although freezing may serve the purpose in the latter instance, it is not always practical and requires a facility that may not be available or reliable in all parts of the world.

All or part of a body may be embalmed. Embalming is a chemical procedure that maintains the integrity of the soft tissues, halts bacterial decomposition and restores tissue turgor (if the embalming fluid is introduced into the tissues under pressure). The active chemical ingredients are formaldehyde and its derivatives, although the processes utilized in a funeral mortuary often involve additional chemicals that are designed to impart a lifelike colour to the tissues (Thiel, 1992). Such additives are not necessary for forensic purposes unless visual identification of the deceased is anticipated.

The embalming of a body prior to its being viewed by family and friends involves several procedures.

Preliminary preparation of the body involves the washing and topical disinfection of body surfaces. The body is positioned and the features set so that a natural appearance is created. Skin lesions, ulcerations or evidence of invasive procedures are dressed and disinfected. If decomposition has commenced, any gas accumulation and fluid leakage is removed.

There are several techniques for *arterial injection*. All have as their aim the total perfusion of embalming fluid through the circulatory system. Arteries used include the common carotid, the femoral and the popliteal. Blood drainage is accomplished through incisions in the large veins, commonly the jugular and femoral.

Commercially available *embalming fluids* include preservatives, disinfectants, anticoagulants, surfactants, perfuming agents and dyes. Buffers, humectants, water conditioners and various inorganic salts may be added to these. Several of these constituents, notably formaldehyde, a potent preservative, are potentially dangerous and need to be used with care (Bhat *et al.*, 1990).

After embalming, the body is dressed, the hair tidied and the make-up and clothing arranged so that the family and friends can view the body if they wish. The 'life expectancy' of an embalmed body depends on the extent to which the embalming fluid has penetrated the tissues and the rate at which the active ingredient, formaldehyde, breaks down to formic acid.

Embalming after autopsy

The preservation of human remains following an autopsy places greater demands upon the skill of the embalmer. As the integrity of the body tissues has been disturbed and the circulatory system disrupted, the viscera must be treated separately. In addition, the embalmer has to rebuild any part of the body that has been altered by the autopsy procedures. Apart from these additional processes, the embalming of a body after an autopsy follows a procedure similar to that outlined above (Hanzlick, 1994).

Refrigeration

Storage of bodies in a purpose-built refrigerator at a temperature of 4°C will delay decomposition for up to 2 weeks. Infectious, infested or decomposed bodies may also be refrigerated in a sealed body bag. A well-equipped mortuary will possess separate refrigeration facilities for these hazardous cases in order to limit the exposure of mortuary personnel to possible contamination. Refrigeration slows down, but does not halt, the bacterial processes, and many organisms, capable of causing infection, are viable at these temperatures. Refrigeration is the simplest and most common method of body preservation used in mortuary facilities today. Separate lockable refrigeration facilities are needed for potential homicide cases or those involving suspicious circumstances to ensure that evidence obtained from the body, which may be subse-

quently required for court proceedings, remains undisturbed.

Freezing

A body, or portion of a body, may be preserved indefinitely if frozen and maintained at a temperature of −20°C. The body needs to be dry to prevent the formation of surface ice crystals, and sealed in order to prevent dehydration. Freezing is a useful method for the long-term preservation of unknown or unidentified remains. If future restoration of appearance for possible visual identification is contemplated, it is preferable to use methods other than freezing. This is because the increased permeability of the thawed tissues to embalming fluid makes it technically difficult to render a lifelike appearance to a previously frozen body. It is therefore important to obtain all visual information such as photographs, and three-dimensional casts of the facial features of a body, prior to freezing.

Plastination

Plastination is a technique whereby the tissue fluids in a specimen are replaced by curable polymers, thus rendering the specimen dry, odourless and easy to store. Extremely realistic appearance and handling characteristics can be given to the specimen with the correct choice of polymers (Aufdemorte *et al.*, 1985). An expensive and tedious process, plastination requires specialized laboratory facilities and technical expertise. It is more suitable for use when the tissues are to be used for the purposes of archival storage or teaching than for routine forensic investigation.

Following formalin fixation, the specimen is dehydrated in alcohol and acetone following the routine methods of tissue processing. It is then saturated with an intermediary solvent that is readily miscible with the polymer. Impregnation with the polymer occurs by immersion of the specimen in a container of uncured polymer that is then placed in a vacuum. The lowering of the vapour pressure that occurs boils the solvent and draws the polymer into the tissues, gradually replacing the solvent. Once the solvent has boiled off completely, the specimen is removed and the polymer allowed to cure. Various polymers are used depending upon the desired characteristics of the completed specimen. Epoxy resin will produce a hard, durable specimen, whereas silicone rubber will produce a more realistic surface texture (Hildebrand, 1968).

Restoration of appearance

The physical appearance of the deceased person becomes important when it is necessary or desirable for the remains to be viewed. This may be for establishing identity or for the consolation of the deceased's relatives at the funeral service. The viewing is frequently performed by persons who are unfamiliar with death and for whom the death has strong psychological connotations; it must therefore be undertaken sympathetically. Differences in emotional response are largely predictable through reference to a variety of sociological and psychological bereavement theories. These refer to cultural and racial definitions of appropriate reactions, family social structure and the expectation of death as an independent variable. These considerations determine the conditions under which a body may be presented for visual display.

In Western society, the expectation of those viewing the remains are that the body will resemble a peaceful, sleeping person. It is important that the staff of the mortuary are aware of this and that every effort is taken to restore the appearance to that level of expectation. Bony structures of the face must be repositioned using an intra-oral or intracranial approach, and held in place with plaster of Paris, plasticine or paper. Damage to the body that cannot be repaired using standard reconstructive techniques must be concealed beneath drapes. If such damage is on the face, an attempt must be made to repair it with cyanoacrylate adhesive and the area covered with cosmetics (Prahlow and Lanz, 1993). The hair should be washed and arranged in such a way that any marks of injury or autopsy incisions on the scalp are hidden, the face shaved if necessary and the eyes closed. If the body is female, and it is deemed appropriate, standard cosmetics may be applied. It is not always necessary to go to such extreme lengths when the viewing is for forensic or legal purposes, although the psychological effects on the viewers mentioned above should always be borne in mind.

In most developed countries, the bodies of persons who die as a result of trauma, homicide or apparently unnatural causes are subject by law to a physical autopsy. Following this procedure, the technical staff in the mortuary endeavour to restore, as far as possible, the pre mortem physical appearance of the face in order to assist identification. It is helpful to have obtained a photograph or videotape picture of the facial features, taken as soon as possible after death to assist in the restoration procedure. This becomes particularly important if the facial features or underlying structures of the face have been investigated during the autopsy. A pre mortem photograph obtained from relatives may assist if the restoration is for the purpose of comforting the bereaved but cannot be used if identity is in question as it may influence the technician.

Conditions for viewing

From a forensic point of view, the body is viewed for the purpose of establishing identification. It is usual for a relative or close friend to perform this task. Changes following death are so rapid that it is not uncommon for relatives to fail to identify a body. Bereft of facial expression and familiar bodily posture, pale and in a recumbent position, the corpse may bear little physical resemblance to the vital person previously known. In such cases, it may be necessary to rely upon alternate methods of identification.

A body should be presented for viewing in such a way that the distress caused to those involved is minimized. Fear of death and modern social conventions make it difficult for most people to approach a deceased person at any time, and in the atmosphere of a mortuary, they may find themselves unable to cope. Appropriate grieving and counselling facilities, together with appropriately trained personnel, can help to overcome this situation. The physical environment of the viewing room is also important. A 'morgue' atmosphere is to be avoided. This may be done by the use of a neutral decor, lighting which is sufficiently subdued that details of any injuries go unnoticed, and no apparent unusual smell. A pane of glass between the viewer and the body helps to protect and isolate the viewer, who may be overcome and wish to attempt physically to contact the deceased person. The body should be arranged on a trolley and draped in such a way that only the head is visible; the rest of the body should appear normal in outline. The bodies of children and babies can be displayed lying in a cot in normal bed clothing, together with appropriate rugs and soft toys. If a technician is present during the viewing of the body, clean hospital-type clothing should be worn.

The scene described above is an ideal situation that should be available in any large city mortuary. Different conditions, however, may apply in instances of mass disaster or war, when makeshift conditions in temporary mortuaries necessitate mass viewings of multiple bodies for the purpose of identifying victims. Every attempt should be made in these cases to limit the number of bodies viewed by prior selection for age, sex and race. Bodies in this situation are often traumatized and, in such cases, methods of identification other than the visual should be used where possible.

Putrefied bodies pose a problem if visual identification is required for forensic purposes. A method has been devised whereby casts of the faces of putrefied corpses may be obtained which are of sufficiently good quality that recognition is possible (Quatrehomme *et al.*, 1995). The process involves several stages. First, the putrefaction gases are released by degloving the soft tissues from the facial bones and allowing sufficient time for diffusion into the atmosphere. Following this, the now sunken tissues are replaced and injected with two chemicals (Inr-Seal®, Dodge Feature Builder®, Dodge Chemical Co., Cambridge, MA, USA) which restore and remodel the structures subcutaneously. An additional advantage of the injection technique is that sufficient tissue turgor is obtained to resist deformation owing to the weight of the casting materials subsequently used. Considerable skill is required during the injection process and the subsequent modelling of the compound. It should be emphasized that this technique, like others aimed at facial reconstruction, is useful only when recognition of an otherwise unknown individual is required. A positive identification based on such a reconstruction might not be sufficient for some legal purposes.

Duplication of remains

Cases often arise where it is necessary to duplicate forensic evidence prior to or during an investigation. Reasons for this are numerous. It may be necessary for the evidence to be available to more than one investigator, particularly when cases arise that are sufficiently complex to require the opinions of experts who may be separated by vast distances (Haglund and Reay, 1993). An accurate replica may be sent anywhere in the world without compromising the continuity of evidence. Evidence that is fragile, such as burnt bone, or is subject to biological breakdown, such as soft tissue, may be rendered more permanent and robust. The replicated evidence may then be presented in court for demonstration purposes. For example, a model of the skull of the deceased may be shown to demonstrate to a court the trajectory of a bullet through the skull.

A family may occasionally put pressure on a coroner to release a body for funeral purposes before sufficient time has elapsed to allow for a complete investigation. As a result, it may be necessary to replicate body parts so that the investigation can proceed unimpeded by time constraints.

Apart from the investigative aspect, duplicated material can be used for record-keeping, for teaching and research, for the building of archival collections when anthropological collections would raise sensitive issues, and to provide multiple copies of skulls for three-dimensional facial reconstruction.

Traditional methods of replication

The methods described under this heading require a degree of craftsmanship. Experts working in this field are often employed primarily in other areas and are intermittently called to forensic work as the need arises. They may be artists, sculptors or dental technicians. The actual techniques are similar, but the application of the techniques is varied to suit the case in hand.

Plaster of Paris has been the traditional material used for the replication of many types of object for years. Plaster can be used to produce a mould or a model, or both. It is still the material of choice for use in the field if large objects such as footprints or motor tyre tracks need to be replicated in a hurry. It is easy and quick to prepare, requiring a minimum of equipment or expertise, and produces a model that is adequate for many purposes.

Unfortunately, plaster of Paris also has a number of disadvantages that render it unsuitable for the replication of some biological specimens. Its granular nature does not allow the reproduction of fine detail. This becomes important when a bone is reproduced, as muscle markings and other fine surface details are lost, and faint markings, which may betray the presence of an impact on the bone, or damage by animals will not be seen. Skeletal remains are irregularly shaped, often with undercut areas. Although it is possible to design a plaster mould that will overcome this, it would be complicated to construct and the risk of damage to the fragile original such that it would be unwise to attempt such a task. The use of plaster for the finished model, i.e. the positive cast that is taken from the mould of the original, is more common and is in fact the method of choice if fine detail, such as that mentioned above, is not necessary. It is a cheap method of producing working models for three-dimensional facial reconstruction when multiple copies are required, but the models need to be treated with care. Plaster models have low impact resistance and are easily chipped and broken. The chalky surface will be eroded if handled frequently, and this will result in further loss of detail. The larger models such as skulls are heavy unless cast hollow, in which case they become weak and more likely to break during handling.

A more modern approach is to use acrylic resin for the reproduction, although the method of fabrication is more complex. An acrylic model is light and fairly robust, and may be realistically tinted to match the original specimen. With special handling, it can be made dimensionally accurate and can display the fine detail of the original specimen. An acrylic model constructed using the technique described below should satisfy the need for material that will be appropriate for presentation in court.

Method for fabrication of a replica of a skull

The technique to be described will use the replication of a cranium as an example. However, it is suitable for use in a variety of forensic situations, the materials being sufficiently adaptable to allow the replication of compressible and friable objects as well as skeletal or other hard objects (Quatrehomme *et al.*, 1996).

DESIGN OF THE MOULD

It is possible to cast the cranium in a two-part mould, providing that care is taken. A similar technique is used to cast the mandible as a separate entity, but for the sake of clarity, the description will be confined to the cranium only.

Upon presentation of the original skull, time needs to be spent establishing the design of the mould, taking into account the plane of greatest circumference of the cranium. This commonly corresponds to the Frankfort plane, an imaginary line running from the external auditory meatus on each side, passing along the lower border of the orbits and continuing around the occipital region. It is here that the two halves of the mould will meet, thus allowing for easy release of the original specimen and, subsequently, the finished reproduction.

PREPARATION OF THE SKULL

In order to prevent the flow of the moulding material through to the interior of the skull, all apertures (with the exception of the foramen magnum, which will be used as a casting sprue) need to be obliterated in such a way as to enable them to be accurately reconstituted in the final model. Molten dental casting wax is applied to each aperture and, when cool, trimmed to a depth below the external opening, thus allowing the surface anatomy to remain clearly visible. This important step is time consuming but is necessary if anatomical accuracy is to be maintained in the finished reproduction. If any apertures remain open, the silicone impression material will flow into them

and subsequently tear when removal is attempted (Fig. 7.1).

Modelling clay is applied in a strip around the skull at the line of the Frankfort plane. The strip should be between 40 mm and 50 mm wide, with a groove or keyway inscribed around the perimeter (Fig. 7.2).

CONSTRUCTION OF THE MOULD

A room temperature, vulcanizing silicone impression material is used to construct the mould. This material has been chosen for the following reasons. It is easy to handle, having a comparatively long working time prior to polymerization and a flow rate that may be regulated by the addition of differing amounts of catalyst and/or thixotropic agents. Following polymerization, it has outstanding release properties and a high elasticity and strength that allow it to record undercut areas without tearing. Most importantly, it has a linear shrinkage upon polymerization of only 0.2–0.4%, enabling adequate dimensional accuracy to be obtained.

The impression material is brushed directly onto that part of the skull above the clay band, in incremental layers, the first layers consisting of a thin mix obtained by using 5% catalyst mixed with the base

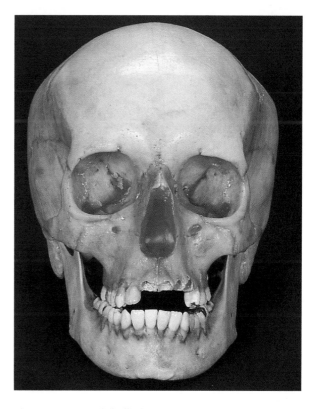

Fig. 7.1 Original skull, showing apertures occluded with red dental wax

material. The painting procedure is repeated several times until an even coverage of about 3 mm is obtained. At this point, polyester wool is placed in the orbits and sealed over with more silicone. This gives flexibility to the mould and prevents damage to the area when the skull is removed. A final layer of silicone, to which a thixotropic agent is added, is applied thickly using a spatula, with the aim of eliminating any undercut areas. Preformed silicone nipples, placed at strategic points, aid in the location of the hard backing, which is applied next (Fig. 7.3). The hard backing consists of epoxy resin to which sufficient polystyrene microfiller has been added to give the appearance of dry cake mix. The mixed resin and catalyst is applied in a 5 mm layer, and left to cure for 24 hours.

The next stage in the construction of the mould consists of inverting the skull, removing the clay divider and repeating the above procedures. A small amount of petroleum jelly smeared around the edge of the first half of the mould will prevent sticking. As

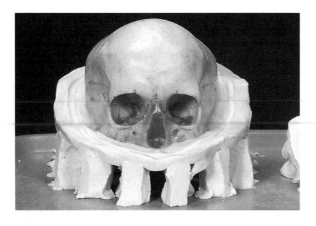

Fig. 7.2 Modelling clay applied around the circumference of skull and supported by clay pillars

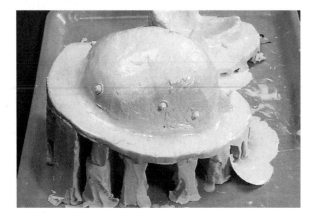

Fig. 7.3 Latex material covering the skull, with attached retention nipples

the foramen magnum will be used as a sprue for pouring the model, dental wax is formed into a plug and placed into it.

Upon completion of the second stage of mould preparation, the two halves are separated and the skull released (Figs 7.4a and 7.4b). The mould must be checked carefully for any air bubbles or tears and for accuracy of detail. The wax plug is then removed from the foramen magnum and replaced with a permanent plug constructed from formastic putty. The two halves of the mould may then be reunited and held in place with strong elastic bands.

FABRICATION OF THE REPLICA

The replica is poured using self-curing acrylic resin. Dental acrylic polymers of various colours are blended to create a resemblance to bone in both colour and texture. The polymers are mixed with acrylic monomer in a ratio of 3:1, which gives a consistency similar to that of glycerine. The mix is poured through the vent hole and the plug replaced. The mould is rotated in an endless and random pattern for approximately 20 minutes so that all internal surfaces are evenly covered prior to the initial polymerization of the acrylic (Fig. 7.5). Final polymerization takes a further 45 minutes, after which time the model may be released from the mould.

Finishing the reproduction skull is accomplished using dental rotary instruments. Flash lines are removed and the apertures carefully reconstituted, using the original specimen as a guide. If necessary, surface colouring may be added to give an aged effect and the teeth polished (Fig. 7.6).

ACCURACY OF THE TECHNIQUE

The reproduced model should be carefully compared with the original using anthropometric callipers. As stated earlier, room temperature vulcanizing silicones have a linear shrinkage of 0.2–0.4%. Additionally, the self-curing acrylic has a 0.18% linear shrinkage. However, since a portion of this shrinkage occurs after it has attained a solid state, it is reflected in residual stress rather than shrinkage. It is doubtful, in fact, whether there is any noticeable effect when a hollow cast is produced, as the exothermic reaction of polymerization will expand the trapped air inside the mould, thus producing positive pressure, which will in turn force the acrylic out toward the periphery. In practice, there is less than 0.2% overall linear shrinkage and an insignificant discrepancy observed when comparing the replica with the original skull.

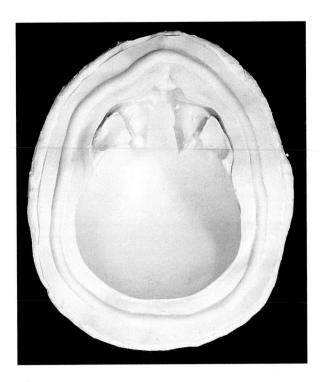

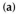

(a)

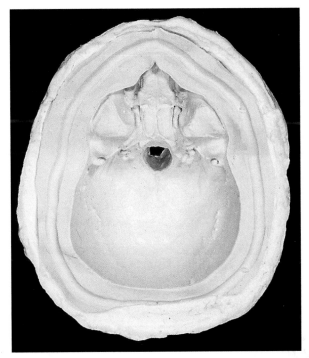

(b)

Fig. 7.4 (a) Superior aspect of the interior of the mould after removal of the skull. (b) Inferior aspect of the mould, showing the aperture of the foramen magnum, which is to be used as a casting sprue

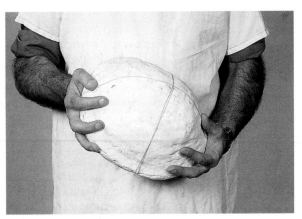

Fig. 7.5 Filled mould rotated randomly to ensure an even distribution of material over the interior surface

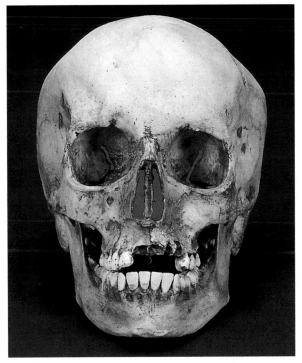

Fig. 7.6 Completed replica skull after finishing (compare with Fig. 7.1 above)

Computer-assisted methods

Computer software packages are now available which enable images to be captured digitally and manipulated at will on a computer screen (Ubelaker and O'Donell, 1992). Unlike traditional methods, many variants of an image can be reproduced easily and quickly, either as a two-dimensional picture or, when attached to a milling machine (CAD-CAM), a three-dimensional model (Vanezis *et al.*, 1989). Although a certain amount of experience with the equipment is needed, there is no need for any specific talent, so the techniques are available to a wider range of investigators. The cost of the hardware and software is, however, considerable and the facilities may not always be available.

The computer programme creates a three-dimensional image from a number of surface measurements, each of which exists in a precise location in space, relative to a fixed source. In order to obtain these measurements, the specimen must be mounted in such a way that it can be rotated through 360 degrees while an interfaced laser projector and video camera record the surface points. The computer then calculates the co-ordinates through triangulation of the points. An image created in this way does not have the detail of a traditionally prepared replica but can be used for many forensic purposes, such as photographic superimposition, as a base for a sculptural facial reconstruction and as a vehicle for the testing of hypotheses in a coronial inquiry. Differing hairstyles, soft tissue outlines and colouring may be added at will to create variations that may assist in identification.

References

Aidan E, Cockburn E. 1984: *Mummies, disease and ancient cultures*. London: Cambridge University Press.

Aufdemorte TB, Bickley HC, Krauskopf BS, Townsend FM. 1985: An epoxy resin and silicone impression technique for the preservation of oral pathology teaching specimens. *Oral Surgery, Oral Medicine, Oral Pathology* **59**, 74–76.

Bhat N, Rosato EF, Gupta PK. 1990: Gynecomastia in a mortician. A case report. *Acta Cytologica* **34**(1), 31–4.

Haglund WD, Reay DT. 1993: Problems of recovering partial human remains at different times and locations: concerns for death investigators. *Journal of Forensic Sciences* **38**(1), 69–80.

Hanslick R. 1994: Embalming, body preparation, burial and dis-interment. An overview for forensic pathologists. *American Journal of Forensic Medicine and Pathology* **15**(2), 122–31.

Hildebrand M. 1968: *Anatomical preparations*. Berkeley: University of California Press.

Iserson KV. 1994: *Death to dust – what happens to dead bodies?* Tucson: Galen Press.

Mann RW, Bass WM, Meadows L. 1990: Time since death and decomposition of the human body: variables and observations in case and experimental field studies. *Journal of Forensic Sciences* **35**(1), 103-11.

Prahlow JA, Lanz PE. 1993: Cyanoacrylate adhesive technique in wound edge approximation. *Journal of Forensic Sciences* **38**(6): 1507–12.

Quatrehomme G, Garidel Y, Grevin G, Liao Z, Bailet P, Ollier A. 1995: Method for identifying putrefied corpses by facial casting. *Forensic Science International* **74**, 115–24.

Quatrehomme G, Garidel Y, Grevin G, Liao Z, Bailet P, Ollier A. 1996: Facial casting as a method to help identify severely disfigured corpses. *Journal of Forensic Sciences* **41**(3), 518–20.

Thiel W. 1992: The preservation of the corpse with natural colour. *Anat-Anz,* **174**(3), 185–95.

Ubelaker DH, O'Donnell G. 1992: Computer assisted facial reproduction. *Journal of Forensic Sciences* **37**(1), 155–62.

Vanezis P, Blowes RW, Linney AC, Tan AC, Richards R, Neave R. 1989: Application of 3D computer graphics for facial reconstruction and comparison with sculpting techniques. *Forensic Science International* **42**, 69–84.

CHAPTER 8

Craniofacial dissection

DL RANSON

Introduction	95	Dissection from the scalp downward	102
Preliminary procedures	97	Removal of the jaws	104
Facial dissection procedures	97	Conclusion	104
Dissection from the neck upward	99		

Introduction

Probably there is no more emotive area of human dissection during the autopsy than the human face. In interacting with each other during everyday life, it is faces to which we relate best. Indeed, where physical injury has occurred to a person, the injury that people fear most is a disfiguring injury to the face. The thought of mutilation of the face fills many people with horror; consequently, there is great sensitivity about the face being interfered with during an autopsy.

Despite these concerns, dissection of the face is a not uncommon procedure during autopsy. It is utilized in a variety of death investigations, particularly in those in which facial injury has occurred or human identification is an issue. At first glance, it may be thought that the dissection of the face will be associated with permanent disfigurement, with a consequent change in the visible identifying characteristics of the face. In practice, such a degree of disfigurement of the face rarely results from the autopsy dissection. In situations in which complaints are made that the face has been altered as a result of the autopsy, a careful examination of the allegation usually reveals that there was facial damage, disfigurement and alteration prior to commencement of the autopsy. In many forensic cases, the family will not have seen the body of the deceased prior to the autopsy and, as a result, they can confuse the effects of the autopsy procedure with the injuries the deceased suffered prior to death.

RECONSTRUCTION

As described in Chapter 3, reconstruction of the body is an important phase in the autopsy procedure. Reconstruction of the postcranial portion of the body and reconstruction of the head and neck, including the face, are critical tasks, which, because of the sensitivity given to facial injuries, must be carried out with the utmost attention to detail. The restoration of the face to a form that can be recognized by family and friends is also discussed in more detail in Chapter 7. Given that a complete and thorough dissection of the face is not inconsistent with satisfactory reconstruction of a body after autopsy, there should be no reluctance on the part of the pathologist or dentist to carry out such a dissection.

When dissection of the face is limited to the soft tissues only, little alteration in facial outline should be expected. However, where the dissection involves not only the soft issues but also the facial skeleton, restoration of facial shape and form can be more difficult. In this situation, it may be prudent for the pathologist or dentist to obtain photographs of the body prior to autopsy and also photographs of the individual in life prior to craniofacial injury and death.

The jaws and teeth have a major part to play in contributing form and structure to the visible face. As a result, if the maxilla or mandible has to be removed as part of the facial dissection for the purpose of analysing injury or obtaining information from the dentition relating to identity, the work of rebuilding the face on completion of the autopsy is made more difficult. A variety of prosthetic devices can be used to assist in reconstruction of the face when the jaws have been removed at autopsy for further specialized examination. The facial skeleton may be remoulded with a supporting structure of wire and plaster of Paris, and if this is combined with dental prosthetic structures such as dentures or wax bite blocks, a satisfactory appearance can be achieved.

AIMS OF FACIAL DISSECTION

The soft tissues of the face need to be examined carefully in a variety of autopsies, including those performed for both clinical and forensic purposes.

In the clinical autopsy, it may be necessary to dissect the soft tissues of the face in order to identify pathology in salivary glands, muscle and soft tissue. Skin pathology may need to be explored, and where skin tumours have invaded the deeper structures, facial dissection may be required in order to determine the extent of direct tumour spread. Examination of the structures within the lining of the mouth, including the tongue, the nose, the nasopharynx and the oropharynx, will require a degree of facial dissection. In the forensic autopsy, soft tissue dissection of the face may be required in order to identify areas of trauma. Again, oral structures may need to be dissected, and the region of the lips, the nose and the eyes may require specific examination. The forensic autopsy often involves an examination of the subcutaneous tissues of the face in order to identify areas of bruising corresponding to sites of externally applied force. Given the nature of the forensic autopsy, injuries to the face are a common feature of the pattern of trauma in cases of interpersonal violence.

In addition to soft tissue dissection, examination of the bony tissues of the face may be required. Again, in the clinical autopsy, pathology in the overlying soft tissues may have spread to involve the underlying bony tissues of the face. Specific regions of the facial skeleton of the skull may need to be dissected in some detail. Bone tumours invading the skull, including the dental structures, may require detailed dissection, involving removal of portions of bone in order that the extent of disease can be determined. Specific structures, such as the sinuses and the deeper regions of the nose and orbits, require special dissection techniques. In the forensic autopsy, it may be necessary to examine the bony tissues of the face in order to determine the extent and nature of trauma to the face. Fine fractures of the facial skeleton may be difficult to determine on X-ray. For this reason, facial dissection should be carried out in all autopsies where the deceased has suffered a facial injury.

Gross trauma to the facial skeletal structures is a feature of many forensic autopsy subjects. Firearms injuries to the face are particularly destructive of the facial skeleton, and the exploration of these injuries can involve the dissection and removal of large portions of the mandible and the maxilla.

In autopsies in which the identification of the deceased person is unknown, it is necessary to make a detailed record of the mouth by means of detailed charts, photographs, radiographs and descriptions of the dentition so that these can be used for comparison purposes. In many cases, it may be possible to obtain this information by direct visual inspection of the inside of the mouth. However, it may in some cases be necessary to disarticulate the lower jaw (mandible) in order to expose the dental structures. Similarly, in some cases it may also be necessary to remove the maxilla.

THE DAMAGED FACE

Where the face and head are already grossly damaged and deficient in structure as a result of injury, the effect of the dissection to exposure the facial structures for the pathologist's examination may pose little future cosmetic problem. Indeed, where the face has been partially destroyed by fire, formal reconstruction may be impossible. In these cases, the skill is related not so much to not disfiguring the face and planning to allow for the subsequent reconstruction as avoiding damaging the friable carbonized remains during the dissection. Such bodies often cannot be reconstructed to a level that restores their appearance to that before the injury, and in the case of extensively burnt and charred bodies, there may be no generally visually identifiable structures remaining. Stabilization of such charred remains with waxes, glues and resins is an essential aspect of dissection in these cases. Where the skin of the face has been largely burnt away, it is essential not to put too much dissection stress and traction on the remaining tissues. The oscillating plaster saws cause particular problems in this regard and can shatter brittle tissues such as charred bone.

In cases where the body has been exposed to high temperatures, the shortening of the musculature that occurs as a result of the effects of heat results in the lower jaw becoming fixed in position. To avoid damaging potentially friable dental and facial structures, the muscle holding and fixing the mandible in position must be cleanly incised prior to attempting to open the jaws. In grossly charred and carbonized remains, even this process can be difficult, and the temporalis muscle often has to be excised without prior removal of any remaining surface skin on the head. Gaining access to the infratemporal fossae is even more difficult in these cases as fixation of the mandible precludes access to the oral cavity via the mouth. The freeing of the lateral and medial pterygoid muscles may then require an approach that includes direct lateral dissection of the cheeks or an inferior approach through the floor of the mouth, involving removal of the tongue.

Preliminary procedures

In practice, the extent and scope of the examination and dissection of facial structures must be seen in the context of the rest of the autopsy. The examination of the head and central nervous system, in particular the brain, is often linked to the dissection procedures involved in facial dissection. Similarly, examination of the upper airways and the upper part of the gastrointestinal tract, including the mouth and oropharynx, may involve procedures that occur contemporaneously with some of those used in facial dissection. As mentioned in Chapter 3, it is essential that the procedures performed at the autopsy by different specialists are co-ordinated so that there is minimal interference by one specialist with the tissues and structures that are the concerns of her colleagues.

The detailed dissection of the tissues and structures of the neck is linked to the examination of the soft tissues and hard tissues of the face. In practice, the dissection of the neck in the routine autopsy can be seen as preliminary to the more extensive procedures involved in facial dissection. Prior to detailed dissection of the face, it is often useful to have concluded the remainder of the macroscopic autopsy. As with dissection of the neck, the prior removal of the thoracic organs and brain allows blood within the soft tissues of the head and face to be drained. This results in the soft tissues of the face becoming relatively free of blood, allowing the pathologist to obtain good visualization of both soft and hard tissues during dissection.

Facial dissection procedures

In order to adequately expose the facial structures, it is essential that the body be opened in the correct fashion. Traditionally, opening the head initially involves opening the scalp. This is usually accomplished by an incision that extends in the coronal plane over the top of the head just posterior to the vertex, extending down on each side of the head to just behind each external ear (Fig. 8.1) Prior to making this incision, it is important to ensure that the hair is first parted forwards and backwards on each side of the line of the incision. If this is done, the sutures from eventual closure of this incision will be hidden by the deceased's hair when it is combed back.

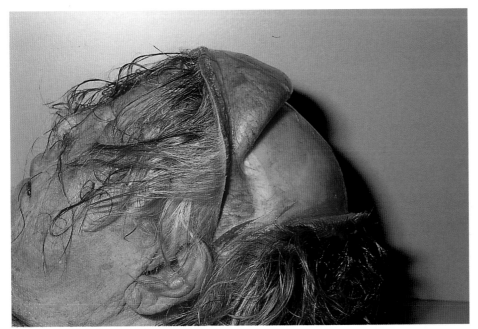

Fig. 8.1 Full thickness incision in the scalp, with initial reflection of the anterior and posterior skin flaps

When the scalp is being dissected forwards and backwards on either side of this incision, it is important to examine the soft tissue of the scalp and the underlying cranial vault. Haemorrhage in the deep scalp can be associated with blunt force injuries to the head, underlying skull fractures and hair avulsion trauma (particularly in infants). Following exposure of the vertex of the skull, the temporalis muscle over the temporal bone must be cleanly dissected free from the surface of the skull (Fig. 8.2).

In the routine autopsy, the cranial vault would then be opened using a hand saw or oscillating orthopaedic or plaster saw. The cuts in the bone are made over the mid-part of the front of the mid-forehead approximately 2 cm above the supraorbital ridges. This saw cut in the bone is continued on either side across the frontal bone and into the posterior portion of the temporal bone. The direction of the saw cut is then changed and orientated more superiorly so that the saw passes through the parietal bone on either side of the head posteriorly. The saw cut should cross the posterior of the skull vault just above the occipital bone in the midline. The removal of the brain will not be described further here. However, it should be noted that it will sometimes assist in the subsequent facial dissection if the brain has been previously removed from the cranial cavity. This opening of the cranial vault prior to facial dissection is not always appropriate, and where multiple facial fractures are present in conjunction with cranial vault fractures, it may be useful to leave the skull unopened, at least during the initial phases of facial dissection.

It is not usually possible to dissect the face without including the neck and the region of the thoracic inlet as part of the general dissection field. There has been considerable debate regarding the skin incision needed best to expose the structures of the upper chest, neck and lower face. A variety of incisions have been suggested for this. These include a single mainline incision extending from the midline of the neck anteriorly over the larynx down to the pubis, and a wide yoke incision that extends over the front of the shoulders crossing the midline in the upper part of the chest.

Where a detailed facial dissection is to be performed, I would suggest that the above methods of opening the trunk of the body are not suitable. Instead, the best incision is one that commences behind each ear and passes down the posterolateral part of the neck on each side before moving anteriorly to pass just inferior to the supraclavicular fossae on each side and then medially to join in the midline of the upper chest. It is important to ensure that the incision runs in the posterior part of the neck on each side and only moves anteriorly once it has reached the top of the shoulders where they join the neck (Fig. 8.3). If this is done, the incision will not usually be apparent to family and friends who wish to view the front of the body after autopsy. However, if the incision is made too far back on the neck and extends too far on to the front of the upper chest, the amount of skin forming the neck flap will be excessive and will make the subsequent facial dissection more difficult.

In practice, the dissection of the face is accomplished by a variety of procedures that can be performed in a range of sequences. While some areas of dissection have to be performed before others, in

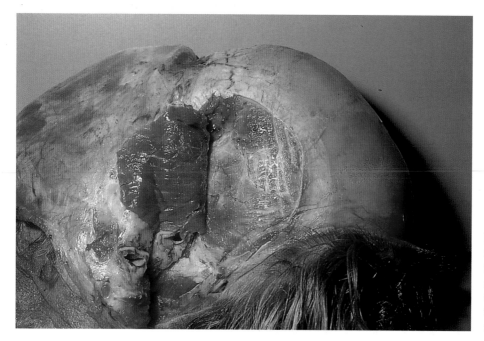

Fig. 8.2 Reflection of the temporalis muscle from the side of the skull and cutting of the cartilaginous portion of the external auditory meatus

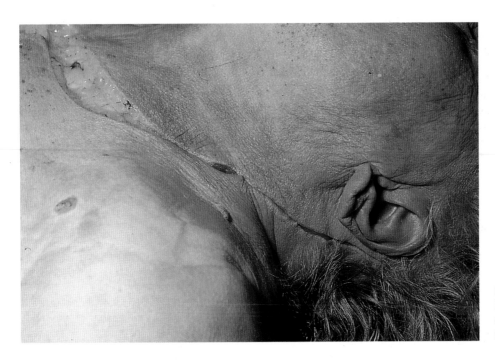

Fig. 8.3 Site of the lateral neck incision extending from behind the ear

many cases the prosector has considerable freedom to organize the dissection to meet the needs of the operating environment. For the sake of simplicity, I have described the dissection process in two stages (dissection upwards from the neck and dissection downwards from the scalp). However, many prosectors will combine these two approaches or rely predominantly on one with a few modifications.

Dissection from the neck upward

In order to expose the lower part of the face, it is necessary to dissect the skin flap formed by the meeting of the incisions in the skin on each side of the neck that have originated from behind the ears. This dissection exposes the tissues at the front of the neck. If the thoracic organs have been removed prior to neck dissection, the amount of bleeding that will occur during dissection of the anterior neck structures will be reduced. The removal of the thoracic organs in this way involves separating them from the anterior neck structures at the level of the thoracic inlet. Care should be taken in reflecting the anterior neck flap upward towards the mandible. In many forensic autopsies, it is necessary accurately to examine the structures of the anterior neck to look for signs of neck compression. This will involve examining the layers of soft tissue at the front of the neck and dissecting free each of the strap muscles on either side of, and at the front of, the larynx and hyoid bone.

Once this anterior neck dissection is complete, the neck skin flap can be dissected up over the outer surface of the mandible, and the underlying neck structures, including the tongue and floor of mouth, can be removed (Figs 8.4 and 8.5). Removal of the tongue and larynx is not essential at this time. However, if it is important to examine the palate prior to upper facial dissection, removal of the tissues of the floor of the mouth will facilitate this. In order to complete examination of the superficial surface of the mandible, particularly in its posterior and lateral parts, it is necessary to extend the lateral neck skin incisions so that they join with the coronal incision in the scalp over the vertex of the head. It is useful to mark where these incisions join so that the anterior and posterior skin flaps can be correctly aligned with each other during facial reconstruction. Once the lateral skin incisions in the neck have been joined with the scalp incision, it is possible to bring forward the lateral edges of the facial skin flap that has been formed. This involves cutting through the cartilaginous part of the external auditory meatus on each side and dissecting the skin and muscle free from the lateral or external surfaces of the body of the mandible (Figs 8.2 and 8.6). Again, if the assessment of soft tissue injury is relevant, it is important to carry out this dissection in layers. It must be remembered that there is no deep fascia in the face. The facial muscles insert directly into the skin and, as a result, dissecting the musculature free from the overlying subcutaneous tissues can be difficult.

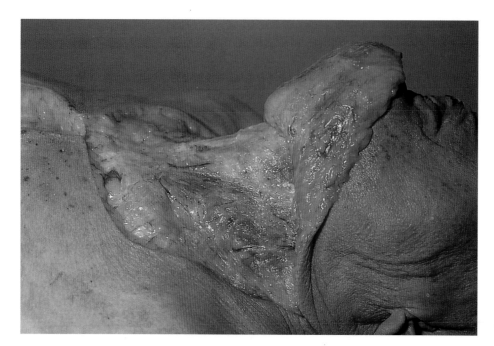

Fig. 8.4 Initial upward reflection of the neck flap

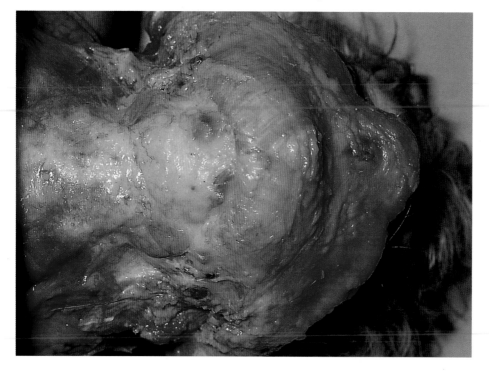

Fig. 8.5 Further reflection of the neck flap to the level of the lower border of the mandible

It is important to remove all of the soft tissue from the mandible in order to be able adequately to examine the bone. Bringing the neck skin flap up over the front of the mandible exposes the gingiva, which must be incised completely around the jaw to permit the skin flap to be extended over the area of the mouth. The lateral edges of this skin flap are then dissected medially towards the nose and the soft tissue

extension of the gingiva/buccal mucosa at the angle of the jaw is separated from the overlying skin. When this has been done, the neck skin flap can be dissected further over the lower part of the maxilla, exposing the zygomatic arches and the inferior and lateral borders of the orbits (Figs 8.7, 8.8 and 8.9). It is important at this point in the dissection to leave the skin flap attached to the distal part of the nose. The

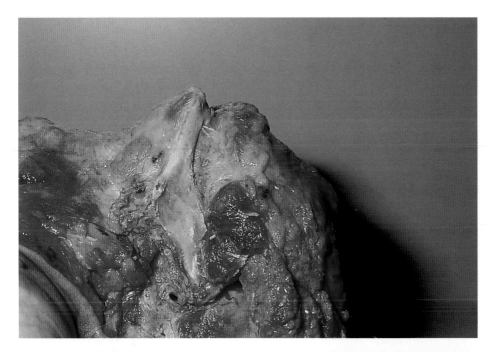

Fig. 8.6 Dissection of the soft tissue from the lateral surface of the mandible

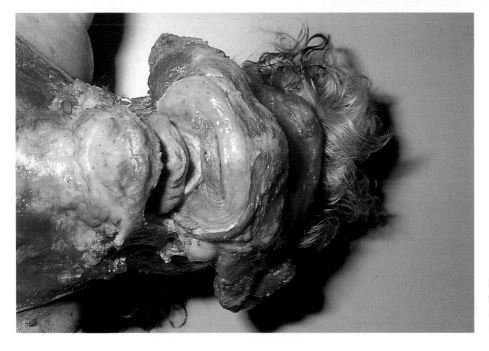

Fig. 8.7 Extension of the dissection of the neck skin flap up to the inferior maxillary border

inferior and inferolateral portions of the nose need to have the skin dissected free in order to expose the bony portions of the nose and the anteromedial region of the maxilla. However, the skin must be left attached to the cartilaginous tip of the nose to ensure adequate repositioning of the facial skin during reconstruction of the face.

In some cases, it may be necessary completely to remove the skin from the face. In such situations,

reconstruction of the face can be difficult unless steps have been taken to ensure that the facial skin can be repositioned accurately. This is best accomplished by marking the undersurface of the skin flap with coloured inks or sutures and similarly marking the corresponding adjacent surface of the underlying facial skeleton.

Before the upper part of the maxilla can be adequately explored, the upper skin flap of the head,

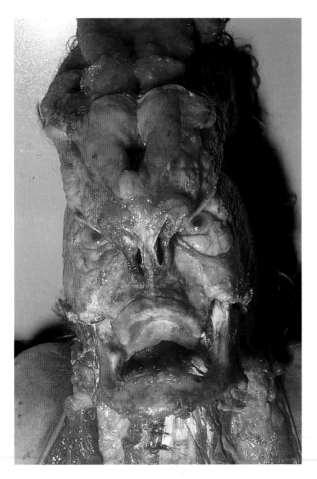

Fig. 8.8 Dissection of the lateral skin flaps, exposing the anterior maxilla

being the anterior scalp, needs to be dissected downwards.

Dissection from the scalp downward

With the opening of the scalp described above, the incisions in the skin are first continued on either side to join the lower neck incisions behind the external ears. At this point, the skin of the anterior scalp, the face and the anterior neck is separated from the remainder of the skin of the body. The scalp and forehead skin flap is then dissected forwards and downwards to the superior rim of the orbit anteriorly and to just above the zygomatic arches anterolaterally (Fig. 8.10). Careful dissection of the region of the surface of the zygomatic arch is now required on each side, associated with lateral dissection of the skin carrying the external ear. With transection of the external auditory meatus in its cartilaginous part, the superior and lateral skin flaps are dissected inferiorly and medially towards the lateral edge of the orbits. This is most easily accomplished if the lower neck skin flap has already been dissected to the level of the upper maxilla and inferior orbital rim.

In order to examine the region of the orbits, the skin must be dissected free from the superior, lateral and inferior orbital edges. The medial edge of the orbit is more difficult to expose unless the facial skin flap is completely removed from the body. In some cases, however, it is possible to leave the facial skin

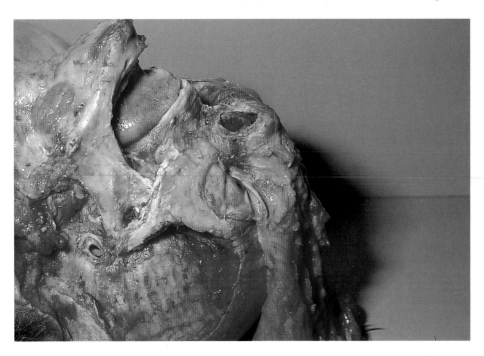

Fig. 8.9 Dissection showing removal of the superficial muscles of mastication

flap attached at the tip of the nose and still expose the entire orbital rim. It is sometimes useful to mark the soft tissue and the corresponding point on the lateral orbital rim at the lateral angle of the eyes with a suture in order to facilitate later reconstruction of the face. In dissecting the skin to the orbital rims, it is necessary to incise the conjunctiva of both eyes completely. Care must be taken not to cut through to the external skin surface of the eyelids as such injuries can be disfiguring. Once the orbital rims have been exposed laterally and superiorly, the skin can be pulled across the face on each side in turn, exposing that eye and permitting dissection of the medial edge of the orbital rim, including the region of the nasion and superior nasal bones. On completion of the dissection of the lower neck/facial skin flap, the skin of the face can be lifted free apart from at its attachment at the tip of the nose (Fig. 8.11).

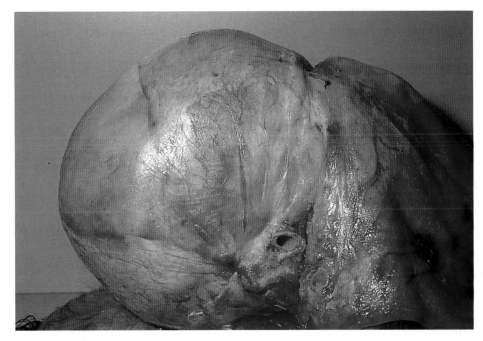

Fig. 8.10 Forward and downward reflection of the anterior scalp flap to the superior orbital ridges

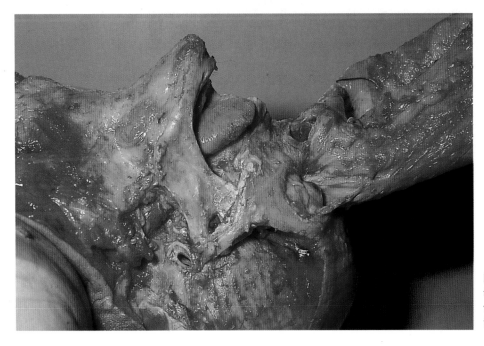

Fig. 8.11 End point of the soft tissue dissection, with tethering of the skin flap at the tip of the nose

Removal of the jaws

The mandible articulates on each side at the temporomandibular joint, which is a condylar synovial joint with the temporal bone. It has two joint cavities with an articular disc, and these need to be completely excised before the jaw can be disarticulated and removed. The mandible is a difficult structure to remove because of the position of its muscle attachments. The temporalis muscle is attached over a broad area, and it is difficult to gain access to it as it passes under the zygomatic arch. The locations of the other muscles that move the mandible (the masseter and medial and lateral pterygoids) are difficult to gain access to from the outside of the facial skeleton, and unless the mouth can be opened, cutting these structures presents problems. Removal of the floor of the mouth can assist with gaining access to the internal muscles of mastication from below when the jaw is firmly closed by rigor mortis or heat contraction of muscles. Jaw retractors/separators can also be of use, but care must be taken to ensure that they do not damage the teeth. A thin, long-handled scalpel can assist in severing these muscles through a partly open jaw, and such an instrument can also be passed behind the zygomatic arch to free the temporalis from the mandible.

Removal of the upper jaw is more problematic. If only the lower maxilla is required for dental examination purposes, a plaster saw can be used to remove the lower maxilla and palate at the level of the floor of the nose. The removal of more of the maxilla can be highly destructive of the integrity of the mid-facial skeleton and associated sinuses, which may be crucial for identification. It can also result in stability problems during reconstruction of the head. Removing the bulk of the maxilla via a pyramidal approach, cutting through the front of the maxilla in the paranasal region and the medial aspect of the orbital floor, works well. A plaster saw with a long flexible blade is an effective tool for this purpose.

Conclusion

Dissection of the face involves prosection techniques that require a high level of skill on the part of the operator. They can be physically taxing and technically difficult, but perhaps the most important consideration is that mistakes can result in facial disfigurement that is difficult to repair. Given the sensitivity in the community with regard to autopsies, great care must be taken to ensure that, where facial dissection is performed, it is carried out in a manner that causes least disfigurement.

Recommended reading

Cotton DWK, Cross SS. (eds) 1994: *The hospital autopsy.* Oxford: Butterworth-Heinemann.

Fierro MF. (ed.) 1986: *CAP handbook for postmortem examination of unidentified remains: developing identification of well-preserved, decomposed, burned, and skeletonized remains.* Stokie, IL: College of American Pathologists.

Gresham GA, Turner AF. 1969: *Post-mortem procedures: an illustrated textbook.* London: Wolfe Medical.

Hutchins GM. (ed.) 1994: *An introduction to autopsy technique. College of American Pathologists.* Northfield, IL: College of American Pathologists.

Knight B. 1984: *The post-mortem technician's handbook: a manual of mortuary practice.* Oxford: Blackwell Scientific.

Knight B. 1991: *Forensic pathology.* London: Edward Arnold.

Ludwig J. 1972: *Current methods of autopsy practice.* Philadelphia: W.B. Saunders.

Ranson DL. 1995: *Anatomical figuring: forensic body chart resource.* Melbourne: Victorian Institute of Forensic Medicine.

CHAPTER 9

Scene photography

K BYRNE

Introduction	105	At the scene	111
Equipment considerations	105	Specific techniques	117
Maintenance	109	Conclusion	120
Exposure and techniques	109		

Introduction

The old adage 'a picture tells a thousand words' is never more applicable than in the courtroom environment. Investigators, courts and juries all appreciate and expect clear and informative photodocumentation of a scene. Poor photodocumentation misleads and confuses the viewer. It is for this reason that the photographer must adopt a methodical and consistent approach, and responsibly choose the appropriate equipment, composition and lighting.

Every endeavour must be taken to ensure that each photograph is an accurate representation of the scene at the time it was taken. This chapter discusses equipment considerations, correct exposure and the actual photographic procedure.

Equipment considerations

Who uses the final image influences the choice of equipment. Court, legal and medical requirements, as well as record-keeping and storage obligations must all be considered. Sturdy, quality equipment is paramount and can be thought of as an investment. This section outlines the options available in photographic equipment and some advantages and disadvantages of each system.

CAMERA CHOICE

For the purposes of this chapter, camera format can be broken down into three sizes: large, medium and small. Large-format cameras, also known as view cameras, are mainly used in commercial and architectural photography, and are generally considered too large and cumbersome for scene work. They produce negatives or transparencies that are upwards of 4×5 inches (10×13 cm) and, as such, have excellent image detail. This may be useful where poster size enlargements are required.

Medium-format cameras, such as Hasselblad and Bronica, are strong and reliable. Although portable, they are not as compact as a 35 mm or small-format system. Again, the large negative size allows good image detail.

Small-format, or more specifically 35 mm (there are smaller formats), cameras are portable and easy to handle. The image size is smaller, and image detail is thus less than that of medium or large-format cameras. In recent times, however, improvements to emulsion technology have meant that modern 35 mm film format now has excellent resolution. There are up to 36 frames on each roll of film, and it is possible to buy 35 mm film in bulk from photographic suppliers. This format camera is the camera of choice for many biomedical and scientific applications. This means that there is a large choice of specialist lenses and accessories available to the user.

A single lens reflex (SLR) system is advisable as it has a mirror and a pentaprism; what is viewed through the camera is what the camera sees. Some cameras have a viewfinder system in which the scene to be photographed is viewed through a small window. The camera is seeing a slightly different view, which may inadvertently result in the cropping of vital information.

Both medium and small-format systems are used extensively in scene photography. Once a camera format is chosen, there are many other options to consider: automatic or manual components, metering systems, lens and flash compatibilities, and the availability of a cable release for long exposures.

A fully automatic camera theoretically enables the user to photograph a scene without having to worry about exposure. In practice, however, it is essential to have a good understanding of correct exposure and to be able manually to operate a camera. For example, difficult lighting situations, even when appropriately identified, will often cause problems owing to inherent limitations of the camera. Problem lighting situations require compensatory adjustments and are covered later. The photographer at the scene often has only one chance to capture the information, particularly with 'transient evidence', and an automatic camera is almost certain to be restrictive and result in disappointing images. A manual camera gives the user control over the aperture, depth of field and shutter speed, and is therefore much more versatile. Many cameras come with the option of using either automatic or manual mode.

The availability of a cable release and 'B' or bulb setting on a camera allows for long exposures (i.e. longer than 1 second). This can be extremely useful in low light conditions. When purchasing a camera, it is best to look at the whole unit, i.e. lenses and flash unit, to ensure compatibility.

CHOICE OF LENS

A lens of high quality, capable of resolving fine detail and as free of distortions as possible will optimize accurate results. As with choosing the camera, this choice involves a gamut of options. Scene photography requires a variety of focal lengths to document both the overall scene and close-up detail. This can be accomplished in two ways: using a selection of fixed focal length lenses or using a zoom lens. With the latter, the focus stays constant as the focal length alters. The advantage of a zoom lens is its ability to cover a range of views without the inconvenience of changing lenses. It may also be argued that this type of lens allows more rapid documentation of the scene and is therefore more efficient than using fixed focal length lenses. It is, however, more difficult to be certain of the focal length used for any particular image recorded with a zoom lens. This is a serious shortcoming because such information becomes vital in the interpretation of a scene. Investigators often require exact details involving focal length to reconstruct the scene and calculate distances.

The use of fixed focal length lenses requires a decision physically to change lenses to alter the focal length. Such changes are easy to document, and the photographer will be able to recall with certainty the lens used for the production of a particular image. Given that scene photography requires overall views, medium or orientational views and close-up views, a minimum of three fixed focal length lenses is required.

To define some of the terminology, it is best to start with a 'standard' lens, generally the lens of choice for medium or orientational views. Ray (1994) defines the idea of a 'normal' or 'standard' focal length as one that takes into consideration the correct perspective in a photograph, viewing distance and a comfortable viewing cone of vision. A useful guide is the measurement of the diagonal of the format. For example, 24×36 mm format (35 mm film) has a diagonal of 43 mm. Ideally, a standard lens would then be 43 mm; however, a 50 mm lens with a field of view of some 47 degrees is generally accepted as the standard for this camera format.

Ray (1994) points out that although the human eye has a field of view of some 120 degrees for horizontal, binocular and stereoscopic vision, a visual cone of only about 50 degrees is seen distinctly in static viewing. This means that, from a given point, a photograph taken at eye level with a standard lens will result in a view similar to that of an observer or witness at that point. This is useful to demonstrate the view a particular person may have had when viewing a crime scene. Altering the focal length of the lens from that point will alter the image size. By selecting a longer than standard focal length lens, the image size will increase. Conversely, by selecting a shorter than standard focal length (sometimes called wide-angle) lens, the image size will decrease. The perspective will not change.

A shorter than standard focal length (or wide-angle) lens is one whose focal length is significantly less than the diagonal of the format in use. It can be used to provide overview photographs of a scene. It is advisable to avoid very wide angle lenses as geometric distortion and vignetting can become a problem. For a 35 mm camera, a 35 mm lens with a field of view of about 63 degrees is recommended.

A longer than standard focal length lens with close focusing capabilities is required to obtain a large image of a small object or examine details. A 105 mm macro lens for a 35 mm camera–lens system may be used, for example, to document the entry wound of a gunshot injury. Black deposit on the skin surface surrounding the injury may give some idea of how far away the firearm was when it was discharged. The longer than standard focal length allows greater working distance and hence working space. For example, directional lighting with lamps placed close to the specimen can be introduced to demonstrate a fracture effectively. A 1:2 magnification is possible with these lenses, and larger magnifications are achieved by the addition of extension tubes. Extension tubes and close-up photography techniques are covered in detail in Chapter 10.

FILM CHOICE

The choice of film is as important as any other equipment selection so far mentioned as the quality of the end image is only as good as the weakest link. A film capable of handling a varied range of lighting conditions in the field, while still being of high resolution, capable of accurate colour rendition and readily available, is critical.

At present, most scene photography is documented on colour negative film to produce colour prints, as they are easy to handle in the court environment. Ray (1994) states that the usual nearest distance of comfortable viewing for the human eye is about 250 mm. With this in mind, the photographs will need to be enlarged to facilitate the optimum conditions for pre-

sentation to a court or jury. It is therefore important that the film selected maintains high quality even after enlargement. In districts where slide presentations are preferred for court, transparency film is required. Colour slides (transparencies) are first generation images, i.e. the film is the final rather than an intermediary image, as is the case with colour negatives. As such, there is no problem with 'subjective' printing. Slide film also has superior image stability over a long period of time, particularly if stored in archival slide pages. Table 9.1 describes some of the terminology and characteristics of the different film types.

The best way to decide on a film is to collect a variety of different ASA films from different manufacturers and test each one under the same conditions (extreme and general) to compare their performance. Once a film (or films) has been decided upon, its use and storage recommendations should be detailed in the photography department's protocol of procedures.

ARTIFICIAL LIGHT SOURCES

When daylight is inadequate, the photographer must rely on artificial light for the correct exposure. The main artificial light source in scene photography is the electronic flash. As electronic flash is a daylight-balanced light source, it is sometimes used

Table 9.1 Film characteristics

Negative film	Produces an image on film in which the colours or tones are a reversal of those in the actual scene. It has a greater exposure latitude when compared with slide film. The negative is printed on to paper to produce a positive image. This is a two-step process, and there may be some subjectivity in the printing process, which could lead to an unwanted colour variance in the final image
Reversal film	Produces a slide or, as alternatively termed, transparency. It is a single-stage positive process to produce the final image in which colour rendition is accurate. Images are projected. Reversal film has a lower exposure latitude compared with negative film and is generally more expensive
Instant film	The film packaging contains the chemicals to process the image. It lacks the quality and latitude of most conventional films but is quick and convenient. Its archival qualities are questionable
Film speed	The ASA (American Standards Association) or ISO (International Standards Organization) number indicates the speed of the film. The higher the number, the faster the film, and the faster the film, the more visible are the grains (particles of silver or pigments) in the image. Low ISO speeds generally have improved grain and resolution characteristics
Colour balance	Daylight films are manufactured to produce best results in bluish light such as daylight or electronic flash. Tungsten films are manufactured to produce the best results when used in the red/yellow light of incandescent sources

in conjunction with daylight to fill in shadows. At night, a flash may be used as the main light source. Electronic flash units come in small powerful, reliable and portable models, available in both automatic and manual modes or a combination of both. An automatic flash has a sensor that shuts off the emission of further light when the proper amount of light required for the exposure has been emitted. The automatic flash does not cope with all problems. A dark-coloured bullet casing on a white-tiled kitchen floor is one such problem. The sensor will emit light to illuminate the white surface and result in underexposure of the subject of interest, in this case the bullet casing. Such problems will be discussed further below. In manual mode, the flash puts out a maximum burst of light each time it is fired. The exposure is controlled by altering the aperture depending on the flash-to-subject distance. Guide numbers supplied by the manufacturer with each flash unit may be used to obtain the camera exposure provided the speed of the film is known. The guide number is divided by the flash-to-subject distance in order to calculate the appropriate f number. In some modern units, TTL, or through-the-lens metering, is available. These units need to be matched with a compatible camera sensor through the lens that shuts off the unit when enough light has reached the film plane. A greater choice of apertures is available with this system.

Other available light sources include large floodlights and studio lights. It is advisable to become familiar with all the different light sources used by scene investigators. This may mean adding film balanced to different colour temperatures to the kit. A handheld light meter, to measure the light correctly and calculate the correct exposure, is essential.

As with any light source, the direction and behaviour of the light is an important consideration. Versatility of the flash head, i.e. its ability to tilt and swing, and the option to remove the flash from the camera body altogether are favourable attributes. These options allow the photographer to direct the flash head towards a nearby surface (ideally, a white wall or ceiling) and bounce the light back toward the subject. This bounce flash technique is useful when photographing a reflective surface such as a kitchen sink and will be discussed later.

The power source to energize the unit may be internal, external, reusable or disposable. Internal batteries are convenient and readily available, and eliminate the need to carry a power pack; however, they are slow to recycle. External battery packs have many advantages: they recycle quickly and, when properly charged, have extensive flash capabilities. A disadvantage is carrying a battery pack and connection cord, which may be heavy and cumbersome.

ACCESSORIES

Motor drives

A motor drive is simply a mechanical attachment that winds the film on and resets the shutter. The main advantage is that the photographer can concentrate on the image, taking several photographs and maintaining the camera's position without having to wind the film on manually.

Filters

There are numerous types of filter available. Only a few are commonly used in scene photography. A skylight or UV filter will both protect the lens and help to filter out haze. A polarizing filter will remove or reduce reflections from non-metallic surfaces such as water or glass. A magenta filter can be useful to balance fluorescent light to daylight slide film.

Extension tubes and extension bellows

The extension tube is used to achieve 1:1 and higher magnifications. It is placed between the lens and the camera body to mechanically alter the lens-to-film distance, thus increasing the image size. The tubes come in different sizes, and different magnifications are possible by using different tubes or by stacking. Tubes are generally made of metal and are sturdy for scene photography.

The extension bellows work on a similar principle and consist of a lens board with a bayonet mount, an adjustable tube made of opaque cloth and a focusing rail. Extension bellows are more versatile but also more expensive and fragile than extension tubes and will consequently only very rarely be used at any scene.

Camera case

A good camera case of the correct size, with lots of compartments, can be a real asset. Ease of access to equipment and a case that is easy to move about are two important criteria when making a choice. They come in both hard-case designs and soft-case coverings. Soft cases hold more equipment, and the top opening flaps allow easy access. It is advisable to have a waterproof top and bottom. Most cases are designed to be carried over the shoulder, leaving the photographer's hands free in the process. Metal or hard case designs are usually fitted with solid foam and provide the best protection for transporting equipment in all types of weather. They are usually silver in colour to reflect the heat of the sun, and most are lockable. These can be used in place of a pair of steps for the photographer to stand upon. It is, however, slightly more difficult to access equipment quickly compared with a soft-case design.

Once at a scene, many photographers have found that a photovest with numerous pockets is also of great use.

Tripod

A good tripod is invaluable to the photographer. Ideally, a tripod will be so heavy that it will be almost immovable in order to prevent any possibility of camera movement. A compromise, however, is a portable, but sturdy, tripod. It needs to be stable for long periods of time with the heaviest lens. There are many features available in tripods, and prices vary accordingly.

Ladder

A sturdy but lightweight ladder can be of use to obtain 'above' views of a scene. Some photographers take their own boxes, or indeed their camera cases, to a scene for this purpose.

Maintenance

It is vital that equipment be in excellent condition for scene photography: there is often only one opportunity to capture the information. Equipment needs to be kept away from dust, moisture and extremes in temperature. Cameras should be cleaned with compressed air and a blower brush. Avoiding the mirror during this process is vital as it is easily damaged and should not be touched under any circumstances. It is recommended that cameras and lenses be taken to a reputable camera dealer to be cleaned and checked once a year. Battery contacts should always be cleaned with a very fine sandpaper prior to installing new batteries. In order to protect lenses, a UV or sky-light filter should be attached to them at all times. The optical surface of the lens is highly susceptible to damage and should therefore be cleaned only with cleaning fluid and lens tissue available from photographic suppliers, following the manufacturer's instructions.

Exposure and techniques

BEHAVIOUR OF LIGHT

To understand exposure, it helps to have a fundamental understanding of the behaviour of light.

This is a complex subject, and the author's intention here is to outline some basic principles that will assist in general photography; Ray (1994) goes into more detail.

The brightness of a subject depends on both the amount of light that falls on it and how it reflects that light. The intensity of the light reaching the subject is governed by the power of the light source and its distance from the subject. This relationship between the intensity of light and the distance is covered by the 'inverse square law'. Jacobson *et al.* (1988) explain this. The rule states that the intensity of illumination is inversely proportional to the square of the distance from the light source to the subject. Put more simply, if a lamp is moved twice the distance from the subject, the light intensity falling on the subject will be a quarter of what it initially was. This concept is important to both selecting the appropriate light source and assessing lighting conditions in a given situation.

When light falls on a subject, one of three main things can occur: it may be absorbed, reflected or transmitted. Light is absorbed in most situations. However, it is almost totally absorbed with non-reflecting black surfaces such as velvet. A fire scene with black charring is therefore a good example of a situation in which a large amount of light will be absorbed. Such a scene will require additional light (Fig. 9.1).

Objects also reflect light. When light strikes a mirror or other shiny, smooth surface, it is reflected at the same angle as the angle of incidence. This is a very important rule when using a flash on a camera. If photographing a reflective surface with the light source perpendicular to the surface, it will be reflected directly back into the lens, resulting in a hot spot in the image and possibly obscuring information. Understanding this rule will enable the photographer to remove the flash from the camera and place it at an angle to the subject to avoid the above problem. Light falling on a rough surface will scatter in a more or less haphazard fashion. Light that is neither absorbed nor reflected is transmitted.

A basic understanding of the way in which light behaves in a given situation will enable the photographer to make informed decisions about the exposure required and the direction of a light source.

EXPOSURE

Factors governing the determination of exposure include the diaphragm or aperture, the shutter speed and the film speed. Inspection of the diaphragm of a lens will show that, as the f stop number is increased, the diaphragm decreases, allowing less light to reach the film plane. Conversely, as the aperture ring is rotated

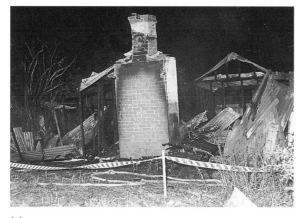

(a)

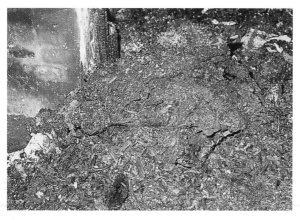

(b)

Fig. 9.1 (a) Exterior of a burnt residence. (b) The photographer has deliberately overexposed this image to reveal detail in the dark subject. However, the human remains are still difficult to find in this photograph

to a smaller f number, for example f5.6 or f2.8, the diaphragm is more widely open allowing more light to reach the film plane and thus influencing its intensity. Opening up the aperture one f stop allows a factor of two, or twice as much light to reach the film plane. The shutter limits the amount of time that light is permitted to reach the film and therefore indicates the actual exposure time. For a given film speed, the exposure can be adjusted by varying the shutter speed and the aperture, as described by the reciprocity law: Exposure = Illuminance × Time (Jacobson *et al.*, 1988).

Under the law of reciprocity, for a film of any given speed, a long exposure with a small diaphragm opening is equivalent to a short exposure with a large diaphragm opening. This is maintained provided that each such combination transmits the same total amount of light to the film. Vetter (1992) points out that when this reciprocal relationship is carried to extremes, the density does not remain constant. This

phenomena is identified as a reciprocity effect or reciprocity law failure. Manufacturers provide some information with the film packs. However, reciprocity failure is rarely a problem in routine scene photography.

The aperture controls not only exposure but also depth of field. When a lens is focused at a certain point, there will be a zone both in front and behind that point that also appears acceptably sharp on the film.

LIGHTING

Available light is the main light source in scene photography. Light is measured at the scene by the meter, hand held or 'in camera', and an overall 'average' illuminance is calculated. For a scene with highlights and shadows but predominantly midtones, the appropriate shutter and aperture combination will ensure an overall correct exposure. In most cases, this amount of light will be adequate. However, in situations in which the lighting ratio is extreme, important shadow detail may be obscured, so alternative techniques may be required. A high lighting ratio, i.e. a large difference between illumination falling on the darkest and on the lightest areas of the scene, may require an additional light to 'fill in' the shadows. Such a situation may arise on a bright sunny day, with a lighting ratio as high as 20:1. The technique of combining sunlight and the light from electronic flash is called 'synchro-sun'.

Synchro-sun is relatively simple and involves obtaining a standard exposure based on sunlight and the synchronized shutter speed. The correct ASA number should be set on the flash. Once this is completed, the f stop for the scene exposure is located on the dial, noting the flash-to-subject distance. The flash is then positioned at this distance for a 1:1 lighting ratio. For a 2:1 lighting ratio, the flash would be positioned at the distance indicated on the dial for the next largest f stop.

In situations in which daylight is not available, or is simply inadequate, the usual light source is electronic flash. Basic factors affecting exposure when using electronic flash are the light output of the unit, the distance from the flash to the subject and the ASA rating of the film. Flash units vary in their output capabilities. Manufacturers generally supply a guide number when the unit is purchased, which can be used to calculate the exposure at any flash-to-subject distance. The f stop is calculated by dividing the guide number by the flash-to-subject distance. Prior to taking any photographs, the correct ASA should be selected on the flash and the shutter sync speed selected on the camera. The manufacturer will mark the speed with an X or a lightening bolt symbol to ensure that the shutter is completely open before the flash is fired.

Using the flash attached to the camera, often called 'on-camera flash', is fast and convenient. There are, however, many situations in which removing the flash from the camera will result in superior images, for example to improve texture and demonstrate shape by the modelling nature of the light (Fig. 9.2). Emphasizing texture and pattern in footprints and tyre tracks are two situations in which this technique may be used. The exposure for the 'off-camera flash' technique is still calculated by measuring the flash-to-subject distance, as outlined above.

Most portable flash units are a reasonably small light source and may produce hard shadows. A solution to this is the bounce flash technique. It involves directing the flash towards a wall or cardboard reflector (preferably white) and bouncing the light back towards the subject. In this way, the entire surface of the reflector becomes a larger light source. The light falling on the subject will be less unidirectional, shadow edges will be less abrupt and 'softer', and the illumination will be generally more even. Problems involved with this technique include an overall decrease in contrast and a significant loss of light. The light has to travel a longer distance, so intensity is lost and light is scattered. This may necessitate a larger aperture, thereby limiting depth of field. The light may also assume the colour of the reflecting surface, so a white wall or ceiling is the best choice. Exposure calculation can be difficult owing to a variety of possible reflecting surfaces. The flash-to-subject distance is measured from the flash head to the reflective surface and then to the subject. Camera and flash systems using TTL metering technology automatically calculate the correct exposure, cutting the flash off when sufficient light has reached the film plane.

Another option with electronic flash is the ring flash. This is a circular flash tube that attaches to the lens. It is particularly useful to photograph cavities such as the oral cavity in odontological documentation. As it is a direct 'on-camera' light source, care needs to be taken when photographing very shiny surfaces as circular highlights may obscure information.

At the scene

The photographs taken at a scene are a permanent record of that scene at the time the images were taken. The photographs help to refresh the memories of both investigators and witnesses. They also assist the investigators and the jury in understanding, and possibly reconstructing, a certain sequence of events. As new evidence comes to hand, different aspects will be reviewed, so photographic documentation is vital. The images taken at the scene will also form part of the brief for new investigators or for second opinions from colleagues.

The main aim overall is to ensure that the photographs taken will be admissible in court. In order to be admissible, the photographs should be a true representation of the crime scene at the time the incident was reported. Duckworth (1983) notes that care must be taken not to add or subtract from the scene, subject or item of evidence before it has been photographed as found. Hunt (1984) also says, 'The object of the photograph must be relevant to the case. The photograph must be instructive or stress a particular point. The photograph must not appeal to the emotions or tend to prejudice the jury.'

WHEN A PHOTOGRAPH MAY BE INADMISSIBLE

Some photographs are damning to the defence. In order to make the photograph inadmissible, the

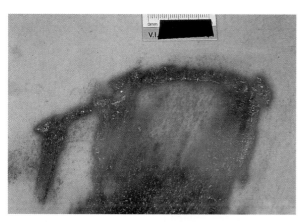

(a)

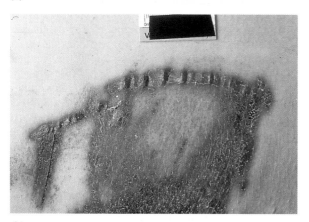

(b)

Fig. 9.2 (a) A single flash on the camera, documenting an injury. (b) A single flash at a 45 degree angle to enhance the texture of the injury

defence need only create a doubt as to the integrity of the photograph. In one scene, the photographer took the overall photographs of a kitchen in a house where a homicide took place. Unbeknown to the photographer, while he was taking photos in the bedroom, an inexperienced investigator left her handbag on a chair in the kitchen. When the photographer returned to the kitchen to take several more photographs, the presence of the handbag went unnoticed. Later, the inconsistency of no handbag in one shot and its sudden appearance in the next cast doubt on the integrity of the photographs, and they were disallowed in court.

Another example concerns the photographs of a suspect in a homicide. The circumstances involved a stabbing murder of a person in their kitchen. The suspect was held at a local police station. The photographer attended this station and took routine photographs showing the face, hands, arms, any injuries and possible bloodstains on the suspect's body or clothes. One photograph showed four blood droplets on the suspect's left foot. Since she had no apparent injuries to explain this blood, this was vital documentation. The photograph, however, was deemed inadmissible owing to the inclusion in the photograph of a tattoo around the ankle. The tattoo, it was argued, cast aspersions about the character of the defendant. As a result, the prejudicial effect on the jury is greater than the probative value to the court. Had the tattoo been cropped out of the image, the photograph would probably have been admissible in court.

PREPARATION

It is vital that equipment be checked prior to attending a scene. Adequate film is required. Ensure that accessories and extra batteries are available. Back-up camera and flash equipment should also be taken to a scene. Most photographers have at least one horror story concerning the breakdown of equipment. A colleague happily quotes that, in 15 years' experience, he knows of 1000 mistakes that can be made with his Bronica medium-format camera, which has three moving parts. Even the most experienced photographer can forget to check a setting on the camera, with the dreaded result of incorrectly exposed film, or, worse still, no images at all. Early detection will occasionally enable the photographer to retrace and rephotograph. Camera settings need to be checked and then checked again. Generally speaking, however, you get only one opportunity at a crime scene – there is no room for error. A fresh roll of film should be loaded and equipment packed in such a way to keep it clean and protected during transit.

Another, seemingly worldwide, phenomenon is that homicides come in batches. A crime scene squad may be quiet for a couple of days and then suddenly have four consecutive homicides, invariably at 2 a.m. on the darkest of nights in extreme weather conditions. It is these situations which push equipment maintenance to the limit. Battery power for the electronic flash units will be one of the first things to run out, and it is also vital to have adequate film. Automated equipment has its limits, and a thorough knowledge of camera equipment and theory is essential. The electrical components of a camera are susceptible to breakdown in wet or humid conditions. If the photographer has enough knowledge, he or she can easily convert to fully manual controls and continue unhindered.

POLICIES AND PROTOCOLS

A methodical and logical approach to a scene will ensure that every aspect is covered, and a department policy or protocol is advisable to ensure continuity within the department. There are some mandatory criteria that should be included in that protocol. A standard log book or data record of the scene photographs is essential. Scene information to be recorded includes: the date and time; the identity of the photographer; the exact location; the film and camera used; the number and a brief description of photographs taken; and the weather conditions. The log book must also include the chain of custody from exposure of the film, delivery and reception from the processor to storage or distribution of the final product.

Once at the scene, photographers need to communicate with the officer in charge and identify themselves, explaining their requirements. Preserving the scene to ensure the integrity of the photographs is one of the primary duties of the officer in charge. There are always many conditions to consider prior to entering a crime scene. For example, the weather may dictate the priority of photographs or equipment required. Other conditions include potentially explosive or unstable structural environments, the likelihood of additional crime occurring in the area and legal and political issues (Duckworth, 1983). The photographer may need to identify certain items, such as perishable food and trace evidence that is easily destroyed, and prioritize the order of photographs accordingly. Duckworth (1983) also suggests that the photographer be aware of potential interference by the media and the public. Personal experience and the experience of co-investigators will greatly assist in dealing with these situations.

Much care must be taken not to destroy evidence. This cannot be overstated. It is relatively easy accidentally to stand on tyre marks or a footprint in the middle of the night or even during daylight. This applies not only to the photographer but also to the team of investigators visiting the scene. This situation highlights the importance of quality photographs taken quickly and accurately. In the event that items are lost or damaged at the scene or in transit, it is possible that these photographs will be the only record of evidence available.

TAKING THE PHOTOGRAPHS

The basic rule of scene photography is to document from the general to the specific. An overall view shows the scene in its entirety. For the purposes of this chapter, overall photographs are those taken with a wider than standard lens, for example a 35 mm lens on a 35 mm camera. As the main purpose of these images is orientation, landmarks such as trees or signposts are included in the composition. In one scene, a skeleton was discovered amongst shrubs in a disused paddock. The overall scene photograph usefully showed where the skeleton was in respect to the fence and surrounding plants. If a house is the location of a crime scene, overall photographs are taken showing the front, back and both sides of the house, and neighbours' houses if appropriate. Aerial photographs may also be requested and are essential if the crime scene is a large area. Once inside the house, part of the photodocumentation will involve overall photographs of each room.

Orientational photographs refer to those images which are taken with a standard lens, for example a 50 mm lens on a 35 mm camera. As the standard lens has a field of view close to that of human vision, several views of the scene should be taken at eye level to demonstrate the general appearance of the scene to the investigator and witnesses. The standard lens is the best one to use when moving into the scene to concentrate on certain areas. With reference to the skeleton in the paddock, for example, the orientational photographs may reveal that one plant appears to be growing through the neural canal of one of the vertebrae. This image records some aspects of the time frame of the case. The size and type of plant now becomes more important. If, in the house scene described above, the front door was the site of forced entry, it would already be included in the overall photographs. The photographer would then move forward to concentrate on the door itself. Tool markings or a forced lock can be isolated in each photographs. For further detail, it is important again to change lenses.

Finally, close-up photographs are those which are taken with a longer than standard focal length. When using a 35 mm camera the lens of choice would be a 105 mm lens. The tool markings on the door from the aforementioned scenario should be photographed both with and without a scale. The scale must be parallel to the lens, the scale and the subject both being in the plane of focus. This will enable an accurate 1:1 enlargement of the markings to be matched with a possible tool at a later stage. The inclusion of a scale in the photograph may occasionally be thought to obscure further evidence, so a second shot is taken without a scale. The perspective in a photograph depends mostly upon viewpoint and is another important consideration. A lens does not give perspective: perspective is a result of its spatial position, or viewpoint relative to the subject (Ray, 1994). A common fault is to leave a shorter than standard (or wide-angle) lens on for the close-up images after taking the overall photographs. In a three-dimensional scene, the resultant images will make the relative size of the objects and the apparent space between the objects appear different from those of the true situation.

SCENE PHOTOGRAPHS OUTSIDE

In any scene, whether it is a building structure or a plot of land, all views need to be photographed. In the case of a building, all walls need to be documented, compass directions being very useful for orientational purposes. As mentioned, all views are taken at eye level. Any points of access or entry are documented, as are any vehicles (and their number plates) parked outside the premises. Mail or newspapers in the crime scene area are all photographed as they may give some indication of the time period involved. Tyre tracks and footprints are best photographed using a single flash at a 45 degree angle to emphasize the pattern of the tread. Figure 9.3 exemplifies the process that may be employed.

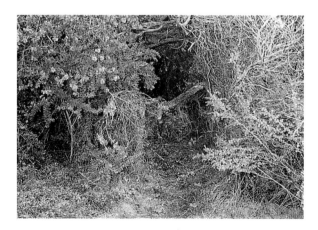

Fig. 9.3(a)

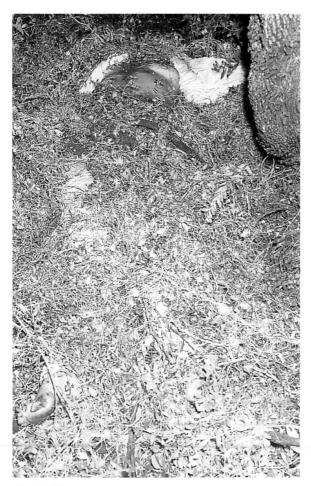

Fig. 9.3(b)

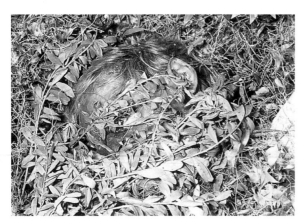

Fig. 9.3(c)

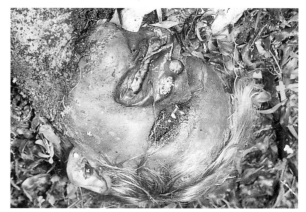

Fig. 9.3(d)

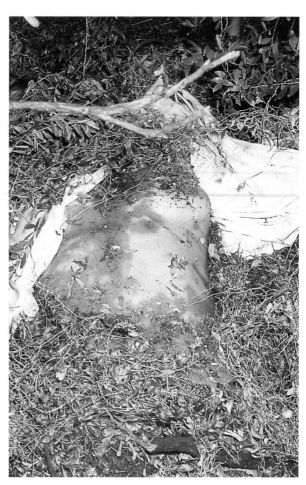

Fig. 9.3(e)

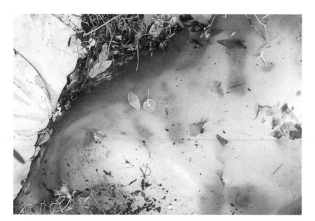

Fig. 9.3(f)

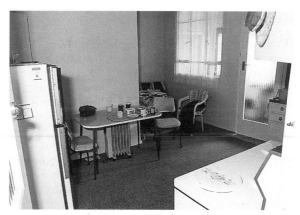

Fig. 9.4(a)

Fig. 9.3 The body of a murdered victim was found beneath plant debris and undergrowth along a nature walk. The individual had been missing for 2 weeks. (a) An overall view of the area where the body was discovered. The body was found behind the branch in the centre of the photograph. A closer view (b) reveals that the body was obscured by plant debris. Different views are required to orientate the body in relation to the structures surrounding it. A still closer view (c) shows a view of the face partially exposed. (d) The effect of decomposition, mummification and insect activity on the exposed areas, highlighting the difficulty of visual identification in these cases. A medium-distance view (e) of the chest area orientates the viewer to a close-up (f) of a point of interest – the button

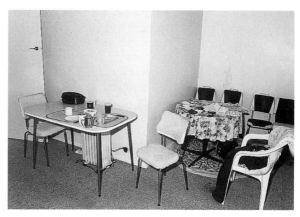

Fig. 9.4(b)

SCENE PHOTOGRAPHS INSIDE

Once inside, a sequential set of photographs is required to orientate the viewer yet again. The general layout should be clear and include views both into and out of the room or rooms where the crime occurred. To document the interior of a room comprehensively, it is best to stand in a corner of the room facing the opposite corner and take the photograph at eye level. If this is done for all four corners, the room should be covered. If the room is a long rectangle or an odd shape, it can be divided and extra shots taken, ensuring that there is an overlapping area in each shot (Fig 9.4). Avoid capturing investigators in the photographs. All latent fingerprints are photographed prior to being lifted. Positive evidence such as blood splatter, a bloody knife or writing on the wall are obvious subjects to include in the photographs. What is not immediately obvious is the need to document what is *not* there – the negative evidence. The *lack* of signs of a forced entry may be just as important as a blatant break in. Although it is ideal to obtain background information to have an idea of what to photograph, it is vital

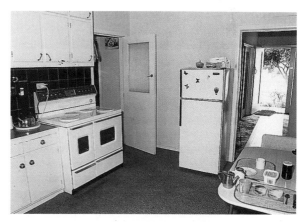

Fig. 9.4(c)

Fig. 9.4 Parts (a)–(c) demonstrate the documentation of an unusually shaped room

to keep an open and clear mind. Once a mindset develops about a sequence of events, important documentation in the form of photographs that should have been taken from specific angles and views may be overlooked.

DOCUMENTING HUMAN REMAINS

Documenting a victim at a scene is approached in the same way as is the entire scene, i.e. overall, orientationally and close up. The overall photographs of the inside of the room will already show the victim's position with respect to the surrounding objects. Gerberth (1996) refers to the 'chalk fairy' who, while the first officers are securing a scene, suddenly has the irresistible impulse to draw chalk lines around the body. This is, of course, completely undesirable and may, by adding to the scene, mean that any photographs of the body with these lines are 'inadmissible' to show the state of the body when it was found. All sides of the body, including the view from directly above, are photographed. Orientational photographs are best taken by using three photographs to document the whole body: the head and chest area in one photograph, the torso in another and finally the legs in the third. Care is taken to ensure there is an area of overlap in each photograph. Figure 9.5 shows how this may sometimes be problematic.

Consider a body, lying on its back in the kitchen with a stab wound to the chest, a ligature around the neck and the hands underneath the back. Facial photographs will be taken for identification and documentation of any injuries. A photograph of the upper chest, head and neck area will demonstrate both the stab wound and the ligature. The photographer will then concentrate on the neck area, from top, front and both sides, taking the photographs both with and without a scale and changing lenses for close-up shots. The same will then be done for the stab wound area, systematically covering each point of interest. Any clothing, tattoos and jewellery are also photographed.

All these photographs are taken without interfering with or moving any evidence, including the body. Once the body has been cleared by the coroner or medical examiner and the investigator in

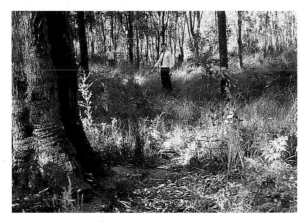

(a)

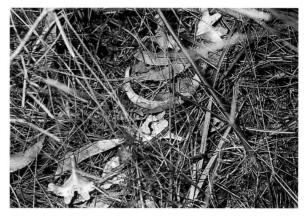

(b)

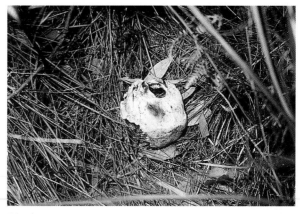

(c)

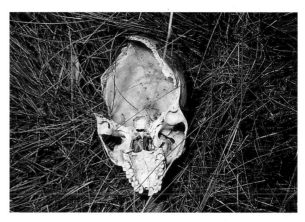

(d)

Fig. 9.5 In this case, the remains of a young individual were found in a wooded area. The remains had been scattered by animals and covered a large area. Although it is normally not ideal to have police personnel in the photograph, (a) demonstrates that, in reality, long grass may obscure police markers. (b) Body remains camouflaged by leaves and grass. (c) Part of the skull discovered. (d) The rest of the skull discovered 15 m away

charge, more photographs can be taken. The body can now be rolled over to photograph the back. In this example, the victim may have had the hands tied behind the back. Close-up photographs would be taken documenting the type of material and the knot used. Once the body is moved, the area underneath should be photographed to record any trace evidence and to document the condition of the surface beneath. A very porous surface, for example, can mask splatter patterns and the extent of blood loss. Bloodstains can be difficult to photograph, particularly if they are on a dark surface, for example dark green carpet. In this situation, it is possible to photograph the stains using black and white film with a red filter over the lens. The red, bloodstained area will show up as a lighter area on the resultant print. Once the scene has been cleared and the body removed, evidence that has been partially obscured can be documented. This includes contents of rubbish bins (Fig. 9.6), the fridge and the contents of drawers.

AT COMPLETION

After attending a scene, the films taken need to be processed as soon as possible. If they are processed within the department, the time and name of the person accepting responsibility for the film should be noted in the log book. If films are processed by a commercial laboratory, the management should be approached so that the film is handled by a limited number of people and security of the negatives and the prints is ensured. Once the prints are returned, they are sorted and delivered to the appropriate investigators. Camera equipment should immediately be cleaned and restocked, and batteries recharged, in preparation for the next job.

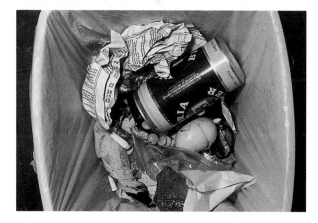

Fig. 9.6 The contents of a rubbish bin. In this case, some tablets are visible

Specific techniques

Scene photography will almost always test the photographer in some way. It seems that most scenes are attended in dark situations with difficult access. This section addresses some specific techniques to enhance textured patterns, the use of lighting and how to illuminate large dark areas. Aerial and digital photography will also be covered. This section does not pretend, however, to cover the myriad of specific techniques available to the photographer but merely outlines some common ones.

ENHANCEMENT OF TEXTURED PATTERNS

Understanding the behaviour of light, and using this information, enables a textured surface to be enhanced. Latent fingerprints, tyre tracks and footprints can all be photographed using this method. By taking a single flash or studio light off the axis of the camera and angling it at 45 degrees to the subject, the tops of the ridges will be highlighted, leaving the indentations darker and clearly showing the pattern. With a constant light source, for example a torch or studio light, it is easy to select the optimum angle. A 45 degree angle will usually enhance a pattern; however, a more oblique angle will sometimes show more. It is often necessary to move around the object at different angles to enhance different aspects of the pattern (Fig. 9.7).

Using high-contrast lithographic black and white film can effectively document latent fingerprints or lip prints on a glass surface. It involves the same technique as above. A single light source is angled at the prints until they are clearly visible through the camera lens. It is best to have an assistant to change the angle of the light until it is in the correct position. The angle can sometimes be quite oblique – 15 degrees for example – to obtain the best result. Prior tests are useful with a specific light source so that the exposure can be estimated. In any case, it is advisable to bracket heavily, i.e. to take the same view with various exposures, with this technique. Lip prints can be photographed in this way.

DIFFICULT LIGHTING SITUATIONS

There are many difficult lighting situations in scene photography, one of the most challenging being the scene where the single light source is simply inadequate. An example of this is a large open area at night or a burnt-out concert hall. There are a few options; two available to the photographer are painting with light and a multiple flash technique.

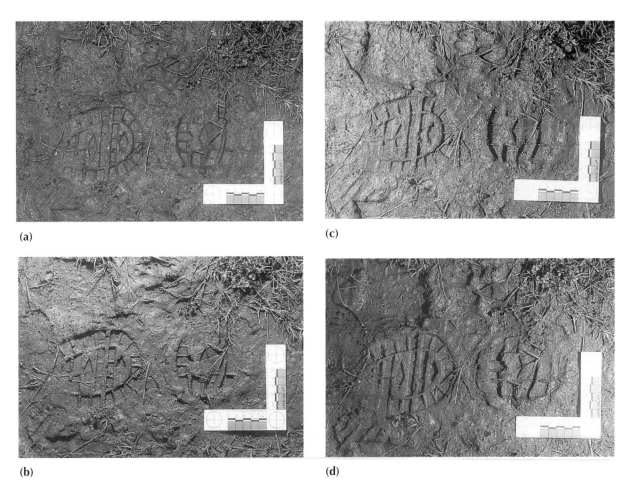

(a)

(c)

(b)

(d)

Fig. 9.7 (a) A single flash from directly above a footprint. This lighting is 'flat' in that texture is defined. It is difficult to ascertain whether the pattern is indeed raised or indented. (b) A single flash obliquely from the top of the photograph. The resulting shadows accentuate the pattern. (c) A single flash from the left side of the photograph. (d) A single flash from the right side of the photograph. Viewed together, the photographs allow a comprehensive assessment of the pattern

Painting with light

There are some equipment considerations with this method. The photographer will require a sturdy tripod, a cable release, a portable flash unit, a small piece of lightproof cloth such as black velvet and a torch. The camera is mounted on a tripod with the cable release attached, and the view is composed through the camera. A wide aperture setting of f2.8–f3.8 is recommended, and the shutter should be on B (bulb) setting. The photographer should ensure that there are no strong lights directed towards the lens (street lights, for example, should be avoided if possible). It is helpful to have at least one assistant with this technique. To determine the viewing area of the lens, the assistant can walk away from the subject with a torch in his hand; once the torch light can no longer be seen, this point is marked.

The idea is to leave the shutter locked open on the camera and, section by section, expose the film. As the portable flash is fired from a predetermined marker (for example, left of the camera), that section of the scene is illuminated and recorded on the film. The assistant then repeats this process by moving to the area right of the camera and so on until the whole scene is covered (Fig. 9.8). Duckworth (1983) points out that care must be taken not to stand between the lens and the flash, or silhouettes will appear on the negative. As long as the assistant is out of view behind a subject inside the scene area, for example a car, the flash can be directed upwards but back towards the camera. This will help to separate the subject from the background. To avoid stray light entering the lens while the assistant moves to the next position, a loose lightproof cloth is place over the lens. Once all sections of the scene are covered, the shutter is closed. This technique is possible with a single operator leaving the shutter open and quickly

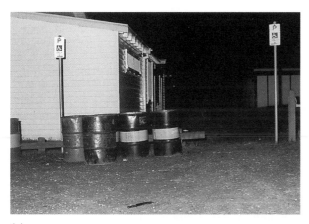

(a)

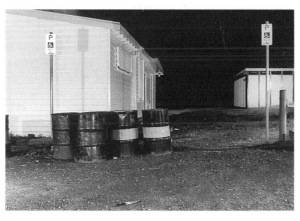

(b)

Fig. 9.8 (a) Photograph taken a night with a single flash. (b) The same view using the 'painting with light' technique. Note the extra detail visible both in buildings and in the foreground. The tell-tale signs of this technique are the multiple shadows that are formed

moving from position to position firing the flash. Some stray light may enter the lens (as the lightproof cloth cannot be used with a single operator), but good results are still possible.

Multiple flash technique

As with 'painting with light', the multiple flash technique is used to illuminate a large area in low light conditions. The same principles are involved in both techniques. The main difference is that painting with light requires only one flash whereas 'multiple flash' requires just that – multiple flash units and some way of synchronizing those flashes. Slave units attached to flash units can be triggered by another flash being emitted. This can be difficult if long distances or large objects obstruct the slave triggers. With a TTL system and the proper interconnecting cords (long

cords are available), a number of dedicated flash units may be simultaneously controlled. Radio slave units can be purchased, and although they are expensive, they work well. They are, however, contraindicated in some situations, for example where unexploded terrorist bombs may be present. Radio slave units work by emitting a radio signal with a primary flash, allowing numerous units to be triggered simultaneously. Correct exposure can be established by using a flash meter to measure the light falling on the subject. To be thorough, this should be checked from different angles to ensure that the direction and distance of each unit are correct.

AERIAL PHOTOGRAPHY

Aerial photography provides an opportunity to document a scene from an alternative viewpoint. The aerial photograph helps to orientate the location with respect to size and surrounding structures. As with all scene photography, the key to success is thorough planning, with access to the appropriate equipment and a clear set of objectives. Although the same basic principles apply to aerial as to any other scene photography, there are some special considerations. These include the direction of the sun, avoiding blurred images and coping with haze.

When the sun is high, illumination is greater and the shadows will be shorter. This is ideal as there is less chance of important information being obscured by shadows. Blurred images are a problem owing to the speed and vibration of the aircraft and the turbulence of air current. To avoid blurred images, the fastest shutter speed possible is recommended, preferably 1/500 or faster. Depending on the available light, a faster film may be required to enable the use a faster shutter speed. Leaning on the structure of the aircraft for support should be avoided as vibrations are transferred directly to the camera.

Haze can have an overall lightening and often bluish effect on photographs. This can be lessened by using a haze or a UV filter. If using black and white film, a yellow or red filter will prevent blue light reaching the film, thereby reducing the effects of haze.

Both vertical and oblique views are possible, and the choice of the view depends on the information required. Vertical photography results in map-like images that can be analysed for size, shape and measurement. If both the focal length and the altitude of the aircraft are known, the scale can be calculated:

$$\text{Scale} = \frac{\text{Lens focal length (in)}}{\text{Altitude of aircraft (in)}}$$

It is again good practice to keep accurate records, including case number, time, aircraft, pilot, location, altitude, latitude, longitude, film, frame number, exposure and lens. This will enable accurate calculations on the photographs if required.

Oblique photography enables a greater area of coverage to be documented. Taken from the side, a scene looks more familiar and structures are often easier to recognize than with vertical views.

Equipment considerations are similar to those in standard scene photography. Medium- or small-format cameras are generally preferred for aerial work, and the choice of lens depends on the scale required in the image. This needs to be ascertained prior to the flight. Communication is of utmost importance. It is critical that the pilot has a detailed brief, understanding the altitude and the views required. Helicopters and slow-flying high-wing planes are the best choice of aircraft for aerial photography. In some helicopters, it is possible to remove the door and decrease obstructions to the view. In any aerial photography, especially if there are open doors, it is imperative that equipment is secured and that a neck or hand strap is used with the camera. The photographer should also be secured in an appropriate safety harness. The most important factors are planning and communication. With a concise plan, the appropriate equipment and an informed pilot, aerial photography can be a smooth process producing informative and useful images.

DIGITAL IMAGING IN SCENE PHOTOGRAPHY

The advent of digital cameras has caused some controversy concerning their forensic applications. The new digital cameras are becoming more compact, with increased resolution and storage capabilities. They are not, however, the panacea to every photographic ill: they have both advantages and disadvantages.

Advantages include the obvious instantaneous nature of the photographs and the fact that there is no need to process film or print images. It is possible to transfer images almost instantly to another location, be that to investigators in the central office or across the country. The information transmitted can vary from a suspect amongst the onlookers to an image for a second opinion from a specialist consultant.

The main disadvantages are the present cost of this technology and the susceptibility of digital imagery to tampering. As Robson (1993) says, 'many people feel that because the source is electronic, items key to a case could be added or deleted'. One of the biggest hurdles to digital images is explaining the technology to the judge and jury. If they are apprehensive about the reliability of the images, the case is fraught with problems. There are some secu-

rity measures to be addressed before a legal environment will wholeheartedly embrace this technology.

Regardless of whether the system is digital or traditional, the photographer still needs to understand lighting, exposure and composition principles. If this knowledge is lacking, the images will be inferior. Digital technology should be viewed as another visual communication tool available to the photographer.

Conclusion

This chapter has dealt with essentials of scene photography. Every scene will challenge the photographer wishing accurately to document the information around her. The photographer has a major role in scene investigation. Many people, including the judge and jury, will rely heavily on the images presented to them. Well-maintained, quality equipment and a wide knowledge base are essential. This knowledge, and some lateral thinking, can assist in identification matters in otherwise baffling cases, as in the one described in Fig. 9.9. Although a daunting res-

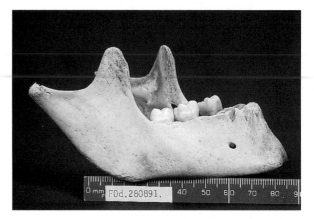

(a)

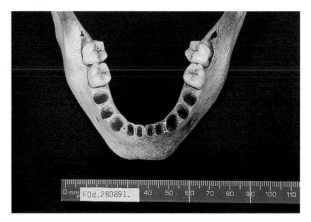

(b)

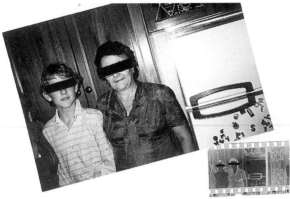

(c)

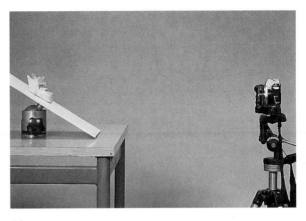

(e)

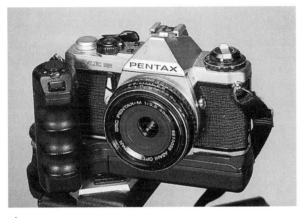

(d)

Fig. 9.9 A young surfer disappeared. Three years later, a jaw (a, b) was found washed up on a beach. Superimposition techniques were used to ascertain whether the jaw was that of the person who had been lost. A family photograph taken shortly before the surfer's disappearance, with its corresponding negative, was obtained (c) along with the camera used to take the photograph (d). Using the negative inserted into the original camera and the fridge as a reference point, the perspective, angle and distances of the family photograph could be recreated. In the studio, the jaw was photographed using the same measurements with the original camera (e). The resultant photograph was then used for superimposition, and the jaw was positively identified, to the satisfaction of the Coroner, as that of the surfer.

ponsibility, forensic photography, if done well, is both rewarding and appreciated.

References

Duckworth JE. 1983: *Forensic photography*. Springfield, IL: Charles C. Thomas.

Gerberth VJ. 1996: *Practical homicide investigation: tactics, procedures and forensic techniques* (3rd edn). Florida: CRC Press.

Hunt SM. 1984: *Investigation of serological evidence*. Springfield, IL: Charles C. Thomas.

Jacobson RE, Ray SF, Attridge GG. 1988: *The manual of photography* (8th edn). London, Boston: Butterworth Scientific.

Ray SF. 1994: *Applied photographic optics* (2nd edn). Oxford: Focal Press.

Robson S. 1993: Is the jury still out? Electronic vs. traditional photography. *Law Enforcement Technology* **20**(6), 36–8.

Vetter JP (ed.) 1992: *Biomedical photography*. Stoneham, MA: Butterworth-Heinemann.

Also useful are the unpublished papers of the International Forensic Photography Workshop, Dade County Medical Examiner, Forensic Imaging Bureau, 1994, Miami, Florida, USA.

CHAPTER 10

Photography of remains

A HENHAM

Introduction	123	Perspective	131
Equipment considerations	123	Background	132
Equipment for close-ups and macrophotography	126	Orientation	132
Film	126	Cropping	133
Lighting	127	Scale	133
Exposure	128	Colour	133
Focus and depth of field	130	Macrophotography	134
Identification	131		

Introduction

Specimen photography generally has the advantage over photography in the field in that the photographic environment can be controlled in order to make the most of the material. To do this successfully, the photographer has to consider the aims of the photography and then select the appropriate equipment and techniques. Standardized methods are useful for efficiency but are limiting if used to the exclusion of a flexible approach.

Factors to be considered include equipment such as cameras, lenses, lighting, light meters and accessories for normal range photography, with a slightly different approach for macrophotography. The type of film, its exposure and process should also be chosen according to the aims. A good understanding of perspective, colour balance, focusing techniques, orientation and scale are essential to obtain the best results.

Equipment considerations

Appropriate equipment is essential for producing high-quality photographic records of specimens.

While no one piece of equipment will be suitable for all tasks, it is not necessary to have shelves filled with expensive, state-of-the-art products in order to achieve results. Excellent results can be obtained using a small number of carefully selected, quality items. The most important factors are to choose equipment that is most suited to the bulk of the work and fully to understand its capabilities and limitations. This approach not only allows better control over the photographic procedures but also, with an understanding of basic photographic principles, will allow adaptation of some equipment to specific tasks.

CAMERA

Considerations in camera choice should include format size, focusing and metering methods, and the availability of lenses and other components.

Format should be considered according to the end use of the photographs. Medium or large-format cameras should be considered where extremely high definition enlargements are required. However, 35 mm single lens reflex (SLR) cameras are the most practical for general use, particularly for the close-up work needed in specimen photography. The cost of materials and processing for 35 mm format is also considerably less than that for larger formats. For these reasons, most of this discussion refers to 35 mm format.

Camera systems such as Nikon are often used in medical photography owing to their wide range of specialized components, available accessories, and durability. Fully automatic cameras should not be considered, as control over exposure and focusing is essential.

The assumption is normally made that all photography is film based, but digital camera technology is now available. At present, the equipment capable of producing high-quality images is significantly more expensive than traditional systems and requires the use of considerable computer hardware. The scanning process requires the camera to be attached to a computer, and scanning can be relatively slow. Stand-alone digital cameras are at present inadequate in comparison with the standard 35 mm SLR. For these reasons, digital cameras cannot be regarded as entirely suited to specimen photography. However, rapid technical progress is being made, and the situation is likely to change in the near future.

LENSES

The lens, more than any other aspect of the camera system, will affect the quality of the final image. Quality lenses are essential to attain good image sharpness and accurate colour reproduction. The main factors to consider when selecting a lens include focal length, focusing range, maximum and minimum apertures, resolving power, distortions and compatibility with existing equipment.

Lenses should be interchangeable to allow for the use of different focal lengths, and no one lens will give the best results in all circumstances. Unfortunately, the lenses that offer everything, for example a wide-ranging zoom, compromise on quality.

The focal length of a lens affects the angle of view and working distance, and this indirectly affects image size and perspective. Thus the focal length should be chosen according to the size of the subject and the available working distance.

A 50 mm lens is useful as its angle of view is closest to that of normal human vision. However, longer lenses, such as 100 mm or 200 mm, with greater camera-to-subject distances, create less distortion and allow more flexibility in the placement of lights and accessories. This is particularly useful in macrophotography. The perspective distortion and small working distance associated with wide-angle lenses make them of little use for specimen photography, other than for particularly large subjects such as skeletons.

Zoom lenses can be useful for general work where accuracy is not critical, but they are not recommended for forensic and medical work. Inherent optical distortions in zoom lenses make them unsuitable for work where accuracy is required, particularly in the reproduction of straight lines. Also, variable focal length lenses make standardization difficult and later recollection of exact focal length, for example in court, almost impossible.

LIGHTING

Factors to consider in lighting equipment include power output, source colour temperature in relation to film, the physical size of the unit and the actual light source, modelling lights and attachments such as diffusers. The portability and adaptability of equipment, working space and the size and characteristics of the subjects should also be taken into account.

Relatively powerful units are needed. This allows the use of smaller apertures to increase depth of field as well as reducing ambient light exposure. It also allows short shutter speeds that reduce the risk of movement during exposure.

The size of the source should be chosen according to the size of specimen to be photographed. For example, a 3 cm square light represents a very small source in relation to a large specimen such as a skull. On the other hand, it would act as a large source when photographing minute bone fragments. The physical size of the light may also be a factor, depending on the size of the room and the working distance between the camera and subject.

Portable studio flash units are the preferred form of lighting for specimens as they give high light output with little heat and eliminate the need for long exposures. The colour temperature of flash, matching that of daylight, allows the same film to be used in the studio as outside. Thus adjustments can be made to the power output without changing the colour temperature. Most reputable brands of studio flash have a wide range of accessories, such as diffuser soft boxes, barn doors to direct the light more accurately and fibreoptic attachments for macro work. Flashes with built-in modelling lights are strongly recommended as they allow the lighting to be assessed and adjusted before exposure. If units with modelling lights are not available, a small torch strapped to the flash may help by showing where shadows and highlights are situated on the specimen.

While tungsten lights can be relatively inexpensive and have the advantage of allowing exact visualization of the image, they can be inconvenient in use. This is due to their heat output, and the long exposure times they require compared with an electronic flash.

In addition, the colour temperature of the globes does not remain consistent over their lifetime.

The choice of daylight temperature or tungsten sources should be considered in relation to film type.

Most built-in camera flashes are lacking in power and size, and their fixed position makes them unsuitable for specimen photography. Small, portable electronic flashes are limiting when attached directly to the camera but will allow some degree of control, and therefore improved results, if positioned off the lens axis. This type of set-up is acceptable for use with small specimens and when portability and speed are the key issues. This arrangement is achieved using extended sync cords, and flash brackets designed for the purpose, which are not difficult to design and construct. According to Le Beau, 'While multiple flash brackets have been commercially available for some time, only the Lepp ... Bracket has stood the test of time for production of 35 mm colour slides on location. The Lepp system is a bracket that holds the camera with two mini-flash units set at desired positions above, below, in front, behind, or on both sides of the lens' (Le Beau, 1992). It is advantageous to use flashes with heads that can be swivelled and tilted as this allows greater flexibility and adaptation of the lighting. In order to give some modelling, one of the lights should have reduced output. This is best achieved by placing a $0.3\times$ neutral density filter over one flash.

Power packs are a convenient method for powering portable flashguns as they are rechargeable and have a faster recycling time and more power than batteries.

Ring flashes that attach to the end of the lens provide effective on-axis lighting for photographing cavities. Some types that allow segments of the ring to be turned off individually will provide some modelling, but ring flashes generally produce very flat lighting. This, combined with their low power output, make them unsuitable for most other subjects.

LIGHT METERS

A hand-held incident light meter, reflected light meter or camera meter can be used, depending on the type of lighting in use. Built-in camera meters are adequate when using either continuous light sources or dedicated flash systems, as long as their limitations are recognized.

It is necessary to use a hand-held flash meter for metering the output from portable studio flashes as the short flash cannot be read by normal meters. If standardized lighting conditions are used, there is no need to meter for every photograph. Initial testing can be carried out and the results assessed to establish the correct exposure. However, to maintain flex-ibility in illumination as well as accuracy of results, it is essential to have a light meter.

ACCESSORIES

Flash accessories, such as soft boxes for diffusing light, come in varying sizes and shapes to suit a wide range of subjects. Although not essential, they provide a convenient and quick method of changing the quality of a light source. For example, a 50 cm square soft box replacing a standard reflector will provide diffused, even lighting for medium-sized specimens.

A sturdy tripod should be used to produce accurate and repeatable results as it allows for better control in fine-tuning the framing and for making adjustments to focus, supports or lighting. A tripod is particularly important when using a continuous light source as exposures are likely to be longer.

A permanent specimen photography set-up can easily be arranged by attaching a copy stand to a table designed for the task. The stand should be rigid, as well as horizontally and vertically adjustable (Fig. 10.1). Various types of table are commercially available but they are also relatively simple to make. An average specimen table consists of a glass top that is supported about 30 cm above a black, white or coloured background. The size of the table top should depend on the average size of the specimens to be photographed and allow room for attachments such as supports or reflectors. For ease of use, the table height should be lower than an average table.

This system creates a shadowless background, giving the impression that the specimen is floating. It is convenient and allows for easy standardization while

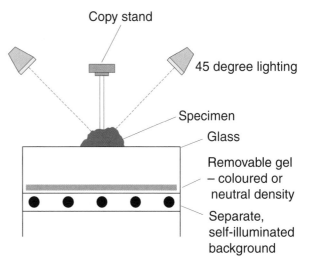

Fig. 10.1 Diagram of the components and geometry of a specimen copy stand, showing the separately illuminated background

also offering some flexibility. It is best for photographing flat or semi-flat specimens or for recording one plane of a specimen. In most cases, a three-dimensional effect is best achieved by shooting the specimen from an angle of about 60 degrees using a tripod, rather than from directly above.

High-quality images of specimens can rarely be obtained without the use of appropriate supports, backgrounds, stages or other similar pieces of equipment.

One or more suitable backgrounds are essential and should be given very careful consideration. Other necessary items may range from plasticine and cotton wool, to specifically designed clamps or tables. Plasticine is useful for raising small specimens, such as teeth, away from the supporting surface in order to render the background out of focus. Other examples include electricians' stands, which are very handy for holding scales in position or for holding small specimens at the correct angle. Fishing line can be used to support a specimen and should be anchored outside the field of view. Inverted, round container lids of varying sizes are very good for supporting curved specimens such as skulls. Pencils cut to different sizes provide good supports for positioning scales at the correct height.

Equipment for close-ups and macrophotography

Extra consideration needs to be given to equipment that is required for close-up work or macrophotography.

A normal lens is designed to perform optimally at infinity and becomes optically inefficient when trying to focus at less than 50 cm, which is their normal minimum focusing range. This problem can be overcome with the use of either a specialized macro lens or accessories that allow the normal lens to focus at a closer range.

Most manufacturers produce 'macro' or 'micro' lenses that give a reproduction ratio of up to 0.5× or 1.0×. Strictly speaking, these are close-up lenses as the prerequisite for a true macro lens is that it is able to magnify the object. In specimen photography, where close-up work is frequently required, a macro lens should be considered as a versatile alternative to a standard lens.

Being specifically designed for close-up work, a quality macro or micro lens will produce images that are sharp from edge to edge, as opposed to the lesser-quality lenses that will produce only a centrally sharp image at close range. An added convenience is that the lens reproduction ratio is usually engraved on the barrel. Macro lenses are available in a range of focal lengths, 50, 100 and 200 mm lenses being the most common. The increased working distance of the longer lenses makes them more convenient to use.

Zoom lenses that give the option of internal macro focusing are optically a very poor alternative to a true macro lens. Although often referred to as 'macro zooms', most give a maximum reproduction ratio of only 0.5×. Such lenses should not be considered for quality specimen photography as critical sharpness and fine detail cannot be obtained.

Magnification is achieved either by changing the focal length of the lens using supplementary lenses (diopters) attached to the front of the main lens or by increasing the distance between lens and camera using bellows or extension rings.

Specialist photomacrographic systems that are available in 35 mm and large format are convenient to use as they are rigid, provide a permanent set-up and have a range of accessories specifically designed for macrophotography.

LIGHTING

Lighting requirements for macrophotography follow the same general photographic principles but in a smaller format.

The use of normal-sized lights should not be considered, as their large size in proportion to a macro specimen results in very diffuse lighting, making small highlights and sharp shadows impossible to achieve. In addition, a physically smaller light source is better for macrophotography as the small working area makes large sources awkward to use and takes up much of the limited space available.

Miniature electronic flashes or tungsten lights can be used very effectively, but fibreoptic light is the preferred form of lighting for macrophotography. Fibreoptic lights are directional, small, flexible and cold, making them an excellent choice for macrophotography. The fibreoptic attachments available for many modern studio flashes are very convenient as the output can be easily varied without a change in colour temperature. Care should be taken when using variable-intensity tungsten sources as colour balance can change significantly with intensity, but some have filters that can be used to correct the colour balance.

Film

No one film, whether colour or black and white, will produce the best results in every instance. In general, film should be chosen according to the characteristics of the subject and the intended use of the image. Results will vary considerably depending on film characteristics which include speed, resolution, colour balance, spectral sensitivity and exposure, and processing requirements.

The first consideration should be whether the end product is intended to be prints or slides. If both are required, it is often best to use two camera bodies loaded with transparency and negative film respectively. It is costly to obtain high-quality prints directly from slides. Prints derived from slides, by the production of internegatives, although much cheaper, will give excessive contrast and loss of detail. Similarly, slides obtained from prints will not have the same quality as originals. In addition, loss of quality occurs in the production of black and white prints from colour originals, so if black and white reproduction is required, for example for publications, it is advisable to shoot black and white film as well.

Two major differences should be noted between negative and transparency films. First, exposure accuracy varies. While an adequate print may be obtained from a negative that is up to two stops over- or under-exposed, the lesser latitude of transparency film may produce unusable results, as it only tolerates less than a one stop error. Second, the different processing procedures can produce great colour differences. In the printing process, the variations depend on both the content of the photograph and the subjective input of the printer. Transparency film has a one-step process and gives more accurate colour rendition as subjectivity is not involved.

To avoid severe colour casts, film must be matched to the colour temperature of the lighting – either daylight or tungsten. In instances where the film and source cannot be matched, filtration must be used to correct the colour balance. An 80A filter is used with daylight film under tungsten light, and an 85B with tungsten film under daylight conditions or with flash.

Reciprocity failure is the decrease in film speed that occurs at very high or low levels of illumination. Colour casts or incorrect exposures can occur due to reciprocity failure. In practice, this varies between films, and the manufacturer's information sheet should be checked to give the required adjustments.

In specimen photography, slow or medium speed films are best because of their ability to produce higher resolution and better rendition of detail than fast films. A fine-grain film is particularly important if large prints are required. For this reason, lighting with a good power output is essential to allow correct exposures while avoiding long shutter speeds or large apertures.

A wide range of films is available, so the best way to select the most appropriate film for use is by testing under the conditions in which the bulk of the material will be photographed.

Lighting

The quality of the final image is dependent more on lighting technique than on any other single aspect of the photographic procedure. It is often mistakenly assumed that lighting a specimen effectively merely involves illumination. However, as in any form of photography, variations in lighting can significantly alter the appearance of a specimen. Therefore, just as portraiture calls for specific lighting that will emphasize a subject's better features, specimen photography requires the use of lighting techniques that best illustrate the relevant information. Choice of lighting should depend on specimen characteristics, such as size, shape, contour, colour, opacity, and the specific areas of interest.

It is often easiest to think of lighting in terms of shadows and highlights. Harsh highlights and dark shadows both cause loss of detail. If used effectively, shadows and highlights can convey a large amount of information, from which pathology and other details can easily be evaluated. Shadows and reflections should, in general, be minimized and used only to show the specific identifying features.

The main considerations relating to a light source are its quality and its direction in relation to the subject. The quality of a light is usually discussed in terms of how direct or diffused it is.

Diffuse illumination is essentially lighting from a source that is large in comparison with the subject. For example, a 1 m square light would be a large, diffuse source for photographing a skull; however, the same source illuminating a car would be small and direct, giving less even illumination. Diffused light can be produced by passing it through a fine cloth or tissue. However, it is more convenient to use a portable soft box or to bounce the light off a large reflective surface. An undiffused light source that is very big in relation to the subject will also create diffuse illumination. In macrophotography, a small semi-opaque tube or a polystyrene cup with its base removed can be placed over the specimen to provide diffuse, even illumination. The light from a diffuse source is relatively flat and has soft shadows. If the lighting is too diffuse, its lack of contrast tends to make the subject look more two-dimensional, with less surface definition. This is clearly demonstrated in Fig. 10.2.

Light sources such as bare flash lights or those with only a narrow reflector bowl attached are usually referred to as direct. These produce hard-edged, deep shadows and therefore give a more three-dimensional image with a high degree of contrast.

The basis of a photographic lighting set-up is a main light source, often referred to as the 'key' light. When positioned correctly, the key light can be used to cast shadows that show shape and contour. In most instances, a direct key light is preferable for the photography of bones owing to their inherently low contrast. A key light alone will generally produce a brightness ratio between the highlights and shadows that is too great for photographic film to record effectively, especially when using transparency film. Shadows thus need to be lightened, either by using a second light source or by using a reflector to bounce the main light back into the shadow area. Care needs to be taken not to produce a confusing second set of shadows when using two light sources (Fig. 10.3).

Each specimen should be lit according to its features: there is no one formula for correct lighting. Texture is best accentuated by acutely angled lighting, effectively skimming the light across the surface. Again, fill light must be considered (Fig. 10.4). In some instances, a departure from standard lighting techniques will show information more clearly. An example of this is the use of transmitted light shone through bones to demonstrate fractures (Fig. 10.5).

While a fixed copy set-up with 45 degree lighting will give an acceptable result, the quality of the final image can generally be extensively improved if the set-up allows for small adjustments in lighting ratio and position.

Exposure

Light meters operate by measuring either the light reflected from the subject (reflected light meters) or the light falling onto the subject (incident light meters). Built-in camera meters take reflected readings and operate in the same way as hand-held reflected light meters. While meters are capable of measuring light intensity very accurately, the calculated exposure assumes that the subject is of average brightness levels. For this reason, if both types of meter are used to measure an image that is effectively mid-tone, the readings will be the same. However, a reflected light meter reading can be greatly influenced by very dark or very light areas, causing the subject to be metered incorrectly. For example, a bleached bone will reflect more light than a subject of average brightness. The reflected meter, assuming it to be mid-grey, will give a reading that will result in underexposure. Similarly, dark areas surrounding an average specimen will indicate to the light meter the need for more light

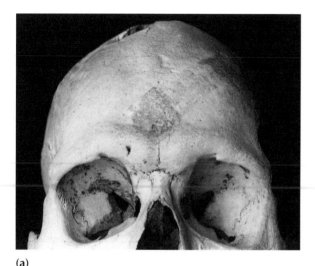

(a)

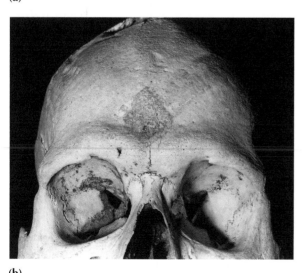

(b)

Fig. 10.2   A skull, demonstrating brow shape. (a) Diffuse lighting. (b) Direct lighting

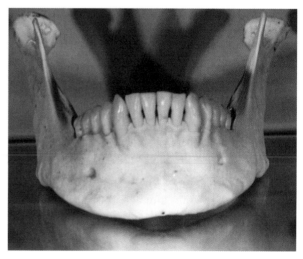

Fig. 10.3   Photograph of the mandible, demonstrating poor lighting and background selection. Note the unwanted reflection below specimen and the confusing double shadows

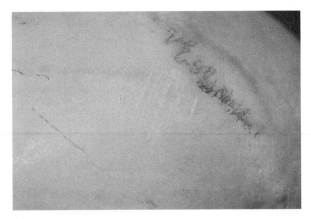

(a)

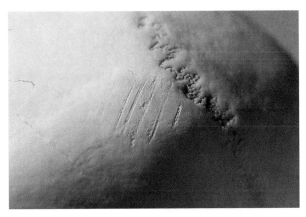

(b)

Fig. 10.4 Photograph of a tool mark in the bone, between the suture and the fracture of the skull. This demonstrates texture by lighting: (a) flash on camera, (b) low-angled lighting

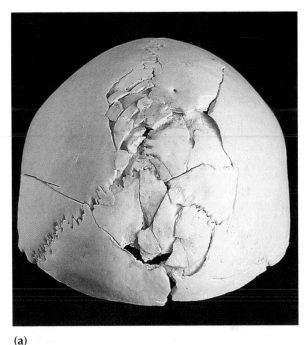

(a)

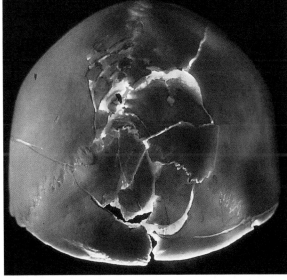

(b)

Fig. 10.5 Photographs of skull fractures. (a) Normal lighting. (b) Transmitted light

than is required to expose the specimen correctly, resulting in overexposure.

Accurate reflected readings can be achieved in two ways. The use of a spot meter, either in the camera or attached to a hand-held meter, allows measurements to be taken from the small, relevant areas of the specimen that contain the most important information. Kodak manufactures a grey card that simulates the reflectivity of an average subject. Taking meter readings from such a card at the position of the specimen can also eliminate exposure problems.

Incident light readings are the most popular method of metering as they are not influenced by the subject. However, they cannot be used in some situations, for example when metering transmitted light. When photographing very dark specimens, it may be necessary to increase the exposure slightly in order to show sufficient detail, but lightening the specimen too much may give false results. It should also be noted that the f number changes with change in focal

length when using zoom lenses. This can cause problems with exposure unless camera metering is used.

Camera exposure meters work well for measuring continuous light sources and when using dedicated flash units attached to the camera. It is important, however, to be aware of the exact system they use for calculating the reading. For example, some cameras measure the light by averaging the brightness levels across the whole frame. Most modern, high-quality cameras have more sophisticated methods, such as centre-weighted, matrix or spot metering, which may be selectable.

Many modern cameras have through-the-lens (TTL) flash metering, which meters the exposure of a dedicated flash while the flash is firing. The calculated exposure is then provided by terminating the flash output once the correct level of illumination has been reached. This method is more accurate than standard automatic flash metering but still requires consideration of the exact subject being photographed.

In many instances, the most appropriate and effective technique is to use manual camera settings combined with hand-held metering and standardized methods. Once the lighting has been metered, the exposure may need to be adjusted for other factors, including filters on the lens, lens extensions or reciprocity failure of the film. TTL metering, whether for flash or continuous light, has the advantage of taking into account light loss due to filters or lens extension.

Bracketing of exposures should be considered in specimen photography as slight inaccuracies in exposure can sometimes result in loss of information. This is particularly necessary when using slide film because of its small exposure latitude. It is highly advisable to take notes of exposure readings and then compare them with the photographic results in order to determine the best exposure for various groups of subjects. For example, earth-stained bones will require significantly more exposure than those that are sun-bleached.

Focus and depth of field

Depth of field is influenced greatly by the point at which the lens is focused as well as by the aperture used.

In most instances, obtaining maximum depth of field is the priority. However, a limited depth of field can also be used to advantage in specimen photography. A photograph may be made clearer if those parts of the specimen which do not add useful information are rendered out of focus. Similarly, an out-of-focus background helps to create a less 'busy' image.

The need for fine control of depth of focus makes an auto focus lens unsuitable for specimen photography.

In general photography, the maximum depth of field will be achieved by focusing at a point one third inside the area of the relevant part of the subject (Fig. 10.6). In macrophotography, focusing should occur halfway into the subject (Fig. 10.11). Depth-of-field scales on the lens barrel can usefully indicate the exact depth of field at a each aperture.

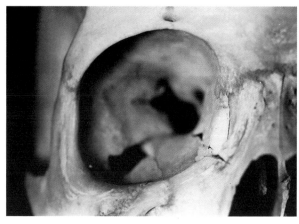

(a)

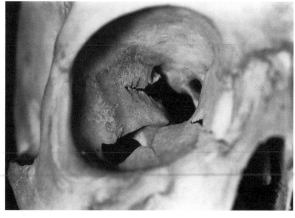

(b)

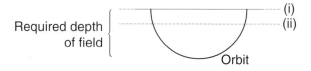

(i) Plane of focus in photograph (a)
  – inadequate depth of field obtained
(ii) Plane of focus in photograph (b)
  – optimum depth of field obtained

(c)

Fig: 10.6 Photographs of the orbit demonstrating the increase in depth of field caused by changing the point of focus. (a) Focusing at the front of the specimen, on the orbital rim. (b) Focusing one third of the way into the orbit. (c) Diagram illustrating the planes of focus for these photographs: (i) inadequate depth of field, (ii) optimum depth of field

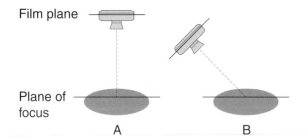

Fig. 10.7 Diagram showing that, in order to maintain the maximum depth of focus, the film plane of the camera should be parallel to the selected plane of focus on the specimen. (a) Correct. (b) Incorrect (the camera at an angle)

Maximum depth of field over the entire frame can only be maintained if the film plane is parallel to the plane of focus (Fig. 10.7)

It is well known that using smaller apertures will increase depth of field, but stopping down to the smallest apertures should be avoided as it degrades the image by diffraction.

Identification

The inclusion of an identification number on the scale is the easiest and most reliable method of recording identification. It is useful to have an area on the scale specifically for this purpose.

The type of scale used is influenced by the intended final use of the film. Any photographs for court use should have scale and identification, but those intended for publication or teaching should have a scale without identification. For evidential purposes, the specimen should be photographed from the same viewpoint both with and without a scale. This is in order to reduce the likelihood of allegations that a relevant part of the specimen has been concealed by placement of the scale.

Perspective

Perspective distortion can greatly alter the information in photographs. Perspective is affected solely by the position of the camera in relation to the subject. Therefore, different focal length lenses will only produce a change in perspective if the magnification of the image is maintained (Fig. 10.8). Note that perspective distortion decreases with the 105 mm lens because of its greater working distance.

It is imperative to minimize perspective distortion, particularly when photographing three-dimensional

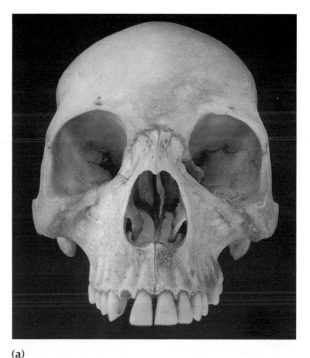

(a)

(b)

Fig. 10.8 Photographs of the same specimen taken from the same working distance and showing perspective distortion of the skull. The choice of lens greatly influences the degree of distortion. (a) Wide-angle lens. (b) Standard lens

objects such as skulls. If the photographs are to be used for measurements, it is necessary to use a long focal length lens. A rule of thumb for obtaining acceptable perspective distortion is to position the camera at least ten subject diameters away (Williams, 1984). For this reason, it is essential to have an adequately sized room, and a stepladder for vertical work.

Zoom lenses often increase perspective problems as they encourage the user to remain at a fixed distance from the specimen. Such lenses encourage the photographer to frame the image by changing the focal length rather than by consciously selecting the correct focal length and then positioning the camera.

The angle at which the specimen is viewed should be directly 'above' rather than oblique, otherwise the resulting image will not allow accurate interpretation of features, owing to alteration of their relative sizes and the apparent space between them.

Background

The background of a subject plays a crucial role in specimen photography. Alteration of the colour or brightness of the background can dramatically change the appearance of the final image, and such effects are often underestimated. An inappropriate background, particularly a cluttered one, may lead to photographs not being admissible in court.

A background should be unobtrusive and provide suitable contrast for the specimen. It should be clean, textureless and non-reflective as well as being chosen according to the subject and the lighting. Wall-mounted paper rolls, available from professional photographic outlets, provide a convenient and relatively inexpensive seamless background. They are available in a variety of tones, colours and widths, and take up little space when not in use.

A mid-grey background is very useful as it suits a variety of specimens and does not cause the exposure problems associated with very light or dark backgrounds. A black background can give effective results by providing contrast, and also does not show shadows. However, care is needed to ensure that the shadowed edges of the subject do not become lost, and black should never be used for dark subjects. In some instances, rim lighting is necessary to show separation between the subject and a dark background. Black velvet draped over the specimen supports will provide a totally black surround for the specimen under controlled lighting (Fig. 10.9). Although dark subjects stand out well against a white background, flare can occur if it is overilluminated. Coloured backgrounds should generally be avoided as they can be distracting and create false impressions. They can also produce colour casts, especially if this colour is reflected in areas of the subject. If coloured backgrounds are to be used, they should be approximately two stops less bright than the subject or they will look washed out.

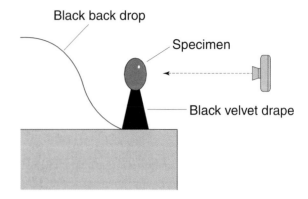

Fig. 10.9 Diagram demonstrating the use of a black velvet drape and backdrop to provide a totally black background for the specimen

For best results, the background should be positioned some distance away from the subject. Such separation provides several advantages. First, an adequate separation will render the background out of focus and therefore not distracting. Second, lighting can be more flexible as separate lighting can be used for subject and background. In particular, edge or back lighting can be difficult to achieve without this space. Third, background shadows can be avoided, either by careful positioning of the main lights or by separate background lighting. If shadows are cast on the background, they will be softer than if the background is close behind the subject.

Shadowless backgrounds can also be produced by supporting the specimen on glass above transilluminated Perspex. A permanent set-up, as illustrated in Fig. 10.1, is a convenient method of producing effective and standardized results. By placing filters over the background light source, the colour and density of the background can be changed. Care must be taken to avoid background flare by masking the area around the specimen with black card, just outside the field of view.

Orientation

Standardized methods are required to ensure that photographs can be easily orientated without confusion. Orientation should be considered in terms of the relationship between the camera and the subject, the areas of interest on the specimen and the specimen in relation to the standard anatomical planes.

The film plane should be positioned parallel to the plane of focus. Framing should always be in line with either the horizontal or the vertical plane of the body as photographs taken from random angles are usually confusing. All views must be orientated in this manner for consistency, in particular for comparisons between overall and macro views. If diagonal framing is needed to demonstrate a particular feature, it should be in addition to the standard orientation views.

The placement of the scale in a photograph has much influence on the orientation of the final image. To maintain standardization, the basic rule is to place the scale horizontally at the bottom of the frame. Similarly, placing shadows at the bottom of the subject by illuminating from above helps to orientate the image. This is particularly important in photographs taken on specimen boxes, which give the impression of a specimen floating in air.

Orientation of the area of interest on the specimen is best achieved by photographing an overall view and by including easily recognizable anatomical reference points in the photograph.

Cropping

Care should be taken in framing and cropping the image to include all the necessary information, with reference points, while at the same time excluding unnecessary or distracting information.

Depending on the model of camera, some viewfinders will show slightly under or over 100% of the recorded image. It is necessary to know the equipment and carry out tests to determine the exact field of view.

Peripheral cropping of about 10% of the image occurs in automatic printing machines, so allowances need to be made when shooting negative film unless it is to be hand printed.

Although some image cropping may be carried out during printing, the best results are obtained by accurately cropping at the shooting stage and thus using as much as possible of the negative.

Scale

As a scale may be of the utmost importance, it is advisable to use those specifically designed for photography. In addition, a custom-designed scale can incorporate information about the department or institute.

Scales that are matt plastic and predominantly grey are recommended as they have an average reflectance and therefore require an exposure similar to that of the subject. Very light, dark or non-neutral colours should be avoided as they can have a marked influence on exposure and colour balance. Shiny scales should also be avoided as they tend to cause flare.

Extra-strong, self-adhesive backing and an area on the scale for labelling are also important considerations.

Scales of 30, 50 and 150 mm in length, with accurate millimetre increments, are a useful series and allow the most appropriate choice of scale for the specimen.

Correct placement of the scale is important in the overall composition of the photograph and is vital for accuracy of measurement. The position of the scale must be at same level as the plane of focus (Fig. 10.10).

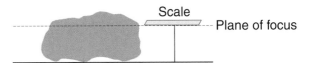

Fig. 10.10 Diagram demonstrating the correct placement of a scale at the selected plane of focus for the specimen

Colour

Colour variations between photographs result from a number of factors. No film can exactly reproduce colour. A distinct colour bias is seen in many film types, and to a lesser degree between different batches of the same film. Films are manufactured to suit certain subjects. For example, some render skin tones more accurately, others suit more general outdoor conditions, and some give highly saturated and high-contrast results. The best way to determine the most appropriate film is through testing in relation to the particular type of specimen.

In addition to the choice of film, the colour of a photograph can be influenced by external factors such as ambient lighting, reflections, processing and printing. When significant ambient light exposure occurs, for example from overhead fluorescent tubes or incandescent dissecting lights, colour casts will result from the mismatch in colour temperatures. Ambient exposure can be overcome to a great extent by using lighting that is powerful enough to allow a fast shutter speed and small aperture. It also helps to reduce the level of ambient lighting by switching lights off or ensuring that they are a sufficiently far from the subject. Light bouncing off surrounding objects such as tinted walls or even the photographer's clothing can introduce colour casts. Walls and other surrounds should therefore be neutral – preferably white or grey.

As previously mentioned, the print process plays a important part in the colour of the final result. Problens with the correct print colour are particularly common in medical photography owing to many subjects being 'non-standard' and thus difficult for the processing technician to judge. A standardized colour reference strip, such as that produced by Kodak, when photographed at the beginning of the film, can help to reduce subjectivity and bias when printing medical material.

A cause of major colour imbalance is the use of daylight film with tungsten light and vice versa. This can be easily corrected with the appropriate filters. If the exact colour of the subject is of primary importance, flat lighting will produce the best results.

Macrophotography

Macrophotography is defined as photography that produces an image on film that is bigger than the object size. Although there is no precise magnification at which it becomes photomicrography, it is usually considered to occur at between 40× and 80×. More accurately, it is the point at which an image begins to lose resolution, a factor that depends greatly on the equipment.

Different pieces of equipment can be used to achieve this magnification, and they should be chosen according to the results required as well as the time available.

Low-power macrophotography can be achieved using a reversal ring that mounts the lens backwards onto the camera, making a normal lens more optically suited to close-up work. For example, on a 35 mm camera, a wide-angle lens used in reverse will give a magnification of approximately 2×. This allows excellent quality images to be achieved. However, the working distance is very short, and it should be noted that the automatic 'stop-down' features of a lens will be lost.

Supplementary lenses of varying power, attached to the front of the lens, can be used to give magnification. Their advantages are that they are inexpensive, simple to use and require little or no alteration of exposure. They can also be stacked by placing the highest power diopter closest to the lens in order to give a further increase in image size. However, some loss of image quality will occur. Unless very high quality diopters dedicated to the lens are used, the results will be acceptable only at small apertures.

Magnification is also increased by increasing the distance between the lens and the film plane. This is achieved by using extension rings or bellows, which can produce quality images without distortion problems, at up to 1× reproduction. However, when using non-specialized lenses at magnifications greater than 1×, the lens should be reversed.

Extension rings are available in different lengths, of which several can be used together, to give a wider range of possible magnifications. Alternatively, a single variable length extension ring is available for some brands of camera. Bellows are another form of variable extension, giving the convenience of being able to alter the magnification easily by small exact amounts. Some brands of bellows also have the advantage of a tiltable lens plane to produce an increased depth of field. When using bellows, it is important to determine that the aperture control is operating when the shutter is depressed as some types require a dual cable release (one each for the shutter and aperture) in order to operate correctly.

In many instances, it is desirable to calculate the image magnification (m) prior to setting up the photograph. This can be achieved using the formula:

$$V = F (m + 1)$$

where the focal length (F) and the amount of extension (V) are known.

Another useful formula can be used to calculate the object distance from the lens (U) before setting up the camera:

$$U = F (1 + m)/ m$$

Enlargement from slide or negative should be considered in calculation of the final magnification. For example, an additional magnification factor of 5× is present when a 35 mm image is enlarged to a 5 × 7 in print. It must be remembered that lack of magnification at the shooting stage cannot be corrected at printing, as excessive enlargement causes severe loss of resolution.

Metering in macrophotography is not as straightforward as in normal photography. Metering through the camera is convenient and does not require exposure adjustments, but the use of such systems in macrophotography is not always possible. First, at high magnifications, the camera meter may not be sensitive enough to measure the small amount of light present. Second, many cameras cannot meter for shutter speeds longer than 1 s, and with continuous light sources, shutter speeds of several seconds are often required. For readings from fibreoptic flash or other non-dedicated flash sources, a hand-held meter must be used.

Metering for macrophotography using a standard hand-held meter poses two problems. First, the area that a normal meter measures is very large in comparison with macro subjects and therefore cannot be accurate. Second, the very small working distance leads to inaccurate positioning of the meter. For these reasons, a spot meter is required.

A spot meter can measure an area of only 1 degree from a distance, making the readings far more accurate. It should be noted, however, that spot meters include a fixed focus lens, designed for metering from long distances. At short distances, this image may be out of focus, meaning that the area being measured is larger than the 1 degree indicated. This can cause gross inaccuracies if adjacent areas are lighter or darker than the specimen. To correct this, a dioptre should be attached to the meter to focus the image.

Incident spot meter probe attachments are available for some meters and are very useful as their small size allows them to be positioned at the specimen even with very small working distances.

Depending on the set-up and magnification used, adjustment to the initial exposure reading may be required. The amount of light reaching the film plane depends on the inverse square law; therefore, the further the lens is from the film plane, the more exposure is needed. To calculate the required increase in exposure, two formulae can be used:

$$\text{Exposure factor} = (v^2) / (f^2)$$

or:

$$\text{Exposure factor} = (m + 1)^2$$

The exposure factor is the factor by which the measured exposure must be multiplied. Dioptres do not require any compensation in exposure. If the required exposure is greater than 1 s, further compensation may be needed to account for reciprocity failure.

Focusing is a critical aspect of macrophotography, as depth of field becomes more limited with increase in magnification. In some cases, if depth of field is particularly important, it may be necessary to sacrifice magnification on the film.

Greater depth of field can be gained using smaller apertures but, in macrophotography, the need for more light often prevents small apertures being used. In addition, at high magnification, the diffraction that occurs with small apertures may considerably decrease the resolution. It is therefore advisable to conduct tests for a particular lens in order to determine its aperture of maximum resolution.

Focusing techniques will also have an influence on image sharpness. Depth of field will be maximized by focusing at a point halfway in to the depth of the specimen or area of interest (Fig. 10.11). Focusing is best carried out by changing the working distance rather than by adjusting the lens-to-camera distance, as in normal photography. This is achieved by moving the whole camera backwards and forwards, preferably on a focusing rail. Fine focusing is done by moving the specimen on an adjustable stage. These methods not only aid focusing but also ensure that the distance between the lens and the camera is kept constant, thereby maintaining magnification. A clear focusing screen facilitates focusing in low light levels, and a camera with one of these screens is therefore very useful.

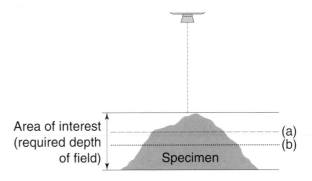

Fig. 10.11 Diagram indicating the optimum plane of focus for macrophotography

A rigid tripod or copy stand is essential for macrophotography to allow accurate focusing and to prevent movement during long exposures. Even small vibrations within the room that are not normally noticeable may degrade the image. To minimize the risk of movement, a cable release is essential. Other means of decreasing vibration include separating the macro table from other equipment (in particular fan-cooled light sources), using a room that is away from busy areas, remaining still during exposures and, of course, keeping the exposure time to a minimum.

As with any photography, lighting in macrophotography should be arranged to show the most important aspects of the subject. Direct or diffused lighting should therefore be chosen for the same reasons. Positioning of lights and reflectors should also follow the same general principles, size being the only difference.

As already discussed, shadows created by direct lighting are not always desirable. However, in macrophotography, this technique frequently helps to give the impression of greater resolution.

Some subjects, particularly highly reflective ones, may only be shown effectively by very diffused lighting. This may be done by surrounding the subject with diffuser material, commonly known as tent lighting.

Further Reading

LeBeau LJ. 1992: Photography of small laboratory objects. In Vetter JP (ed.) *Biomedical photography.* Stoneham, MA: Butterworth-Heinemann, 409–47.

Williams R. (ed.) 1984: *Medical photography study guide.* Lancaster: MTP Press.

References

Botha CT. 1991: Craniofacial characteristics as determinants of age, race and sex in forensic dentistry. *Journal of Forensic Odonto-Stomatology* **9**(2), 47–61.

Clement JG. 1993: Forensic dentistry. In Freckelton IR, Selby H (eds) *Expert evidence*. Sydney: Law Book Company, 3-301–3-463.

Henham AP, Lee KAP. 1994: Photography in forensic medicine. *Journal of Audiovisual Media in Medicine* **17**, 15–20.

Jacobson RE. 1983: *The manual of photography*. London: Butterworth.

Kerley ER. 1977: Forensic anthropology. In Tedeschi CG, Eckert WG, Tedeschi LG. (eds) *Forensic medicine*. Philadelphia: W.B. Saunders, 1101–15.

Langford MJ. 1973: *Basic photography*. London: Focal Press.

Langford MJ. 1980: *Advanced photography*. London: Focal Press.

McGavin MD, Thompson SW. 1987: *Specimen dissection and photography*. Springfield, IL: Charles C. Thomas.

McNamara BL. 1993: Forensic photography. In Freckelton IR, Selby H. (eds) *Expert evidence*. Sydney: Law Book Company, 8-5801–8-5981.

Nelson GD, Krause JL. Jr. 1988: *Clinical photography in plastic surgery*. Boston: Little, Brown.

Palmer K. 1993: Forensic anthropology. In Freckelton IR, Selby H. (eds) *Expert evidence*. Sydney: Law Book Company, 3-901–3-1072.

Peres M. 1992: Close-up photography and photomacrography. In Vetter JP (ed.) *Biomedical photography*. Stoneham MA: Butterworth-Heinemann, 171–99.

Ray SF. 1992: Optics for the biomedical photographer. In Vetter JP (ed.) *Biomedical photography*. Stoneham, MA: Butterworth-Heinemann, 25–47.

Stroebel LD. 1992: Exposure and development. In Vetter JP (ed.) *Biomedical photography*. Stoneham MA: Butterworth-Heinemann, 49–74.

Stroebel L, Compton J, Current I, Zakia R. 1986: *Photographic materials and processes*. Massachusetts: Butterworth.

Vetter JP. 1992: Gross specimen photography. In Vetter JP. (ed.) *Biomedical photography*. Stoneham, MA: Butterworth-Heinemann, 359–68.

Williams R, Newenhuis G. 1992: Clinical and operating room photography. In Vetter, JP (ed.) *Biomedical photography*. Stoneham, MA: Butterworth-Heinemann, 251–99.

Wood WB. 1993: Forensic osteology. In Freckelton IR, Selby H. (eds) *Expert evidence*. Sydney: Law Book Company, 3-601–3-797.

Woolridge ED Jr. 1977: Forensic odontology. In Tedeschi CG, Eckert WG, Tedeschi LG. (eds), *Forensic medicine*. Philadelphia: W.B. Saunders, 1116–53.

CHAPTER 11

Craniofacial photography in the living

T DOBROSTANSKI, CD OWEN

Introduction	137	Film	142
Principles of craniofacial photography	137	Positioning the subject	143
Photographic equipment	138	Dual-camera system	144
Perspective and viewpoint distortion	139	Photographic rig	144
Subject lighting	139	Light source	146
Exposure controls	141	Face-aligning system	146
Aperture and depth of field	141	Photographing the subject	147

Introduction

A photographic record of facial features can be a very useful adjunct to the diagnosis and treatment of patients undertaking orthodontic treatment or facio-maxillary surgery. High-quality photographs may be used to monitor the growth patterns and developmental changes in children, to assist in treatment planning and to provide a record for comparing the preoperative and postoperative conditions. Cranio-facial photographs may also be used in teaching, research and the identification of abductees, run-aways and deceased people.

Many factors must be taken into consideration when taking craniofacial photographs of a patient. Craniofacial photographs may be taken either as a 'one-off' set of views to be included in a patient's medical record or as part of a series, illustrating the growth patterns of the face over a period of time. In both cases, the photographs should be standardized. Changes in magnification, camera position or the subject's head position will render the photographs useless for comparison purposes. To minimize these problems, a specialized photographic rig should be used and specific protocols established in order to provide consistent and reproducible photographs.

Such a rig has been built at the School of Dental Science at the University of Melbourne. It consists of a rigid stand, with two cameras attached so that their optical axes are at right angles to one another. This arrangement allows a subject's full-face and profile views to be photographed simultaneously. It removes the inconsistencies in magnification, camera positioning and subject placement common to normal hand-held photographs. Before describing the rig in detail, it is worth discussing the fundamental elements involved in taking craniofacial photographs.

Principles of craniofacial photography

Consideration must be given to which standard views are needed to provide an adequate record of the subject. The most common of these are the full-face and profile views; other views, such as from 45 degrees or obliquely from above or below, may be necessary depending on the subject's medical or dental problem.

To provide a useful record of the subject, the full-face view must be taken so that the subject's head fills the frame of the camera when the latter is held vertically. The frame must include both of the subject's ears and extend from the top of the head to just under the chin. The eyes should be horizontal within the frame, and the photograph should be taken at the subject's eye level, the sharpest point of focus being on the eyes. The subject should be positioned in front of a neutral backdrop so that no distracting items or shadows appear in the background.

For the profile view, the subject must be photographed at the same magnification as for the full-face view, the sharpest focus being at the outer canthus of the eye. Again, the camera is held vertically, so that the frame includes the regions from the top of the head to below the chin, showing all of the profile side of the face to a point behind the ear. The Frankfort plane (a line between the lower border of the orbit and the upper border of the external auditory meatus) should be horizontal within the frame, and the subject should be in exact profile, turned neither towards nor away from the lens. Again, the subject should be placed in front of a neutral background, and the picture should be taken from the subject's eye level.

Photographic equipment

CAMERA TYPES

Having established the basic requirements for craniofacial photography, what photographic equipment best fulfils these criteria? There are many different makes and types of camera available. These vary in quality and function, from compact 35 mm auto focus viewfinder cameras, to programmable 35 mm single lens reflex (SLR) cameras. While the small compact cameras may be good for taking photographs of people and scenes, they are useless for scientific purposes. Such cameras usually have a separate viewfinder that introduces parallax error, in which the field of view through the viewfinder is slightly different from the field of view through the lens. This parallax error increases as the camera is moved closer to the subject. In addition, these types of camera generally only have a fixed wide-angle lens (40 mm or less); therefore, the field of view at their closest focusing distance will include more image area than is wanted. As these cameras are usually fully automatic, the operator has very little control over exposure, precise focus and depth of field.

The SLR camera has the advantage of viewing through the same lens that takes the picture, eliminating any parallax error. These cameras have a mirror placed at 45 degrees to the optical path, which reflects the image up to a focusing screen at the top of the camera, where it is viewed via the camera's pentaprism. As the shutter is released, the mirror flips up to allow light from the image to reach the film and prevent any light entering via the viewfinder. Only when this has occurred does the shutter open to expose the film. Once the image is exposed, the shutter closes and the mirror drops back to its viewing position. The optical path is arranged so that the lens-to-viewing-screen distance is the same as the lens-to-film distance. This means that if the image is sharply focused in the viewfinder, it will be in focus on the film. The operator can precisely frame the subject to be photographed and can position the plane of sharpest focus where it is needed. The effect of changing lenses, close focusing using extension tubes or stopping the lens down to improve depth of field can be exactly monitored. With its wide range of lenses and accessories, the 35 mm SLR is most appropriate for clinical photography applications.

LENSES

The image quality of the final photograph depends on the quality of the lens used to produce that image; it is therefore unwise to try to save money by purchasing a lens of dubious calibre. There are many lenses of different focal length available, from ultra-wide-angle fish-eye lenses to extreme telephoto lenses, but for craniofacial photography, a good-quality macro lens with a focal length of 90–105 mm is preferred. A number of manufacturers produce macro lenses in this range. Such lenses can focus on a subject at infinity or, at the other extreme, allow an object as close as 200 mm to be brought into sharp focus, giving a reproduction ratio of 1:2 or 0.5× magnification. With an appropriate extension tube (usually supplied with the lens), magnification ratios from 0.5× to 1× or life size, can be achieved. Some brands of macro lens will focus down to 1:1 without the addition of an extension tube. It is also possible to get 50–55 mm macro lenses that, similarly, will focus on subjects down to a reproduction ratio of 1:2 or 0.5× magnification. When using these lenses at the macro end of their focusing scale, the subject-to-lens distance is extremely short (about 100 mm), reducing even further when approaching a reproduction ratio of 1:1 (about 50 mm). Not only would it be intrusive to the subject to have the lens that close but also problems of adequately lighting the subject with a lens at that distance become insuperable.

Perspective and viewpoint distortion

The relationship between the apparent size, shape and position of objects when viewed from a particular point is called perspective. For example, if the wall of a building is viewed from an oblique angle, the near end appears taller than the far end, even though the two ends are the same height. It is this effect of perspective that provides a visual indication of depth in a two-dimensional photograph of the wall. The variation in heights of the near and far ends of the wall is in direct ratio to their distance from the observer. If the near end is 3 m and the far end 9 m away, the ratio is 3:1. In this case, the far end of the wall appears to be one third the size of the near end; thus the perspective is steep, and the wall gives a strong impression of depth. If the viewing distance is increased so that the near end is 30 m away, the far end will be 39 m away, giving a ratio of 39:30 (or about 1.3:1). From this viewpoint, the two ends now appear to be more similar in size, giving less impression of depth – perspective is flatter.

Perspective is always dependent on viewpoint, whether the scene is being viewed or photographed. If the viewpoint is fixed, changing the focal length of the lens, from wide-angle to telephoto, will not alter the perspective but will alter the final image size on the film. If, without changing the lens, the distance between the viewpoint and subject is altered, perspective and image size changes.

When taking craniofacial photographs, it is possible to use a variety of lenses of different focal lengths, but in order to fill the frame with the subject, the camera-to-subject distance and therefore the perspective must also be changed. Thus if a wide-angle lens is used, the camera-to-subject distance has to be small in order to fill the frame with the subject's face, assuming that a wide-angle lens will focus on a subject that close. The resultant perspective will be very steep, with foreground objects (such as the nose and chin) appearing larger and having greater prominence than background objects (the ears), which appear smaller, giving the face an unnatural, distorted appearance. Viewpoint distortion will decrease as the focal length and thus the camera-to-subject distance increases. This applies to a lesser extent with lenses that have focal lengths up to 100 mm (Fig. 11.1).

The 100 mm lens allows the subject's face to be photographed, filling the frame, at a distance of about 1.5 m. The perspective at this distance gives a more natural impression of the facial features, similar to that seen during normal social contact. All features of the face appear to be correctly proportioned, with no emphasis on either background or foreground objects. Owing to their greater camera-to-subject distances, lenses of longer focal length will give a flatter perspective to the subject, with little apparent size difference between foreground and background objects. This flatter perspective tends to give increased prominence to background objects, resulting in an image that is foreshortened, with less apparent depth. In practice, with their longer working distances, telephoto lenses become impractical in all but large photographic studios.

No single lens can fulfil all photographic requirements. The forensic photographer will need a range of lenses for the different subjects that he or she is required to photograph. Considering all of these factors, a macro lens of focal length 100–105 mm is the most appropriate lens for craniofacial photography.

Subject lighting

Lighting is possibly the most critical aspect of recording an image that the photographer needs to master. Without an adequate level of illumination and careful thought to the placement of light sources, having the best equipment available will produce, at best, only an inadequate record of the subject being photographed. Ideally, the lighting used should be strong enough to allow the use of a small aperture, thereby increasing the depth of field of the image. It should provide even illumination of the subject, so that strong shadows do not obscure important details, and it should be of an appropriate colour temperature for the film emulsion being used.

Colour temperature is a measure of the colour quality of a light source, expressed in degrees Kelvin (°K); it is the temperature to which a perfect black-body radiator would have to be heated to emit light of the same colour as the light source. Although only light sources that have a continuous spectra (that produce light of all wavelengths) can be said to have a colour temperature, those light sources such as fluorescent tubes and electronic flashes that have discontinuous spectra can be given an approximate colour temperature value. Light sources that have a low colour temperature emit light that is rich in colours from the lower or red end of the visible spectrum and are said to be warm. As the colour temperature increases, more blue light is emitted, the spectral distribution becomes more even and the light becomes whiter. As it increases further, blue wavelengths predominate, and the light is often described as cool. Unlike the human eye, which can adapt to changes in the colour of light sources, colour film is very sensitive to colour shifts. Thus in a situation where there is a change in

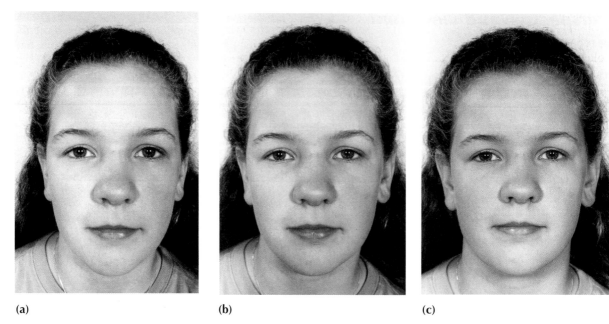

(a) (b) (c)

Fig. 11.1 Anterior face photographs showing the effect of lens focal length on facial distortion. All three views were taken so that the subject's head filled the frame. (A) 28 mm focal length. (B) 55 mm focal length. (C) 105 mm focal length. Note that as the focal length decreases, parts of the face such as the nose and chin, which are closer to the lens, become more prominent

colour temperature from daylight to tungsten, the eye may at first see the tungsten lighting as being yellower than the daylight. The human eye soon adapts to this so that the light appears white. Unfortunately, colour film cannot adapt to this change in light condition. Thus care must be taken to match the light source to the film type being used, daylight film for use with electronic flash or daylight, tungsten film for use with artificial light sources.

The forensic photographer has two main choices of light source for photographing subjects in a studio-type situation: tungsten photographic lights or electronic flash units. Tungsten lamps produce light by passing an electric current through a thin filament of tungsten that emits light as it heats up. The disadvantage of this form of lighting is that it requires long exposure times. Furthermore, these lamps produce a considerable amount of heat, and minor variations in the electricity supply voltage can change their colour temperature (normally 3200°K for standard photographic and quartz iodine lamps, 3400°K for photofloods). Consequently, tungsten lamps are more suitable for still-life subjects or copy work.

Electronic flash units produce light by passing a high-voltage electrical discharge from a capacitor through a gas-filled glass tube, creating an intense but brief flash of light. The duration of the flash may vary between 1/500 s and 1/10 000 s depending on the design of the tube and the controlling circuitry; low-powered pocket flash units generally have longer exposure times. Electronic flash units are designed to produce light that has a colour balance equivalent to daylight and a colour temperature of about 5500°K, so may safely be used with daylight-type colour films. With its short duration, the flash essentially freezes any subject or camera movement. Also, its quick recycling times allow repetitive shots to be taken in quick succession, making it ideal for a wide range of photographic applications.

Portable battery-operated flash units are convenient and have their place, but if they are used without consideration to their placement and how they will light the subject, they can produce quite badly lit photographs. If they are placed on the camera's hot shoe or are positioned near the lens axis, they will produce harsh lighting with strong shadows behind the subject. When this form of lighting is used to photograph a face, it produces what is commonly called 'red-eye', which occurs when the light from the flash illuminates the subject's retina through the open iris of the eye. The only way to eliminate this artefact is to move the light source away from the optical axis of the lens; then the retina will be shaded by the iris, and the resultant photograph will not show this problem. Another problem with this form of lighting is that it tends to obscure facial detail. For example, while one side of the face may be adequately lit, the other side will be in deep shadow, making it hard to determine the exact edge of the face. This lack of edge determination makes exact measurements of facial dimensions impossible. To avoid this unwanted lighting effect, the flash should be repositioned. The flash can be bounced off a light-coloured ceiling or wall, or even a white card, to provide a more diffuse light that will give the subject a more natural appearance.

If a special unit is to be set up for craniofacial photography, the best lighting option is studio flash equipment. These units either have a separate power pack with up to four flash heads operating from it or are mains-operated, self-contained flash heads that can be used independently or synchronized to operate in unison. These units are capable of variable power output. Simpler models may be switchable from full power to half or quarter power, whereas more expensive units have power controls that can be varied by increments as small as one tenth of a stop. An added advantage of studio flash units is that they are fitted with a modelling lamp, allowing the effect of light positioning and output power to be seen. This allows the photographer to place the flash units where needed, confident in the knowledge that the photograph will be properly lit. Studio flash systems can have a wide range of reflectors or diffusers depending on the style of lighting required. These may vary from concentrated spotlights for harsh lighting effects, to large translucent diffusers for very soft, even illumination. One style of reflector that is quite versatile is the umbrella; this can be used either as a reflector or, where the fabric of the umbrella is translucent, as a diffuser.

For craniofacial photography, a soft, even illumination is required and the light should be balanced to give some three-dimensional modelling to the subject, without harsh shadows obscuring important subject details. A minimum of two flash heads with umbrella reflectors are needed, positioned on either side of the camera. If the lights are placed equidistant from the subject, the subject will be evenly lit with virtually no shadows. If one light is moved closer, so that it is stronger than the other, slight shadows and highlights can be introduced to give the subject some three-dimensional modelling. The subject should be placed at least 1 m in front of the background; if it is too close, it will cast shadows onto the background. Where limited space is available and it is not possible to have this separation, it may be necessary to have a third light source that illuminates the background, eliminating any distracting shadows behind the subject.

Exposure controls

A photographer has two methods of controlling the amount of light reaching the film: adjustment of the shutter speed and of the lens aperture. The shutter controls the length of time that the film is exposed; on most modern cameras, there is usually a range of times from about 8 s to 1/2000 s. A focal plane shutter is used on 35 mm cameras and is located just in front of the film. It essentially consists of two blinds, one following the other, forming an adjustable slit that moves across the film and exposes each section as it moves. At slow shutter speeds, one blind opens to reveal the film and the second blind then follows after a delay. For faster exposure times, the second blind starts moving before the first blind has finished its travel across the film, so that a slit of varying width exposes the film.

For craniofacial photography, the main source of light will be electronic flash. In this case, the shutter has to be set at the flash synchronization speed. This is the maximum shutter speed at which the slit is wide enough for the whole area of the film to be uncovered when the flash fires. For cameras with a shutter that travels horizontally across the long axis of the film, the flash synchronization speed is usually about 1/60 s. Where the shutter travels vertically across the long axis of the film, the flash synchronization speed is usually set at either 1/125 s or 1/250 s. The flash synchronization speed is usually indicated on the camera's shutter speed selection dial either by the speed being marked in red or by having an X next to it.

Aperture and depth of field

Electronic flash is the main light source for craniofacial photography. Given this, the shutter speed has to be fixed at the flash synchronization speed. As a result of this constraint, the amount of light reaching the film from the subject has to be controlled by the lens aperture. The aperture works like the pupil of the eye; it may be opened to let more light in or closed down to restrict the amount of light passing through the lens. This is achieved by a ring of thin metal leaves called the iris diaphragm. The diaphragm is operated by rotating a ring on the lens, which, when turned, closes or opens the diaphragm. The aperture ring has click stops at preset intervals that are calibrated to the standard series of f numbers or f stops f1, f1.4, f2, f2.8, f4, f5.6, f8, f11, f16 and f22. A large f number corresponds to a small opening of the diaphragm, and less light is allowed to pass through the lens. Changing from one f number to the next alters the amount of light transmitted by the lens by a factor of two. Therefore, an aperture of f8 will allow half as much light to pass through the lens as an aperture of f5.6 and twice as much light as an aperture of f11. Each f number in the series is related to the next by a factor of the square root of 2 ($\sqrt{2}$ = approximately 1.4). A change in the diameter of the diaphragm by two results in a change to the area of its opening by a factor of $\sqrt{2}$ (area = $(\sqrt{\text{diameter}})^2/4$).

The aperture also has a considerable effect on the sharpness of the image. When a lens is sharply focused on a particular part of a subject, other points in front of and behind that part will not appear as sharp. A gradual decline in sharpness of the image occurs as its distance from the point of focus increases. Within this range of reduced sharpness, there will be a zone in which the decrease in sharpness is too small to be noticed. This zone is referred to as the depth of field of the lens. Depth of field is therefore defined as the distance between the nearest and farthest point of the subject that can be brought to an acceptable focus when the lens is focused as sharply as possible on one part of it.

Depth of field depends on a number of factors that are governed by the way in which a lens produces an image. A perfect lens, when focused on an object, will reproduce each point of the object as a perfect point on the film. If, however, the object is not flat or there are more objects at different distances from the lens, it is possible to focus only on one part of the subject at a time. Each point of the object that is sharply focused will be represented as a sharp point on the image. Those points of the subject which are not in focus will appear as circles of light instead of points on the film. As the distance of any point on the subject from the plane of sharpest focus increases, corresponding points of the image will appear as progressively larger circles or discs of light on the film. It is this confusion of overlapping, circular images (called circles of confusion) that makes the image look blurred. In fact, there is a limit to the size of objects that the eye can resolve. As a result, if the circles of confusion are small, enough parts of an image will appear to be in focus. Reducing the size of the circles of confusion will increase the zone of apparent sharpness or, in other words, the depth of field of the image.

Depth of field increases when:

1. The maximum allowable size of the circles of confusion is large. A lower standard of sharpness is accepted and more distant points on the subject can therefore be said to be encompassed by the depth of field.
2. The lens aperture is small (large f number). A smaller opening of the diaphragm will produce a narrower cone of light that the lens passes from each point of the subject. Thus points that were outside the limits of the depth of field will have their corresponding circles of confusion reduced in size so that they are now acceptable to the eye as points are included within the depth of field.
3. Lens focal length is short.
4. The subject is more distant. Changing to a shorter focal length lens and increasing the subject distance will have the effect of moving the subject a greater number of focal lengths from the lens. Thus their sharp image points are formed nearer to the lens and are grouped closer together, reducing the sizes of their circles of confusion and allowing a greater depth of the subject to be considered sharp.

The degree of enlargement of the final image will also affect the limits for depth of field, so that enlarging the image will increase the size of the circle of confusion. As a result, points that the eye accepts as sharp at one magnification will not appear as sharp at a higher magnification.

For most photographs, the depth of field extends beyond the plane of sharp focus for twice the distance it extends in front of that plane (the 'one third in' rule). As reproduction ratios approach 1:1, this rule no longer applies. At this ratio, the depth of field extends almost equally in front of and behind the focal plane. Careful use of this rule will ensure that sharpness is maintained over the important parts of the subject, letting unimportant parts drift out of focus in the background. Thus, for example, when photographing a subject's face, the point of sharpest focus should be on the subject's eyes, and depth of field will then extend from the tip of the nose to behind the ears. On most lenses, there is a scale to indicate the extent of depth of field at various aperture settings. This, however, should only be used as a rough guide. It is more accurate to use the camera's depth of field preview facility, while looking through the viewfinder, to see exactly how far depth of field extends.

Film

The choice of the film emulsion to be used for craniofacial photography will depend on the requirements of the end user: whether the photographs need to be colour or black and white, or whether they are to be used as prints or transparencies. Other factors, such as the power of the flash units and the depth of field that is required, need to be considered when deciding which emulsion and what film speed will best.

Low-speed films (under 100 ISO) usually have finer grain and higher resolution than films with a higher ISO rating. As film speed increases, graininess in the image increases and resolution decreases. If a slow film is chosen and the subject lighting is inadequate, exposures may have to be made at a lower f number (larger apperture), thereby giving less depth of field.

Consequently, less of the subject area will appear to be sharply focused. The film should ideally be of a speed fast enough to allow the use of an aperture that will give the required depth of field.

If only black and white prints are needed, the choice of a black and white negative emulsion of an appropriate ISO rating is obvious. However, when it comes to colour prints or colour slides, the choice is not as straightforward.

The introduction of colour to the photographic process introduces another set of variables that have to be taken into consideration. A number of factors can affect the accuracy of colour reproduction of the final image. If care is not taken to reduce these variables, significant shifts in colour can result; thus, for example, the skin tones in a series of craniofacial photographs can vary quite markedly. The factors that govern the quality of the final colour image are:

1. *Film type and batch*. Different film types, such as Kodachrome and Ektachrome, have a different spectral response to colour, and variations in colour also occur between films of the same type but from a different batch.
2. *Storage conditions*. Ideally, all colour films should be stored in a refrigerator to avoid unwanted changes caused by heat and humidity.
3. *Film age*. Films that have passed their use-by date should hardly ever be used, as changes in film speed and spectral response can occur with age.
4. *Colour temperature of the light source*. As mentioned previously, unlike the human eye, colour films cannot adapt to changes in colour temperature of the light source. Consequently, if film designed for use with daylight (5500°K) is used with tungsten light (3200°K), the image will have a strong orange colour cast. Conversely, if tungsten film were used with daylight or electronic flash, the image would have a very strong blue colour cast. Colour conversion filters are available to match the type of lighting to the film in use, so for the first example above, a Kodak Wratten 80A filter should be used to convert the tungsten light to the equivalent of daylight.
5. *Process control*. Film processing laboratories must have strict control of the colour developing process. Changes in processing chemicals due to age, oxidization, over- or underreplenishment, the temperature of solutions and the timing of each step in the process are all critical to the quality of the final image. Lack of control over the process can cause colour shifts and changes in maximum and minimum densities of the negative or slide.

Colour negative films require two stages to produce the final viewable image, as against colour slides, which require only one stage. It is during this second stage of producing a colour print that colour casts or shifts in colour can be introduced. Owing to the subjective nature of colour printing and the variance in colour acuity of different operators, significant variations in skin and other tones can be introduced into colour prints.

Colour slides do not have the second subjective stage of producing a colour print and are ready for viewing once processed. Colour slides have a greater density range, are more brilliant and have higher contrast and saturation than do colour prints. In addition, colour slides have a longer life expectancy than colour prints, which can fade when exposed to ultra-violet radiation.

If required, colour or black and white prints can be made from slides quite successfully. With the current advances in computer and scanner technology, it is now possible to scan a film negative or colour slide, adjust the colour balance and print to a dye sublimation printer. These modern printers can give colour or black and white outputs that approach traditional photographic print quality.

To assist in the correct colour rendition of a series of photographs, a grey scale and colour control patches (Eastman Kodak Company, Publication No. Q-13, Kodak Colour Separation Guide and Grey Scale) should be photographed at the start of each film or when starting a new batch of film. This allows the reference points on the grey scale and colour patches to be compared in order to take into account minor variations between batches. In some cases, it is appropriate to include a colour control patch in each image, for example when attempting to show colour variations in bruises.

Whatever the final choice of emulsion, there should be little problem with changes in colour hue and density if the material is stored properly and processed according to the manufacturer's specifications.

Positioning the subject

Correct positioning of the head is the most critical factor in achieving a series of repeatable, consistent craniofacial photographs. Decisions have to be made of whether the subject is to be sitting or standing, whether they use a comfortable 'self-balance' position or whether the 'natural head position' (NHP) is to be adopted. NHP was defined by Broca in 1862 (Marcotte, 1981) as the posture of the head 'when a man is standing with his visual axis horizontal'. The NHP is a reproducible, natural, physiological position of the head that is obtained when a relaxed subject looks ahead at an external eye reference.

Head position is dependent on the craniocervical

articulation, which, as has been shown in many studies, is affected by a host of factors such as:

- visual and cochlear feedback
- climatic conditions
- postsurgical postural adaptations
- ethnicity
- respiratory health
- cervical vertebral morphology
- craniofacial morphology.

Solow and Tallgren (1971) took lateral cephalograms of 120 Danish male subjects aged 22–30 years. They recorded two head positions: one a self-balance position determined by the subject's own feeling of a natural head position, and the other with the subject looking straight into a mirror – the mirror position. All reference points were entered into a computer, and the variability in inclination of the craniofacial and cervical reference lines to the true vertical and to each other in both head positions were reported. They found that, in the mirror position, the head was kept higher than in the self-balance position. Moorees and Kean (1956) demonstrated that the NHP could be adopted by the subject when looking at the reflection of his own eyes in a mirror placed at a distance of 1.5 m. They found that this position of the head was highly reproducible and suitable for use in photographic and cephalometric analysis. NHP has also been found to be highly reproducible in males and females, children and adults, and Caucasians and non-Caucasians, with a variance of only about 4 degrees shown by Cooke and Wei (1988).

Using the NHP alleviates the need for external rods or other methods of holding the subject's head in position. The use of cephalostats with ear rods to fix head position may lead to errors if the external auditory meati are not bilaterally symmetrical; furthermore, the subject's posture may be changed by adapting their position to fit the ear plugs.

Dual-camera system

So far in this chapter, we have discussed the principles of photography and camera systems that are suitable for craniofacial photography. To be able to secure a high level of accuracy, so that consecutive photographs of the same subject are consistent, it is necessary to construct a dedicated photographic system solely for the purposes of craniofacial photography.

To date, there is little information in the literature which correctly describes a suitable stand that can guarantee a high level of accuracy and reproducibility. Most authors have suggested either hand-held cameras or the use of a tripod, both of which have insuperable limitations. Repeated craniofacial photographs of a subject over a period of days, months or years require great precision and must be taken from precisely the same viewpoint on each occasion. Any slight variations, such as those arising from hand-held cameras and changes in the pose or head position of the subject will produce errors. These unquantifiable variations can be of the same order of magnitude as any real changes in the subject.

Photographic apparatus capable of taking two simultaneous full-face and profile photographs, in a constant head position, is essential for creating a faithful photographic record of the subject. Ideally, it should be designed in such a way that more than one operator could take photographs in the series while retaining a high level of interoperator consistency. Such a system should be set up in a room big enough to allow the operator easy access to the controls of each camera. The room should be of sufficient size to accommodate an appropriate illumination system. Such apparatus has been built at the School of Dental Science, University of Melbourne.

Photographic rig

STAND

The system consists of a stand to support two cameras, one recording a profile, the other a full-face image of the subject. The stand is a rigid metal construction that is secured firmly to the floor (Fig. 11.2). This ensures that sequential photographs are taken from the same relative viewpoints. The stand is 2138 mm high, is made of aluminium tubing of square cross-section and is capable of supporting the weight of two 35 mm cameras and their allied equipment. Two horizontal arms, 1675 mm wide and also constructed of tubular aluminium, are secured at 90 degrees in relation to the camera axis and to one other. These are secured to the main frame and are capable of vertical movement on linear bearings. To equalize the weight distribution, the vertical movement is counterbalanced with an appropriately weighted lead block. This arrangement allows fingertip adjustment of the height of the camera arms; a clutch is incorporated into the system to eliminate vertical creep once the height has been set. The extreme limits of vertical travel of the horizontal arms are limited by cushioning stoppers positioned at each end of the vertical runners of the stand. Each horizontal arm is fitted with a horizontally sliding camera platform. The horizontal movement of the platforms allows for precise adjustment of the full-face and profile cameras. The platforms have six rubber-covered locating pins that aid in aligning the cameras. The cameras are mounted so that the long axis of the film is vertical. Once adjusted, the platforms are locked in position.

CAMERAS

Nikon FM-2 35 mm camera bodies, fitted with E2 grid focusing screens, were chosen as the most suitable and reliable. The etched focusing screen has horizontal and vertical grid lines that allow precise adjustment and calibration of the system. To make the system easy to use and operate in a 'hands-free'

mode, the Nikon bodies were each coupled with an MD12 motor drive. The MD12 battery pack has been replaced with a 12.8 V, 2 A, DC external power supply and connected with an appropriately long cable.

LENS

The Nikon 105 mm 1:2.8 Macro Nikor lens was chosen. Using this lens, the principal area of interest – the subject's face – can be centralized within the viewfinder of the camera from a distance of about 1.2 m, thus minimizing any distortion due to perspective or lens aberrations.

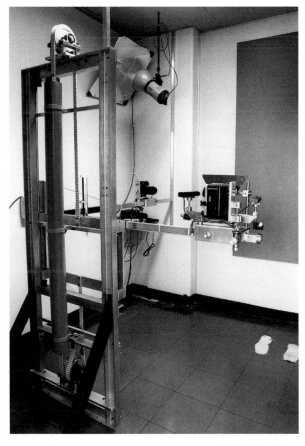

(a)

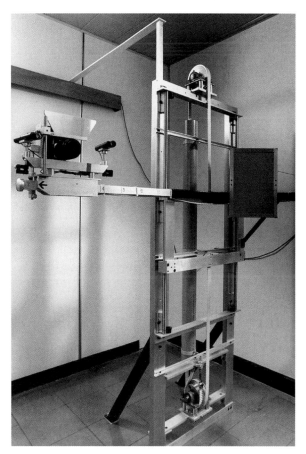

(b)

Fig. 11.2 Orthogonal camera system designed and constructed at the School of Dental Science, University of Melbourne. (a) The two vertically mounted cameras on rigid horizontal arms, which are at 90 degrees to each other. Both cameras are synchronized electronically for shutter opening and film advancement. The two footprints on the floor act as a starting point for subject positioning. (b) The rigid frame, securely bolted to the floor and wall, with a counterbalance mechanism consisting of a counterweight housed in a vertical tube, connected to the camera arms by a toothed belt and braked clutch. The camera arms can be raised or lowered with light finger pressure and, once positioned, stay in place. A mirror is positioned at the internal corner of the two camera arms, mounted at 45 degrees to each arm. This is used to position the subject for left and right oblique views of the face (see Fig. 11.7c, d)

INFRA-RED SHUTTER RELEASE

In order to trigger both cameras at the same time, it was decided that the most suitable way to release the shutters simultaneously was by means of an infra-red triggering device. This consists of a receiver, switchable between two channels, mounted on the camera hot shoe, which triggers the shutter via an electrical contact on the motor drive. The transmitter is a battery-powered, directional, hand-held device that can trigger both cameras simultaneously. Experiments showed that the use of a single infra-red receiver unit to which the two cameras are connected by a cable performed more reliably than having a separate infra-red receiver on each camera body. The infra-red receiver was placed in the hot shoe of the profile camera and connected by a 3 m cable to the full-face camera. The length of the cables that connected the two cameras to the infra-red receiver were initially unequal: that from the receiver to the profile camera was 250 mm long, and that connecting to the full-face camera 3000 mm long. This length difference caused a delay in the triggering of the full-face camera, so that when the flash fired, the two cameras were not synchronized and only one of the cameras recorded the image. It therefore became necessary to equalize the lengths of two cables to ensure the accurate synchronization of the two cameras with the flash units. This was achieved by winding one coil (using 7 m of 0.3 mm copper enamelled wire) on to a soft iron core (3 mm diameter by 35 mm in length) and placing it in series with the shorter cable attached to the profile camera. This device successfully delayed the triggering of the profile camera, thus providing accurate synchronization.

Light source

A two-head, studio-type electronic flash system was used. Ideally, each flash unit was positioned at about 45 degrees in relation to the subject photographed. To avoid harsh shadows from directing the flash tube directly at the subject, umbrella reflectors were used that applied a softer light to the subject. The flash heads and reflectors were placed higher than the subject, one light being slightly closer than the other to the subject. This gave a three-dimensional modelling effect to the image of the subject by the introduction of slight shadows.

Two Elinchrom Prolinca 2500 self-contained studio flash units were used. Their light output, when bounced off the reflectors, was sufficient to permit an adequate f stop of f16 to be used with 200 ISO Ektachrome slide film.

Face-aligning system

The commonly accepted method of head alignment in the NHP is with the aid of a mirror, with a central hole cut out for the lens, placed in front of the full-face camera. There are serious disadvantages to this method. The bulky camera lens obstructs the subject's view of their own eyes, and the subject, in trying to see themself around the hole in the mirror, may drift out of the field of view of the profile camera.

Two strategies were developed to overcome these problems. The first utilized a mirror placed just above the full-face camera and angled down at 5 degrees from the vertical towards the subject, so that they could see the reflection of their eyes in the mirror (Fig. 11.3).

To deal with the problem of the subject drifting out of the field of view of either camera, two conventional projection lecture theatre-style pointers were used. One was placed on each side of the full-face camera and angulated so that the projected beams

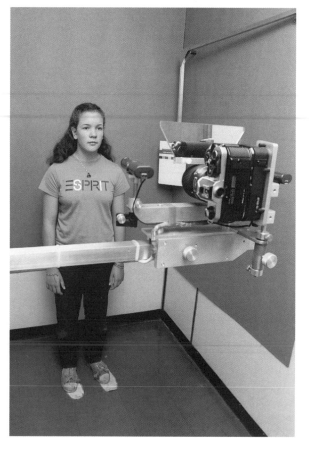

Fig. 11.3 Subject standing prior to final positioning. A mirror mounted at a slight downward angle over the anterior camera helps the subject to adopt the correct position

converged and met at the precise focal plane of the full-face camera lens (Fig. 11.4). The pointers were fitted with special globes with filaments, projecting a horizontal V-shaped image. The pointers were adjusted and calibrated to a known reference point, which was on a white board attached to a swinging arm, bolted to the wall. The arm was set up so that it always returned to the same position when it was swung in front of the full-face camera. This position is the point at which the lens is focused. To calibrate this range-finding system, the two pointers are adjusted so that the horizontal V-shaped images of the globes are brought to focus, forming an X at the reference point. Thus, once the range finder has been calibrated, it is easy to place the subject in the focal plane of the lens. If the two V-shaped images are spread apart, the subject is too close to the lens; con-

versely, if the two V-shaped images overlap, the subject is too far away. Only when the images of the filaments meet to form an X can we be confident that the subject will be in focus.

The profile camera (Fig. 11.5) is set up so that when the subject is correctly positioned by the range-finder, its field of view will include all of the subject's profile, from a point behind the ear to a point in front of the nose. This system eliminates having frequently to check the subject's position in both camera viewfinders, relying basically on the visual information projected by the range-finding system. Once the pointers are correctly adjusted, the system is accurate and requires only occasional adjustment.

Photographing the subject

The subject is shown the rig and the procedure is explained to them. In the case of a child, the parent or guardian is asked to accompany them. To aid in positioning, two cardboard foot shapes are stuck to the floor so that the subject can stand in the area covered by the two cameras. Once the subject is standing on the footmarks, the cameras are raised or lowered until the pointers project their image on the bridge of the subject's nose. The subject is asked to stand up straight, without being ramrod straight, and to look at their eyes in the mirror above the full-face camera, thus placing the head in the NHP. The subject is then asked to move backwards or forwards until the pointers form an X on the bridge of their nose (Fig. 11.6). When the projection of the pointers is X-shaped, the subject is correctly aligned in relation to both cameras and cannot drift out of view of

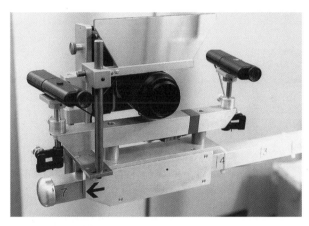

(a)

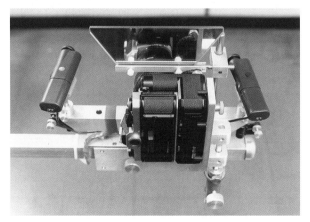

(b)

Fig. 11.4 Front (a) and rear (b) views of the anterior camera showing the mirror for assisting the subject to adopt the correct position and the two pointers which are aimed to converge at the bridge of the subject's nose. The camera can be adjusted horizontally to ensure that the magnification of both cameras is identical

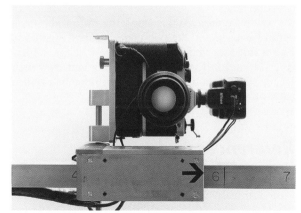

Fig. 11.5 Lateral view camera, mounted vertically with an infra-red remote control and motor drive that allows both cameras to take photographs and wind on to the next frame simultaneously

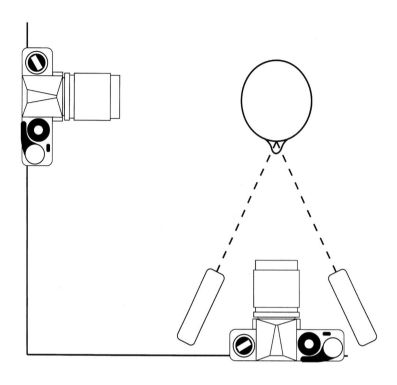

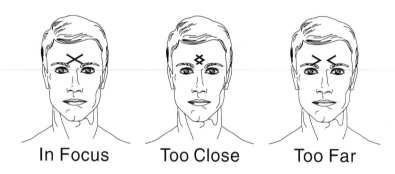

In Focus	Too Close	Too Far

Fig. 11.6 Diagrammatic representation of the range-finding system that ensures the correct position of the subject with respect to both cameras. Projected light beams make a cross on the forehead of the subject when he or she is in the correct position. The studio flash units overwhelm the faint beams from the pointers so they are not seen in the final images

the profile camera. At this stage, the infra-red remote control is used and the two cameras are triggered to give a full-face and right profile view of the subject (Fig. 11.7a, b). If the subject has long hair over their face, a second set of photographs with the hair pulled back off the face may be necessary.

References

Cooke MS, Wei SH. 1988: Intersex differences in cranio-cervical morphology and posture in southern Chinese and British Caucasians. *American Journal of Physical Anthropology* **77**, 43–51.

Marcotte MR. 1981: Head posture and dentofacial proportions. *Angle Orthod* **51**, 208–13.

Moorees CFA, Keen MR. 1956: Natural head position, a base consideration in the interpretation of cephalometric radiographs. *American Journal of Physical Anthropology* **16**, 213–34.

Solow B, Tallgren A. 1971: Natural head position in standing subjects. *Acta Odontologica Scandinavica (Oslo)* **29**, 591–607.

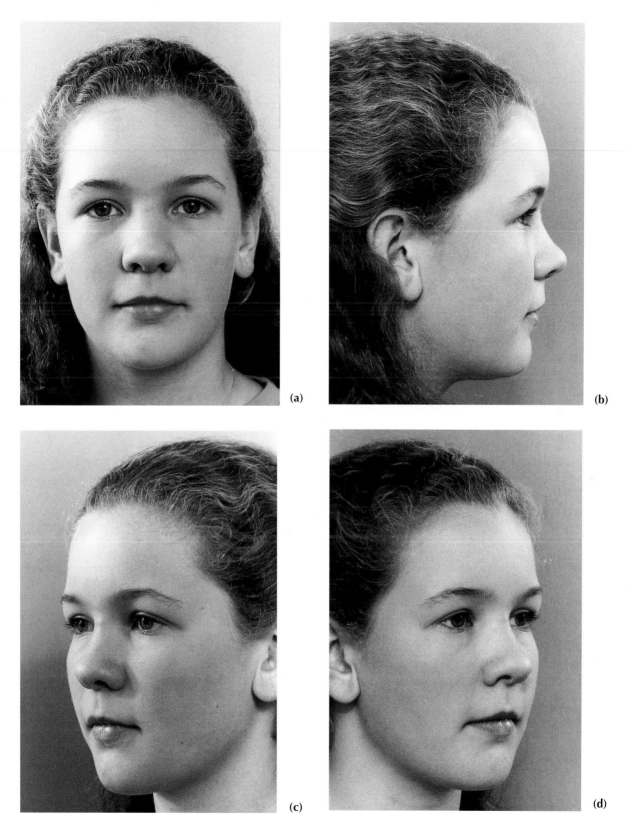

Fig. 11.7 Standard views taken with the orthogonal camera system. (a) Full-face anterior view. (b) Right lateral view. (c) Left oblique view. (d) Right oblique view

CHAPTER 12

Superimposition techniques

JA TAYLOR, KA BROWN

Introduction	151	Reliability	160
Early comparison techniques	151	Conclusion	161
Magnification and skull orientation	155	Presentation of superimposition evidence in	
Photographic considerations	157	a court of law	162
Superimposition comparison and determination			
of identity	159		

Introduction

By definition, to superimpose something is to 'set it or place it on or over something else'. In a forensic context, such a procedure can have many applications, for example in the comparison of tool marks. Craniofacial superimposition is a special technique whereby an image of the skull of a deceased person is compared directly with a photographic portrait of a known individual in order to determine the identity of the skull. It was originally carried out using hand-drawn tracings and has since progressed through the use of still photography, to video and computer technology. Current research is concentrating on the complexities of comparing photographs of living persons, as is required for the identification of surveillance images. Craniofacial superimposition as a means of identification can be used where dental information is not available for comparison. Acceptance of craniofacial superimposition varies and, in some countries, has been considered a less reliable form of identification than dental comparison, although Kashyap and Rao (1987) noted that the lack of adequate dental records in India has meant that superimposition is frequently the only method available for identification.

Early comparison techniques

Artists' portraits, sculptured busts or death masks were once used for comparison to authenticate skulls of historic significance, and alternatively authenticated skulls were used to accredit portraits and sculptures. The earliest work in this field has been attributed to Hermann Welcker (1867), who analysed measurements taken from a skull said to be that of Dante. He compared these measurements with a death mask of the poet housed in Florence and subsequently made direct superimposition comparisons on the purported skulls of Schiller, Kant and Raphael. Lander (1918) seems to have been the first to use a photograph as an ante mortem record for comparison with a skull. Her investigation, however, did not involve the superimposition of one image upon the other, and the only conclusion she reached was that 'It seems improbable that anyone examining the skull would postulate a type of face similar to that seen in the photograph.'

In the early decades of the twentieth century, the English biometric school undertook a series of comparisons of the skulls said to be those of Jeremy Bentham, Sir Thomas Browne, Robert the Bruce, George Buchanan, Lord Darnley and Oliver Cromwell with relevant portraits, busts or death masks (Tildesley, 1923; Pearson, 1924, 1926, 1928; Pearson and Morant, 1934). The accuracy of these artistic representations was difficult to confirm, and the results were open to doubt. Despite these limitations, the authors were, in most cases, able to satisfy themselves of the authenticity of the skulls in question. Various techniques were employed to make these comparisons, but where superimposition was used, it usually involved using a Coradi pantograph to make an outline drawing of a photograph taken of the skull or head in an attitude representative of that in the portrait. This outline was then placed over a pencil tracing of the portrait and the coincidence of the outlines assessed.

PHOTOGRAPHIC SUPERIMPOSITION

The first account of a direct superimposition of a photographic image of a skull upon a photographic portrait appeared in the report of Pearson and Morant (1934) on their investigation into the purported preserved head of Oliver Cromwell. They tested their technique by comparing a photograph of an Egyptian criminal taken immediately following his execution by electrocution with a photograph of his subsequently prepared skull. The photograph contained no scale so the skull photographs were enlarged to fit the size of the portrait; then tracings were made of the photographic portrait and of the photograph of the skull, and these were superimposed. The authors were enthusiastic about the result but acknowledged that such a good outcome would not be possible when comparing a skull with an artist's portrait.

The credit for the first application of this technique in a criminal case has generally been attributed to Glaister and Brash in 'The Ruxton Case' (1937), although Furuhata claimed in 1967 that he had used a similar method for an identification in Japan as early as 1925. The Ruxton case unfolded on 29 September 1935 with the discovery of the mutilated and dismembered bodies of two women in a ravine near Moffat, on the Edinburgh to Carlisle Road in Scotland. An examination of the recovered fragments revealed that considerable effort had been made by their killer to frustrate identification of the victims. Fingertips had been severed, eyes removed and teeth extracted. In the course of this investigation, photographs of two missing persons were obtained. One was the wife of Dr Buck Ruxton, a medical practitioner, the other Mrs Ruxton's maid, Mary Rogerson. Professors Glaister and Brash from Glasgow and Edinburgh Universities decided to use the technique of photographic superimposition to compare the two skulls with the photographs of the missing women.

This was intended not for the purpose of definitive identification but rather as corroboration of other evidence.

They initially made life-sized enlargements of selected ante mortem photographs and full-scale photographs of the two skulls. They used the nasion and prosthion as anatomical reference points, and salient features of each photograph were outlined on linen tracing paper and then compared with the skull image by superimposition. When this confirmed that it was possible to recognize similarities between the skulls and the photographs, direct photographic superimposition was undertaken. Registration marks were placed on each of the negatives of the skulls and portraits. A positive image of the portrait and a negative image of the skull were made; these were then superimposed on X-ray film and positive prints produced from them. Measurable objects – a tiara and a gatepost – depicted in the photographs were used as scales for determining the life-size enlargements. When compared by superimposition of the respective transparencies, a remarkable correspondence was revealed between features on the skulls and features in the photographs.

Meanwhile, police investigations resulted in the arrest on charges of murder of Ruxton. At the subsequent trial, evidence of the superimposition was given. It was emphasized that the identification could not be considered as definitive using superimposition alone. This reservation was appropriate because that was the first occasion when this method had been tested in a court of law. In an attempt to verify the accuracy of the technique, Brash photographed the head of an anatomical cadaver, removed the soft tissues from the skull, which was then photographed, and compared the two images in the manner described. The results were reported as being 'reasonably accurate'.

Many subsequent investigators have modified the technique of Glaister and Brash in various ways, usually by employing different camera systems. Glaister and Brash used a Hunter–Penrose Process Camera with a 16 in Cooke Process Anastigmat Lens to make the full-sized transparency of the ante mortem photograph, which could then be placed over the viewing screen of the camera. Other investigators mostly employed cameras with ground glass viewfinders approximately 6 in square that required a smaller transparency of the ante mortem photograph to fit the viewfinder. They then traced on to the screen salient reference points shown on the photograph to assist in achieving the correct magnification and orientation of the skull. The number and selection of these points varied between investigators. The method of producing the final superimposed print also varied, but this would appear to be a function of available darkroom facilities and personal preference regarding the combination of positive and negative images rather than a significant theoretical modification (Webster, 1955; Sen, 1962; Banerjee, 1964; Basauri, 1967; Furuhata and Yamamoto, 1967; Chandra Sekharan, 1971; Dalitz, 1971; Reddy, 1973; Janssens *et al.*, 1978).

In a variation devised by Gordon and Drennan (1948) to facilitate the superimposition, an outline drawing of a life-sized enlargement of the ante mortem photograph was compared with a machine-made projection drawing of the reconstructed skull, which had been set in the same orientation as the face in the photograph.

Cocks (1970) used a method of superimposition to quantify identification of the fragmented skull of a murder victim. A photograph was taken of the reconstructed skull and compared with a passport photograph of the suspected victim. A system of triangulation was used to demonstrate the degree of correspondence between the skull and the photograph. Corresponding anthropometric landmarks such as the nasion, anterior nasal spine, gnathion and points on the orbits and mandible were determined on the photographs of the skull and the suspected victim respectively. These points were joined to form a series of triangles. The pattern of the triangles from the photograph of the skull were traced on to a transparency, and this was superimposed upon the portrait photograph to compare the patterns. Coincidence of these patterns indicated a 'match'.

Thomas *et al.* (1986) superimposed a projected image upon a photographic print to achieve a comparison. They enlarged a passport photograph of the suspected victim to life size and fixed this to a convenient vertical surface. A transparency of the skull, photographed in a similar orientation, was then projected on to this enlargement. The projector was placed at a distance that produced a projected life-sized image of the skull.

Perhaps the most important contribution to craniofacial photo superimposition was devised by Furue. His system is shown in Fig. 12.1 and has been used in the United States Armed Forces Central Identification Laboratory in Hawaii since 1971 and more recently by Hashimoto *et al.* in Japan (1990). Furue recognized the critical significance of photographic perspective to the accuracy of the comparison of both images. This perspective depended solely upon the camera-to-subject distance, and Furue devised an ingenious system to determine the camera-to-subject distance of the person in the photograph and simultaneously replicate the conditions under which the photographs were taken.

The skull to be identified (Fig. 12.1, A) was mounted on an adjustable stand, placed in front of a backdrop sheet of contrasting coloured cardboard (B) at one end of a bench. A 30 cm grid of 9 mm squares constructed of fine wire mounted on a clear plexiglass sheet (C) was positioned in front of the skull. A mod-

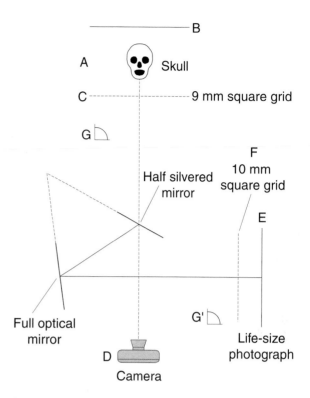

Fig. 12.1 Diagram of the photo superimposition system of Furue

ified 35 mm single lens reflex (SLR) camera (D) was set at the opposite end of the bench. The modification of the camera involved the replacement of the standard split image glass focusing screen with an aerial image focusing screen. To the right of the camera, a life-sized enlargement of the ante mortem photograph (E) was placed directly behind a grid of 10 mm squares (F) constructed from fine wire mounted on clear plexiglass. Two mirrors, one a full optical mirror and the other a half-silvered mirror, were placed at appropriate angles to the left and in front of the camera. The mirrors were arranged such that the full mirror reflected the image of the photograph upon the half-silvered mirror, which reflected it along the central axis of the camera lens. Two 200 W lamps (G, G') illuminated the skull and the photograph independently, and were strategically positioned between the skull and the camera. The image of the skull was transmitted through the half-silvered mirror to the camera and the image of the ante mortem photograph was reflected from the optical mirror and the half-silvered mirror to the camera lens, so that the images of both skull and portrait could be seen through the viewfinder of the camera. Each image could be intensified or reduced by alteration of the distances of the lamps from the skull and photograph.

The distances between the skull, grids, mirrors, photograph and camera were determined according to the distance from which the ante mortem photograph was taken. These distances are critical factors. When these distances were correct, the two grids appeared precisely superimposed, indicating the appropriate degree of magnification and an exact reproduction of the perspective incorporated in the ante mortem photograph. This system enables the skull to be aligned against the photograph before an image is recorded and takes into account the perspective incorporated in the ante mortem photograph. After correct alignment was obtained, an image of the skull was recorded on the camera film following removal of the half-mirror. A negative transparency of the ante mortem portrait was then overlaid onto a positive print of the skull as previously described. A sheet of white film was moved between the transparency and the print to highlight the comparison.

Klonaris and Furue (1980) applied a modification of the superimposition method to compare a maxillary fragment with a dental radiograph of a United States Air Force pilot whose aircraft was lost during a reconnaissance mission in Vietnam. Only a portion of the right maxilla and parts of the ramus and angle of the mandible had been recovered, providing limited material for comparison. An enlarged reverse-contrast transparent radiograph was produced from the ante mortem periapical radiograph. This transparency was placed over a photograph of the maxillary fragment, with a sheet of plain white paper separating the two. Detailed comparison of the two images by wiping one image over the other was facilitated by sliding the paper between the transparency and the photograph.

VIDEO SUPERIMPOSITION

In 1977, Helmer and Gruner in Germany and Brown *et al.* in Australia, unbeknown to each other, introduced a significant modification to the photographic technique of craniofacial superimposition: they substituted video systems for still cameras. This eliminated the time-consuming processes of photographic processing, developing and printing of repeated trial-and-error photographic exposures needed to determine the correct orientation of the skull and the relative enlargement of each image. A plan of the system used by Brown *et al.* is shown in Fig. 12.2. Two video cameras were employed, one focused on the ante mortem photograph and the other on the skull. Each camera transmitted its image to separate monitors, and both image signals were then fed through a special-effects generator that permitted the display of both images superimposed on a third monitor. The immediate display of the superimposed images enabled the operator to adjust the orientation of the skull with greater accuracy to correspond with the position of the face in the photograph. Zoom lenses fitted to the video cameras permitted instant adjustment of magnification of each image to a common scale. The special-effects generator was employed to produce a variety of combinations of the superimposed images displayed on the monitor, permitting detailed comparisons of significant facial features. The superimposition manoeuvres were recorded on videotape for further study or for presentation in a court of law, or photographed by conventional photography (Helmer and Gruner, 1977a, b; Brown *et al.,* 1978, 1981; Brown, 1983).

Most subsequent workers have employed video equipment arranged in a configuration similar to that described above, with minor variations (Koelmeyer, 1982; Dorion, 1983; Bastiaan *et al.*, 1986; Iten, 1987; Loh and Chao, 1989).

The original system developed by Brown *et al.* utilized video cameras designed for amateur use; these were later replaced by semiprofessional Ikegami cameras, with a noticeable increase in image quality. New-generation charged couple device (CCD) cameras offer a further advantage over these older tube cameras in that there is no loss of image quality as the camera ages. Tube cameras tended to 'fade', with unpredictable impact on the transmitted image. The

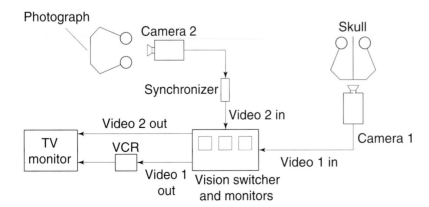

Fig. 12.2 Diagram of the video superimposition system

use of good-quality video and transmission equipment is of paramount importance.

Magnification and skull orientation

There are two factors that require special consideration in both photographic and video techniques for superimposition. They are the determination of 'life-size' magnification and the method of orientation of the skull to correspond with the position of the face in the photograph. To be meaningful, the image of the face must be precisely scaled to the image of the skull, and the 'camera angles' or viewpoints of both skull and photographs must be identical.

MAGNIFICATION

Since the comparison is achieved by overlaying two physically separate images, it is necessary for each image to be of the same relative size. In the past most workers seem to have preferred life-sized enlargements. This is because accurate measurement of the skull is possible and full-scale photographic images were easily produced by using objects evident in the photographs as scales for the enlargement of the ante mortem photographs. Glaister and Brash (1937) utilized a tiara and a gatepost, Gordon and Drennan (1948) a neck tie and Chandra Sekharan (1971) a chair and a saree pattern. Chandra Sekharan correctly pointed out the necessity of these objects being in the same plane as the face to ensure accurate enlargement. Although this can be a useful technique, such photographs are not always available, and the planes of the face and 'scale' object may be difficult to verify, rendering enlargements made from photographs relying on that premise of doubtful reliability.

When no physical objects suitable for reference scales were present in the ante mortem photographs, Simpson (1943a, b) used the interpupillary distance and interorbital width as guidelines for life-size enlargement. Chandra Sekharan (1971) and Reddy (1973) recommended using an arbitrary interpupillary distance of 6 cm. McKenna (1986) considered that reliance on the historical methods for enlargement of the photographs reduced the accuracy of the enlargement, and therefore of the superimposition, to one of 'best fit'. He recommended the use of anterior tooth size as the scale for enlargement, being the most accurate reference points that are 'most likely to be extremely close to the exact plane of focus of the camera' (McKenna, 1986). Loh and Chao (1989) proposed that an ante mortem photograph showing

two people, both full face to the camera, would permit direct measurement of the interpupillary distance of the second person as the scale for enlargement. This technique is of limited practicality as it relies on the availability of suitable photographs and willing associates of the deceased person. The use of an arbitrary or estimated distance is of no greater value than is using a reference object not in the same plane of the photograph.

Earlier, Prinsloo (1953) compared facial proportions in an attempt to determine the similarity between two images and therefore did not enlarge to life size but to a 'size convenient for work'.

In the video technique, immediate alteration of the magnification of both images can be facilitated electronically, thereby eliminating the need to produce separate enlarged prints of the ante mortem photograph and skull. Any determination of magnification must be made within the electronic system rather than measured through the monitor system, as the refractive index of the screen can introduce distortions that will be incorporated into any measurement.

SKULL ORIENTATION

Correct mounting and orientation of the skull is critical for a meaningful comparison by superimposition. Many attempts have been made to establish a standardized method to equate the position of the skull with that of the face in the photograph, ranging from trial and error to the application of mathematical formulae. Glaister and Brash (1937) fixed the original negative of the portrait to the back of the camera to serve as a focusing screen, permitting the direct scaling of both images and orientation of the skull. As a variation, an image of the ante mortem photograph, traced in pencil or ink on the ground glass focusing screen of the camera, has also been used as a guide for determining the orientation of the skull (Webster, 1955; Sen, 1962; Banerjee, 1964; Basauri, 1967; Furuhata and Yamamoto, 1967; Chandra Sekharan, 1971; Dalitz, 1971; Reddy 1973). Gruner and Reinhard (1959) designed an optical bench to hold an outline of the ante mortem photograph in front of the skull to facilitate its correct alignment.

A complex mathematical formula for determining the orientation of the face in a photograph was proposed by Chandra Sekharan in 1973. He defined three possible movements of the head for forward and backward movement, flexion, and extension and rotation, and suggested parameters for aligning these planes to achieve correct orientation of the skull. This method assumed that faces are symmetrical and that measurements made from the midline to the outer surfaces can be used to determine the angle of rotation. All these distances were marked on the photograph, accurately enlarged to life size, and used to determine the orientation of the skull. It is important, however, to emphasize that faces are seldom bilaterally symmetrical (Vig and Hewitt, 1975; Shah and Joshi, 1978; Chebib and Chamma, 1981), thus limiting the reliability of this technique.

Janssens *et al.* (1978) categorized the possible movements of the head in a manner similar to that of Chandra Sekharan. They considered declination (left or right tilt) to be easily compensated for by the positioning of the photograph. They used standard anatomical landmarks on the cranium and face, such as the nasion, prosthion and orbitale, orion, gnathion, glabella, bregma, tragion and gonion, to determine the correct orientation with respect to rotation and inclination. On the photograph, the nasion and prosthion were joined and the photograph adjusted to the vertical. The left and right orbitale were joined, and the intersection of these two planes was designated 'M'. The skull was adjusted until the corresponding planes on the two images were of equal distance. Janssens *et al.* emphasized the necessity for accurate anthropometrical location of these points on both the skull and the photograph. Their definitions of these points, however, do not seem to acknowledge this need for accuracy, although it is nonetheless accepted that the precise location of landmarks on a photograph of a face is difficult to achieve.

Numerous attempts have been made to devise a machine to determine the precise position and orientation of the skull in relation to the face in the photograph. Kamijo and Sakai (1970) designed a remote-controlled clamp for mounting and adjustment of the skull. Movement of the skull during the orientation process could be viewed on a ground glass screen upon which an image of the ante mortem photograph was simultaneously projected. A remote-controlled electronic optical bench was designed by Ishibashi in 1986. The apparatus had a fixed attachment to the camera and was driven by five independent gears that controlled movement in three planes and two axes of rotation. All movements were recorded.

A novel departure from previous systems was introduced by McKenna (1986). Termed a 'goniometer', it provided for the planetary movement of the camera (video or still) about the skull, which was so fixed that a defined anatomical reference point, for example the midpoints of the upper central incisor teeth, represented the centre of rotation of the camera. The camera could traverse horizontally (360 degrees) and vertically (200 degrees) around the skull. However, the camera-to-skull distance was fixed at 1 m, and this failed to recognize the significance of perspective distortion.

Brocklebank and Holmgren (1989) described a system for the support, orientation and photography of the skull. Three-point fixation of the skull was achieved by horizontal fixing pins screwed into vertical, threaded connecting rods. These rods were fitted into selectively drilled holes on a circular plate of aluminium that could be adjusted in height only. This mechanism was seated on a pan-and-tilt device, allowing movement in two vertical planes and rotation in the horizontal plane. The whole device was attached to two parallel rails that also carried the attachment for the (still or video) cameras. Camera movement was provided vertically through 28 cm, or horizontally through any length with the addition of supplementary rails.

In 1987 Taylor and Brown developed a system that would simulate the natural movement of the head and be capable of reproducible computer control. This skull mounting and orientation device (SMOD; Fig. 12.3) permitted controlled, reproducible movement of the skull in six degrees of freedom (three perpendicular planes (x, y and z) and three axes of rotation). All movements were per-

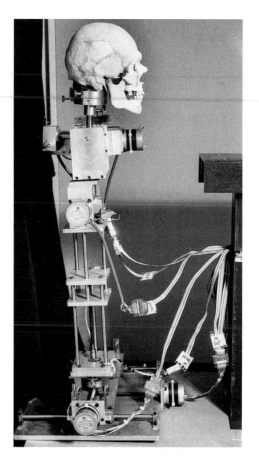

Fig. 12.3 Skull mounting and orientation device (SMOD)

formed by stepper motors controlled remotely from the computer terminal. Precision adjustments could be made in 1 mm steps and 1 degree segments, and incremental data were stored in the computer for future reference.

Photographic considerations

Craniofacial superimposition is a technique employing photographic images, and an understanding of basic photographic principles is essential to produce accurate and reliable craniofacial identification using this method.

A photograph of a person is a two-dimensional representation of a three-dimensional object. The association of the size, shape and position of the objects in the three-dimensional environment and their representation in the two-dimensional photograph is referred to as photographic perspective (Sussman, 1973; Hedgecoe, 1982; Jacobson *et al.*, 1988). The true perspective of a photograph can only be reproduced if another photograph is taken from the same viewpoint and distance. The focal length of the lens of the camera will affect only the size of the image, and not the perspective incorporated in the photograph.

Although few authors have acknowledged the necessity of reproducing the camera-to-subject distance of the ante mortem photograph when making comparative photographs of the skull for superimposition, this factor was recognized by Glaister and Brash (1937). At the Ruxton trial, it was stated, 'Had it been possible to photograph the skulls at the same distance as the heads in the original portraits, the perspectives could have been directly comparable. But it is doubtful if this would have made any appreciable difference in the comparisons.' Glaister and Brash used a camera-to-subject distance of 5 ft (1.5 m) and at this distance, changes in perspective can have a significant impact on an image. Hashimoto (1992) determined that perspective is of critical importance up to a distance of 5 m. In a study by Titlbach, the effect of distance on perspective relating to craniofacial superimposition was found to be minimal when the photograph of the skull was taken from approximately the same distance and viewpoint as the ante mortem photograph (Janssens *et al.*, 1978).

Gejvall and Johanson (1976) also recognized that 'The skull to be identified and the picture of a head to be compared with it must as far as possible be reproduced from the same angle, and preferably, from more or less the same distance, and the picture of the skull has to be reduced sufficiently to fit the head with which it is being compared.' Correct perspective cannot be reproduced if the viewpoint of the camera is not considered.

Janssens *et al.* (1978) referred to the phenomenon of observed differences in perspective as an 'optical illusion'. They stated that 'Use of the original negative of the photograph and the technical data of the camera (focal length of the lens) would permit the determination of the position and angle of exposure of the camera with greater precision, thereby correcting for the effect of the optical illusion.' Perspective is an optical reality rather than an illusion and was recognized by Iten (1987), who observed that 'three-dimensional objects, for instance a skull, appear differently on two-dimensional photographs depending on the direction and distance involved when pictures are being taken'.

Although much has been published on the topic of craniofacial superimposition little recognition seems to have been given to even basic photographic principles.

The ante mortem photograph is already a two-dimensional image of the three-dimensional subject, so factors such as perspective and lighting are already fixed and cannot be altered.

It is therefore essential to ensure that the plane of the ante mortem photograph is precisely parallel to the image-forming plane of the lens of the camera, preventing new distortions being introduced into the image. This determination of parallelism can be achieved by placing over the lens a diaphragm with a small central aperture and a mirror in the centre of the photograph. This enables the image of the aperture to be reflected back along the axis of the lens system and be viewed in the viewfinder. The correct parallelism can be confirmed when the reflected image of the aperture is seen in the exact centre of the viewfinder.

Taylor (1991) investigated the significance of photographic distortion on the outcome of comparisons made by means of craniofacial video superimposition and found a number of factors to be critical. Casework and research carried out by Taylor and Brown has shown certain factors related to the photographic images used for the comparison which are of vital importance.

In an identification case undertaken in 1990, the skull of a murdered female required positive identification. The police provided numerous photographs of a suspect for comparison by video superimposition. Two photographs, one full face and the other a profile, were professional portraits taken prior to cosmetic surgery. The other photographs, also full face and profile, were routine photographs taken following arrests at various police stations. A quite significant change in facial appearance of the subject was observed over the period represented in the photographs.

The first superimposition was made against the full-face professional portrait. This comparison is shown in Fig. 12.4. Features in the lower half of the skull do not coincide with the corresponding features shown on the skull, in particular the nasal aperture, the upper and lower alveolar ridges and the lower border of the mandible.

The second comparison used a police 'mugshot' profile photograph taken a short time before the disappearance of the suspect. As can be seen in Fig. 12.5, large discrepancies are revealed between the superimposed images. The external auditory meatus is correctly aligned with the tragus of the ear, but the profile outlines of the two images are separated by a considerable distance, which is not consistent with standard soft tissue thicknesses.

The exact conditions under which all the photographs had been taken were ascertained, and the comparisons were repeated with the camera settings and the skull camera distance accurately reproduced.

Figures 12.6 and 12.7 show the new superimposition of the skull against the full-face and profile portraits. The improvement in the alignment of the anterior teeth, the nasal aperture and the mandibular border can be seen in both cases. This clearly demonstrates the significance of the camera-to-skull distance in achieving the correct perspective and thus enhancing the chances of achieving a reliable identification.

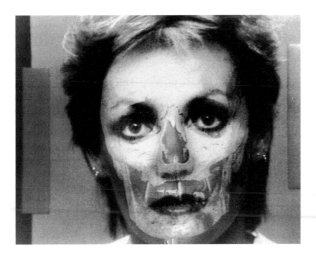

Fig. 12.4 The superimposition comparison achieved using estimated ante mortem photographic conditions (frontal view)

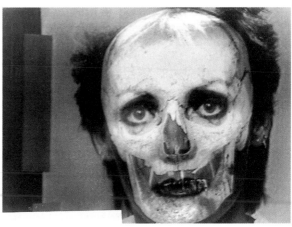

Fig. 12.6 Superimposition comparison achieved when the ante mortem photographic conditions were reproduced (frontal view)

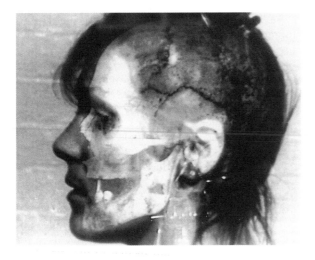

Fig. 12.5 Superimposition comparison achieved using estimated ante mortem photographic conditions (lateral view)

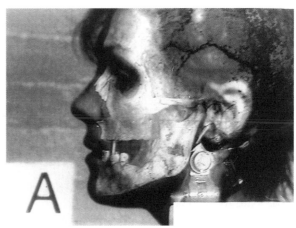

Fig. 12.7 Superimposition comparison achieved when the ante mortem photographic conditions were reproduced (lateral view)

Superimposition comparison and determination of identity

Having achieved correct orientation of the skull and appropriate magnification of the images of the skull and portrait, the next task in the identification process is to compare and interpret the superimposed images.

Determination of identity using craniofacial superimposition is essentially an exercise in determining the anatomical possibility of a skull being that of a person whose face is depicted in a photograph. This demands a thorough understanding of craniofacial morphology and function. The object of the exercise is to decide whether it is possible for the skull, and the anatomical features represented in the photograph, to be those of the same person.

There are essentially two methods for determining the degree of similarity between the two images. Both rely on the location of soft tissue surfaces relative to the underlying bony structure.

The method devised by Helmer (1984, 1987) requires the temporary attachment to the skull of a series of markers gauged to the relevant soft tissue thickness. These are placed at various cephalometric points such as the nasion, rhinion, gonion and gnathion, along a vertical line marked on the skull corresponding to the profile on the photograph. When the superimposition is made, the alignment of these markers with the soft tissue profile in the same plane in the photograph is said to indicate positive identity.

While this offers a simple procedure for assessing similarity, the reliability of this method depends on the availability of accurate soft tissue depth measurements for the population relevant to the racial and geographic origin of the skull. Helmer's use of this method is supported by application of his average soft tissue thicknesses tables. These were determined using ultrasound techniques on a large number of German subjects, taking into account age and general body build (Helmer, 1984). In other situations, use of Helmer's or any other tissue thickness tables is open to challenge unless it can be shown that they are representative of the population being examined.

Even if soft tissue thickness tables are available for a relevant population group, it must be remembered that they are only averages. The object of an identification process is to individualize a person from within a general group. Any one individual in a group cannot necessarily be described by the averages of the whole group. While soft tissue depths may be a useful adjunct to the identification process, it is prudent to rely on known associations between bony structures and related soft tissue points to determine identity. The alternative techniques used by the authors places emphasis on those facial features with the least soft tissue depth and which are less likely to change as a result of growth or weight change. A series of experiments by Taylor (1988) indicated that the features in the middle third of the face, such as the eyes, nose and teeth, were less influenced by any photographic distortions and could therefore be considered more suitable.

Because skin is mobile rather than rigidly attached to the underlying bone, the presentation of any soft tissue feature relative to the underlying bone can be altered owing to the different facial expressions seen in a photograph. Average soft tissue thicknesses in specific locations may be used as a guide but never as definitive measures. These soft tissue thicknesses are recorded perpendicular to the bone surface and are most useful as guides if the photograph depicts the soft tissue directly parallel to the point of measurement. A change in position of the face to a slightly different viewpoint will alter the projection upon the surface of the skin of a specific skeletal anthropometric point.

The location of soft tissue features representative of the underlying bone is relatively well known, and this knowledge is used extensively in plastic reconstruction of the face (see Chapters 14 and 18), but when it is applied to craniofacial superimposition, it must be remembered that these data have been established for the expressionless face and allowance must be made when using such data as a basis for the determination of identity.

It must be remembered that authors differ about the specific definitions for the location of the significant features of the face.

EYES

Krogman and Iscan (1986) place the inner canthus 3 mm medially to the medial wall of the orbit. Drake and Lukash (1978) place it against the medial wall of the orbit, and Caldwell (1981) 2–3 mm lateral to the lacrimal crest and 4–5 mm below the dacryon (junction of the lacromaxillary suture and the frontal bone). Stewart (1983) advises using the anterior surface of the lacrimal sac as the height indicator for the inner canthus.

Slightly differing descriptions also exist for the location of the outer canthus of the eye. Krogman and Iscan (1986) nominated a point 5 mm lateral to the orbit margin. A more realistic working description is perhaps that of Caldwell (1981), who placed the outer canthus 3–4 mm medial to the 'tiny bony tuber' and observed that the upper eyelid crease may extend beyond the bony edge. The 'tiny bony tuber', although not described in many anatomy texts, was referred to by Stewart (1983) as Whitnall's malar tubercle. If present on the skull, it is a very useful landmark for locating the height of the outer canthus.

The actual presentation of both the inner and outer canthi in the ante mortem photograph is, of course, situation dependent but, being a ligamentous attachment, the location of its height will be determinable even if the width of the eyelid opening is not.

EYEBROWS

The orbit can also be used as a guide for the shape and position of the eyebrows. Care must be taken to observe closely the ante mortem photograph to ascertain whether there has been any cosmetic alteration to the shape of the eyebrows and whether any facial expression may have moved the location of the eyebrow relative to the eye.

The eyebrow generally lies 3–5 mm above the upper orbit margin (Krogman and Iscan, 1986) and follows the shape of the orbit and brow ridge (Caldwell, 1981).

EARS

Ears are often not clearly seen on ante mortem photographs as they may be partially or completely hidden by head hair. The cartilaginous ear is at the level of the bony ear (Krogman and Iscan, 1986). Krogman and Iscan (1986) indicated a soft tissue thickness of 10 mm, but Caldwell (1981) pointed out that considerable individual variation is likely.

If the tragus of the external ear is visible on the ante mortem photograph, it is a useful guide for locating the external auditory meatus on the skull. These two landmarks lie at the same height.

NOSE

Caldwell (1981) noted that the nose, particularly the width relative to the underlying nasal cavity, seems to be one of the most variable facial features. The alar will always be wider than the underlying bony cavity, Krogman and Iscan (1986) indicated a distance of 5 mm laterally from the margin of the bone on each side in Caucasian subjects, and Hoffman *et al.* (1991) 6.1 mm wider on each side, although they recommended the use of a multiplicative formula instead of an additive one.

The contour of the nose, and particularly the form of the nasal tip, receives considerable discussion in the literature. The bony nasal bridge can be useful in a profile photograph, as can any nasal deviations visible in the full-face aspect.

MOUTH

Lip form cannot be accurately determined from the skull, although some dental malocclusions tend to produce typical soft tissue presentations; for example, anterior open bites often have thrusting tongues and incompetent lips. Guidelines for lip form suggest that the mouth opening is often as wide as the upper intercanine distances and that the upper lip, at rest, covers approximately the gingival two-thirds of the upper incisors. For these reasons, a photograph showing some anterior teeth will be more useful in a superimposition comparison when these teeth are present in the skull.

Reliability

Controversy over the reliability of craniofacial superimposition has continued since it was first tendered in evidence in a court of law, and some authors still consider that the technique should not be used for definitive identification purposes.

Koelmeyer (1982) described a case in which he claimed to have achieved a 'good' match, using video superimposition, of a skull with a photograph of a person known to be alive. The skull lacked a mandible, which led him to conclude that a complete facial skeleton was necessary for identification but that the technique should be limited to provide exclusion or corroboration only. A case of misidentification was reported by Dorion (1983), in which one skull was identified by two different investigators as being that of two different persons. He stressed that superimposition should not be used as the sole means of identification. McKenna, in 1986, believed that superimposition by video comparison was at that time not as good or reliable as the photographic technique.

On the other hand, many authors have endorsed the capabilities of superimposition as a method of reliable identification. Furuhata and Yamamoto (1967) referred to it as 'useful', Kamijo and Sakai (1970) as a 'powerful method' and Iten (1987) as 'very successful'. Brown (1983) considered that the video superimposition 'appears to provide a much higher measure of reliability' than does the older photographic method. Helmer *et al.* (1989) considered craniofacial video superimposition to be a valid method of identification if performed with the 'utmost accuracy' using high-quality equipment and an ante mortem photograph of good quality.

McKenna (1988) later acknowledged that the technique was 'gaining credibility', but the best measure of its success and reliability is its acceptance by courts of law. Identifications by video superimposition comparison have been accepted by courts in Australia (Brown *et al.*, 1977, reported in 1981; Bastiaan *et al.*, 1986), England (Walker, 1982), Hong Kong (McKenna *et al.*, 1984), Japan (Hashimoto, personal communication, 1988) and Malta (Brown, personal communications, 1989, 1990).

Lan *et al.* (1990) described a system they developed to reduce the level of expert subjectivity in the comparison-making process when identifying an unknown skull using craniofacial video superimposition. All movements required by skull, ante mortem photograph or video camera were computer controlled. A data resource of 52 indices that they considered adequately relevant for identification were compiled from 224 adult Chinese of Han nationality using projected radiographic measurements (Chai *et al.*, 1989). Their technique relied on the placement of 'marking lines' on the images of the face and skull between selected anatomical landmarks. These marking lines were first placed on the image of the face, and the pattern of lines alone was used to align the skull into the correct position. The video camera was placed at a distance of 1 m from the skull. Corresponding marking lines were then placed on the image of the skull without reference to the ante mortem photograph. The computer analysed the two patterns of lines to determine whether any differences fell within the accepted limits of the stored data. The authors claimed that the computer could correct for inappropriate magnification and incorrect orientation of the skull by reference to the stored data and was therefore applicable for comparing two photographs taken from differing viewpoints.

Conclusion

Craniofacial video superimposition can be considered reliable provided that a number of criteria are carefully observed.

It is most important that photographic equipment is employed which provides adequate resolution and detail, and that great care is taken in alignment of the skull. A sound technique, a thorough understanding of cranial anatomy and soft tissue form and relationships, and total professional objectivity are essential elements in avoiding misidentification.

The overall reliability of the technique can be enhanced by the consideration of several additional factors, some of which merely make the comparisons easier to achieve while others impact directly on the accuracy of the results.

The optical performance of the video cameras used should be assessed. Cameras that introduce measurable distortions into the images should not be used. If two video cameras are used, they should produce images of a similar quality so that valid comparisons can be made. Alteration or deterioration of images over time may be a problem with the older-generation tube cameras, and CCD cameras, which are free of this problem, are to be preferred.

The limiting factor in any craniofacial superimposition comparison is the quality of the ante mortem photograph. Lighting, focus, photographic resolution and facial expression can all change the apparent location of some facial features and make accurate comparison difficult. Significant image distortion will occur toward the peripheral areas of the photograph, so it is important that the image of the face is near to the centre of the photograph (Taylor, 1991). It is therefore advisable to base a statement of identity on comparisons with a number of photographs that show the face from a variety of viewpoints.

Selection of a good-quality ante mortem photograph will make the comparison of the combined images more reliable. A poor-quality photograph can, when enlarged by the video camera, result in an image with poor definition that will make determination of particular features difficult. It is advisable to use more than one photograph, showing the face from different viewpoints, if available so that a series of comparisons can be made before a final decision is reached.

The whole area of the photograph must be in close contact with the surface of the easel to which it is attached, and this must be exactly parallel to the image plane of the video camera. If the video camera is moved, this parallelism must be redetermined.

The image of the face in the photograph should be as near to the centre of the photograph as possible. A photograph with the face placed toward the edges of the frame should be avoided as the proportions of the facial features will be significantly distorted. The face should be in good focus, well lit and not in partial shadow. Lighting of the skull should reproduce that recorded in the ante mortem photograph.

If possible, the exact photographic conditions under which the ante mortem photograph was taken should be discovered. Of particular importance is the distance at which the photograph was taken and the focal length of the lens used to record the image. The settings used on the darkroom enlarger to produce the final print may also be important. If these details cannot be discovered, close approximations should be made, although the accuracy of the results is, of course, likely to be affected.

The video camera must be placed at the same distance from the skull as that from which the ante mortem photograph was taken. Easier and more reliable distance determination and parallelism is achieved if the video cameras are mounted on a permanent stable fixed track rather than on movable tripods.

Calculation of the equivalent focal length of the video lens to reproduce the magnification used when the ante mortem photograph was taken is an important procedure. If the exact ante mortem photographic conditions are known, this calculation will enable the superimposition of two images with virtually identical perspective.

Orientation of the skull should reproduce the viewpoint from which the ante mortem photograph was taken. Whatever method is chosen for the mounting and movement of the skull in front of the camera, certain criteria are important. A rigid, reproducible mounting position is essential. A precise movement capable of being executed in small increments, in three planes and in three axes is a minimum requirement. Calibrated, reproducible movement, as achieved with the computer controlled SMOD, makes the superimposition comparison more precise and saves much time.

The ideal craniofacial superimposition involves a comparison made objectively by the assessment of corresponding features. Consideration of the guidelines presented above will generate images of optimum reliability that will facilitate this objective assessment.

Presentation of superimposition evidence in a court of law

The completion of the comparison and the preparation of a medico-legal report do not necessarily mean the end of the matter. In forensic cases, the ultimate test of the experts' work will take place in a court of law. Indeed, at every stage of the process, it is prudent to presume that the matter will be dealt with in a court, requiring the personal appearance and rigorous examination of the expert. General issues regarding the provision of scientific evidence are explored further in Chapter 19; however, in relation to the use of superimposition evidence, special considerations apply.

Ironically, a major difficulty sometimes encountered in the presentation of superimposition evidence results from overexpectation on the part of the court. It is imperative, therefore, that proper consideration be given to the preparation and presentation of such evidence. The Ruxton case, described above, set an important precedent. After legal argument was heard, evidence of the superimposition was tendered on the basis that it was not of itself proof of identification but that it assisted the examiner in reaching his opinion. No case of identification has been achieved by observation of a skull alone.

Superimposition provides a means of comparing and corroborating other evidence, and there must be available a suitable photograph of a known missing person.

How the evidence is presented is almost as important as *what* is presented. This will be determined to some extent by the legal system in operation and the practices adopted by respective courts. The evidence usually needs to be translated into words for the sake of the court record, and any documentary evidence, such as photographs, or a video screening must therefore be described verbally.

Apart from the coronial jurisdictions, the underlying court process in Australia is adversarial. In the presentation of video superimposition evidence, the side calling the expert may want to screen the videotape in court to demonstrate the similarities or differences in the comparison. However, opposing counsel may object on the grounds that displaying the image of the skull in association with a victim's face would be prejudicial to an accused person. If the judge believes that the prejudicial effect on the jury would be greater than the probative value of the evidence, the request to screen the video is likely to be rejected by the court. It has been the authors' experience that South Australian and Queensland courts will not permit a craniofacial video superimposition tape to be screened in court. Such screenings have been allowed in courts in New South Wales, Victoria and the Australian Capital Territory, and have even been demanded in some courts in Europe.

Opinions cannot be conjured out of thin air. They must be founded on facts proved by the expert witness or by some other witness. This places a considerable burden on the expert who invents or discovers a new method or test for a particular situation. Indeed, the first time of presenting a new method in court is critical to its acceptance in that case and also to its future adoption by other courts. The court must first agree to hear evidence of this new method. This is usually considered in a *voir dire*, in which the matter is presented to the judge first, without the jury present; if the judge deems it appropriate, the expert will then be allowed to present it to the jury. The methods or tests so used by the expert must be explained in such a way as to be capable of being understood by the court, which consists largely of laypersons unfamiliar with scientific terminology.

Of course, of great concern for the jury are the results of tests. It is the expert's role to interpret the results of any tests and express an opinion accordingly. That opinion may, however, be subject to certain qualifications. It is thus very important how the opinion is stated and explained. The expert should not be dogmatic or inflexible, especially when the results of certain tests may be capable of more than one interpretation. In such cases, the expert should state first the opinion and then the qualifications that apply.

The expert will be expected to give some guidance to the court with respect to the reliability of the comparison and its statistical probability in response to such questions as 'Is it a recognized test?', 'Is it consistent or inconsistent?' and 'Does it confirm or exclude an identification?' Experts should never respond in a dogmatic, absolute or arrogant manner.

The expert in this field must understand the principles of superimposition and must have an adequate knowledge and experience of the anatomy of the skull, the morphology of the face and the interrelationships of both. Craniofacial superimposition comparison should not be attempted by amateurs. Too often, examples of alleged 'matches' performed by enthusiastic but inexperienced operators have been produced, even showing portions of the skull extending beyond the outline of soft tissues. Such inexpertise does much damage to the reputation of a technique that, when properly used, can be considered reliable and can therefore, with confidence, be presented as evidence in courts of law.

References

Banerjee A. 1964: Camera identifies human skull. *Indian Police Journal* **2**, 42–6.

Basauri C. 1967: A body identified by forensic odontology and superimposed photographs. *International Criminal Police Review* **205**, 37–43.

Bastiaan RG, Dalitz GD, Woodward C. 1986: Video superimposition of skulls and photographic portraits – a new aid to identification. *Journal of Forensic Sciences* **31**, 1373–9.

Brocklebank LM, Holmgren CJ. 1989: Development of equipment for the standardisation of skull photographs in personal identifications by photographic superimposition. *Journal of Forensic Sciences* **34**, 1214–21.

Brown KA. 1983: Developments in cranio-facial superimposition for identification. *Journal of Forensic Odonto-Stomatology* **1**, 57–64.

Brown KA, Hollamby C, Clark BJ, Reynolds L. 1978: A video technique of cranio-facial photo-superimposition. Paper presented at the 8th Meeting of the International Association of Forensic Sciences, Wichita, Kansas, May 22–26, 1978.

Brown KA, Clark BJ, Hollamby C, Congdon IC. 1981: Identification in the Truro murders. An application of the video technique of cranio-facial photo-superimposition as an aid to personal identification. Paper presented at the Seventh Australian Symposium on the Forensic Sciences, Sydney, NSW, Australian Forensic Science Society, 7–14 March 1981, Abstract 65.

Caldwell MC. 1981: *The relationship of the details of the human face to the skull and its application in forensic anthropology.* Tempe: Department of Anthropology, Arizona State University.

Chai O-S, Lan Y-W, Tao C *et al.* 1989: A study on the standard for forensic anthropologic identification of skull image superimposition. *Journal of Forensic Sciences* **34**, 1343–56.

Chandra Sekharan P. 1971: A revised superimposition technique for identification of the individual from the skull and photograph. *Journal of Criminal Law, Criminology and Police Science* **62**, 107–13.

Chandra Sekharan P. 1973: A scientific method for positioning of the skull for photography in superimposition studies. *Journal of Police Science and Administration* **1**, 232–40.

Chebib FS, Chamma AM. 1981: Indices of cranio-facial asymmetry. *Angle Orthodontist* **51**, 214–16.

Cocks FB. 1970: The Barkly Highway murder. *Australian Police Journal* **24**, 173–85.

Dalitz GD. 1971: Superimposition as an aid to identification. A paper presented at the 1971 National Symposium on the Forensic Sciences, Adelaide, SA, 10 February 1971, Australian Forensic Science Society.

Dorion RB. 1983: Photographic superimposition. *Journal of Forensic Sciences* **28**, 724–34.

Drake W, Lukash C. 1978: Reconstruction of mutilated victims for identification. *Journal of Forensic Sciences* **23**, 218–30.

Furuhata T, Yamamoto K. 1967: *Forensic odontology.* Springfield, IL: Charles C. Thomas.

Gejvall N-G, Johanson G. 1976: Solving a mystery death. *OSSA, International Journal of Skeletal Research* **3–4**, 169–81.

Glaister J, Brash JC. 1937: *Medico-legal aspects of the Ruxton case.* Edinburgh: E. & S. Livingstone.

Gordon I, Drennan MR. 1948: Medico-legal aspects of the Wolkersdorfer case. *South African Medical Journal* **22**, 543–9.

Gruner O, Reinhard R. 1959: Ein photographisches verfahren zur schadelidentifizierung. *Deutsche Zeitschrift für gerichtliche Medizin* **47**, 247–56.

Hashimoto M. 1992: A study of the superimposition technique as a positive identification method. *Shikawa Gakuho* **92**, 409–34.

Hashimoto M, Suzuki K, Furue T. 1990: Cranio-facial photo-superimposition. Presented at 241 Meeting of the Tokyo Dental College Society, *Shikawa Gakuho go*, 1454.

Hedgecoe J. 1982: *The photographer's handbook.* London: Edbury.

Helmer RP. 1984: *Schadelidentifizieng durch electronische Bildmischung.* Heidelberg: Kriminalistic Verlag.

Helmer RP. 1987: Identification of the cadaver remains of Josef Mengele. *Journal of Forensic Sciences* **32**, 1622–44.

Helmer RP, Gruner O. 1977a: Vereinfachte Schadelidentifizieng nach dem Super projektionsver fahren mit Hilfe einer video-anlage. *Zectschrift Rectsmedizin* **80**, 183–7.

Helmer RP, Gruner O. 1977b: Schadelidentifizieng durch Super projektion nach dem verfahrer der elektronischen Bildmischung Modifiziert zum Trickbild-Differenz-Verfahren. *Zeitschrift für Rectsmedizin* **80**, 189–90.

Helmer RP, Schimmler JB, Rieger J. 1989: On the conclusiveness of skull identification via the video superimposition technique. *Canadian Society of Forensic Science Journal* **22**, 177–94.

Hoffman BE, McConathy DA, Coward M, Saddler L. 1991: Relationship between the Piriform aperture and interalar nasal widths in adult males. *Journal of Forensic Sciences* **36**, 1152–61.

Iten PY. 1987: Identification of skulls by video superimposition. *Journal of Forensic Sciences* **32**, 173–88.

Jacobson RE, Ray SF, Attridge GG. 1988: *The manual of photography*. London: Focal Press.

Janssens P, Hansch CF, Voorhamme LL. 1978: Identity determination by superimposition with anthropological cranium adjustment. *OSSA, International Journal of Skeletal Research* **5**, 109–22.

Kamijo Y, Sakai K. 1970: Basic study on superimposition with the application of roentgencephalometry. Report II: Postural relationship between soft and hard tissues of the human head and face, a study of special camera for superimposition. *National Research Institute of Police Science Report* 23 March, 10–17.

Kashyap VK, Rao NR. 1987: Importance of dental characteristics in superimposition opinion: a proforma for charting antemortem dental tracts. *Indian Journal of Forensic Sciences* **1**, 133–44.

Klonaris NS, Furue T. 1980: Photographic superimposition in dental identification: is a picture worth a thousand words? *Journal of Forensic Sciences* **25**, 859–65.

Koelmeyer TD. 1982: Videocamera superimposition and facial reconstruction as an aid to identification. *American Journal of Forensic Medicine and Pathology* **3**, 45–8.

Krogman WM, Iscan MY. 1986: *The human skeleton in forensic medicine*. Springfield, IL: Charles C. Thomas.

Lan Y-W, Tao C, Wang Y. 1990: A study on model TLGA-213 skull–image superimposition identification system. Paper presented at the 12th meeting of the International Association of Forensic Sciences, Adelaide, SA, October 22–29.

Lander KF. 1918: The examination of a skeleton of known age, race and sex. *Journal of Anatomy* **L11**, 282–91.

Loh FC, Chao TC. 1989: Skull and photographic superimposition: a new approach using a second party's interpupil distance to extrapolate the magnification factor. *Journal of Forensic Sciences* **34**, 708–13.

McKenna JJ. 1986: A qualitative and quantitative analysis of the anterior dentition visible in photographs and its application to forensic odontology. Thesis for the Degree of Master of Philosophy, University of Hong Kong.

McKenna JJ. 1988: A method of orientation of skull and camera for use in forensic photographic comparison. *Journal of Forensic Sciences* **33**, 751–5.

McKenna JJ, Jablonski NG, Fernhead RW. 1984: A method of matching skulls with photographic portraits using landmarks and measurements of the dentition. *Journal of Forensic Sciences* **29**, 787–97.

Pearson K. 1924: The skulls of Robert the Bruce, King of Scotland, 1274–329. *Biometrika* **XVI**, 18–272.

Pearson K. 1926: On the skull and portraits of George Buchanan. *Biometrika* **XVIII**, 16–256.

Pearson K. 1928: The skull and portraits of Henry Stewart, Lord Darnley, and their bearing on the tragedy of Mary, Queen of Scots. *Biometrika* **XX**, 1–104.

Pearson K, Morant GM. 1934: The Wilkinson head of Oliver Cromwell and its relationship to busts, masks and painted portraits. *Biometrika* **XXVI**, 18–378.

Prinsloo I. 1953: The identification of skeletal remains. *Journal of Forensic Medicine* **1**, 11–17.

Reddy KA. 1973: Identification of dismembered parts: the medico-legal aspects of the Nagaruju case. *Forensic Science* **2**, 351–74.

Sen N. 1962: Identification by superimposed photographs. *International Criminal Police Review* **162**, 284–6.

Shah SM, Joshi MR. 1978: An assessment of asymmetry in the normal craniofacial complex. *Angle Orthodontist* **48**, 141–8.

Simpson K. 1943a: Rex *v*. Dobkin: the Baptist Church cellar murder. *Medico-legal (and Criminological) Review* **11**, 132–45.

Simpson K. 1943b: Studies in reconstruction. 1: The Baptist Church cellar murder. Rex *v* Dobkin. *Guy's Hospital Report* Series 4, **92**, 74–81.

Stewart TD. 1983: The points of attachment of the palpebral ligaments. Their use in facial reconstructions on the skull. *Journal of Forensic Sciences* **28**, 858–63.

Sussman A. 1973: *The amateur photographer's handbook*. New York: Thomas Y. Crowell.

Taylor JA. 1988: Distortion in photography in forensic odontology. BScDent (Hons) thesis, Department of Dentistry, University of Adelaide.

Taylor JA. 1991: Distortion in craniofacial video superimposition. MScDent thesis, Department of Dentistry, University of Adelaide.

Thomas CJ, Nortje CJ, van Ieperen C. 1986: A case of skull identification by means of photographic superimposition. *Journal of Forensic Odonto-Stomatology* **4**, 61–6.

Tildesley ML. 1923: Sir Thomas Browne; his skull, portraits, and ancestry. *Biometrika* **XV**, 1–76.

Vig PS, Hewitt AB. 1975: Asymmetry of the human facial skeleton. *Angle Orthodontist* **45**, 125–9.

Walker A. 1982: A question of identity. *Police Review* Jul, 1406–7.

Webster G. 1955: Photography as an aid in identification – the Plumbago pit case. *Police Journal* **28**, 185–92.

Welcker H. 1867: On the skull of Dante. *Anthropological Review* **5**, 56–71.

CHAPTER 13

Quantification of facial shape and form

CDL THOMAS

Introduction	165	Representations and models	170
Properties of face and skull	166	Conclusion	174
Measurement of faces	167		

Introduction

For humans, the face is a primary means of interaction and identification. People can recognize a familiar face quickly and without conscious effort, particularly when they are in direct contact with the living person. In more difficult and stressful situations, for instance when it is necessary to identify the dead, to sort the guilty from the innocent or to help find the missing, such direct visual identification may be impossible. These situations require the creation of models or representations of the face. These representations may be based on an individual's anatomical knowledge and artistic skills (drawings and sculptures), they may be contained in numerical, computer-based descriptions or they may be a hybrid of the two. Quantitative descriptions of shape may aim, at the extreme, to replace opinion and human judgement, and at minimum to provide a consistent framework in which experts can exercise that judgement. It is the purpose of this chapter to discuss the quantitative aspects of such facial models, their characteristics and applications.

For identification purposes, facial shape is of interest when addressing questions in the areas of:

- offender description – what did he or she look like?

- identification from security camera pictures – which person was it?
- ageing of children's faces – what do they look like now?
- facial reconstruction – what did they look like in life?

Facial shape is also of importance to people working in areas other than identification, including:

- studies of the mechanisms of recognition – how do people recognize others?
- surgery and orthodontics – what will they look like if...?
- access control – is this face in the database of allowable faces?

Much of the current research into face shape and its quantification is being carried out by people interested in the second group of topics. Thus, although these fields are not directly concerned with problems of identification, they are of considerable importance to those interested in this area.

The following sections of this chapter describe some methods for acquiring measurements of faces, the properties of the face and skull that are important for modelling and some representations and models that are in current use. The conclusion attempts to highlight the relevance of the ideas described to identification; to point out areas of application and suggest some possibilities for future work.

Properties of face and skull

Before considering methods for the quantification of faces, an understanding of some of the properties of faces and facial shape is required. Consideration of these properties, in conjunction with details of the particular application, will guide the choice of methods used for quantitative measurement and description.

The appropriate definition of a face varies depending upon the intended purpose. Waters (1992) defines a face as 'the frontal view of the head from the base of the chin to the hair line, and the frontal half of the head from the lateral view'. This is a purely descriptive definition and is not necessarily useful in the case of a male whose hairline is around the occiput! An alternative was offered by Ferrario *et al.* (1992), who used a line 'between the submental soft tissue profile and the prolongation of the mandibular edge, and at the intersection of the forehead profile with a line joining the first point and the lateral eye canthus'. Vanco *et al.* (1995) defined the facial profile in terms of a line perpendicular to Camper's plane and passing 5 mm posterior to the nasion (Camper's plane being a line joining the trageal notch to the lower border of the ala of the nose). The profile was considered to be the soft tissue outline anterior to this line. The latter two definitions are useful as a basis for measurement, but both are dependent on the identification of soft tissue anatomical points, which are not always easy to locate repeatably. In a study involving 100 faces, Sheridan *et al.* (1995) encountered a problem in applying this latter definition because the vertical reference line sometimes excluded more of the forehead than was desirable (Fig. 13.1). Kapur *et al.* (1990) used a complex definition based on cephalometric hard tissue landmarks. This has the advantage of providing a much more repeatable definition of a face but with two sometimes overwhelming problems. It requires a lateral head radiograph and the portion of the profile used is very restricted, its upper limit being on the nose somewhere below the nasion and its lower limit near the point of the chin. In the early work of Lu (1965), a similar definition was used, but in this case the face was defined to be that portion of the profile between the menton and nasion and was thus slightly larger. The exclusion of the brow ridges and forehead from these latter definitions would seem to make them less than useful for identification purposes.

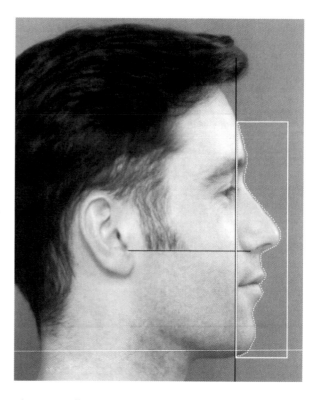

Fig. 13.1   Illustrating one definition of a facial profile. A concept originally presented by Vanco *et al.* (1995) and reproduced from Sheridan *et al.* (1997) with permission of the *Australian Orthodontic Journal*

In the case of manual reconstruction of a face over a skull, the artist creates a whole head. In a quantitative (computer-based) version of such an application, it would be desirable to work in the same manner rather than just model the face on its own. This would ensure that any constraints imposed on the shape of the face by the structure of the skull were adhered to by the model.

There are four billion faces in the world, and probably no two, even those of twins, are really identical. A face has a very complex structure, and the differences between individual faces can be very subtle. For all this, the general conformation of a (normal) face is always the same: the eyes are above the nose and spaced evenly each side of the midline, etc. In view of these two contrasting facts, it must be recognized that the differences between faces are second-order effects.

The surface of the skull is sharply curved in three dimensions and heavily indented and undercut. This complex foundation supports and anchors the muscles of expression, a total of around 100 individual muscles that have all developed from a single sheet in the embryo. This common origin, together with a common nerve supply, may be the underlying reason for the muscle groups in the face acting together for most purposes. The overlying skin is in two layers, the dermis being a viscoelastic material (Larrabee, 1986) with a thin covering of stratified epithelium covered by layers of dead cells (the epidermis). Beneath the dermis lie the subcutaneous tissues, including variable amounts of fat. Muscle tone and skin thickness, texture and elasticity vary between individuals and with ageing. This complexity of structure is reflected in the essentially infinite range of poses and expressions that a face and head can adopt.

In any model of a face, certain properties *must* be represented whereas others may not be needed for all purposes. A full list of properties would include size, surface area, volume, stiffness and other material characteristics, as well as opacity, colour, curvature, movement and the interactions between the various parts. If a quantitative model is to be used to represent changes in the face due to ageing, it must be able to represent changes in the skull and dentition and, most importantly, changes in the distribution and material properties of the soft tissue. Models of facial expression must be able to represent the dynamic response and changes in shape that occur in facial movement and may have to model the non-linear behaviour of soft tissue. Waters (1992) has described the requirements for this in detail.

The previous paragraphs have attempted to list the properties possessed by a face. What faces (and many other biological forms) *lack* are clearly defined edges or vertices, and this lack can have a profound effect on measurement systems used with faces. These are discussed in the next section.

Measurement of faces

Whatever the purpose for which a face is being analysed, the first step in the quantification of its shape is the assembly of a set of measurements unique to that face. The purpose for which the analysis is to be used will be the major determinant of the nature of this raw numerical description. The required accuracy, resolution and speed of response, and the number of dimensions in which measurements are made, are all characteristics of the type of application. This section describes the techniques currently available (or under development and therefore likely to become available in the foreseeable future) for the measurement of faces. These range from the use of images on their own, through the measurement of two-dimensional landmarks, to three-dimensional digitizers and structured light methods that give highly detailed lists of dimensions. Other details can be found in the review of acquisi-tion methods by Altobelli (1994) and the references provided therein.

Methods for measurement and description must record the three-dimensional contours of the face in a way that is accurate. They must be able to resolve the subtle differences between faces, yet be statistically manageable and practical for implementation in the circumstances in which they are likely to be used. The limitations on the applicability of any system stem from a number of considerations. These include the amount of time available (both for data acquisition and for analysis) and the degree of co-operation to be expected from the subject. Student volunteers or patients may be willing to have their heads held steady for several minutes, but bank robbers have been known to fire shotguns at security cameras on entering the bank. Other subjects may have different abilities to co-operate. While orthodontic patients are willing to stand still for a few minutes to have orthogonal pairs of photographs taken (see Chapter 11), they are unlikely to want grids of points drawn on their faces (see below).

IMAGES

The simplest quantitative description of a face is an image acquired under conditions of controlled geometry and lighting. Currently, these may be photographic (see Chapter 11, orthogonal photographic system), radiographic, video or digital still camera images, or obtained from a digital radiography system. The control of geometry and illumination is vital if useful measurements are to be extracted from the images, and this can be achieved by careful alignment of the subject in the camera co-ordinate system and by using standardized lighting (see Chapter 11). Images of all modalities are likely to be used as input to a computer system, if necessary following conversion to a computer-readable form ('digitization'). Photographs and radiographs are converted by scanning television frames by a video digitizer ('frame-grabber'). Once digitized, the morphology of an image becomes infinitely flexible, a characteristic that is both a great strength and, potentially, a great weakness of these methods. A digital image can be divided into sections, and the parts can be moved, copied, rotated and distorted ('morphed') in easily controlled ways. These processes are discussed in detail in the description of the FACE system.

If images are acquired using techniques such as computed tomography (CT) or magnetic resonance imaging (MRI), the data set consists of a series of sections through the head. These sections are two-dimensional images and can be reconstructed (by stacking) to give a three-dimensional representation but no numerical measurements. Features have then to be identified and the dimensions in some way extracted.

TWO- AND THREE-DIMENSIONAL POINT MEASUREMENTS

The most commonly used description of the shape of a face is a collection of measurements of discrete points, lines and angles (Farkas, 1994). The points may be defined by anatomical features (which are in general much better defined on the skull than on the surface of the soft tissue), or they may be artificially imposed on the surface. Bertillon, in 1889, created a method for offender identification that involved 11 linear measurements of the body, only two of which were of the head (Muller, 1977) (Fig. 13.2). This system was used successfully in France, the USA and elsewhere before being supplanted by fingerprinting early in the twentieth century. The success of 'Bertillonage' suggests that lists of linear measurements (including measurements of body size) can be used to identify individuals. The measurements were augmented by written descriptions of the eyes, hair colour and of the profile of the nose. Bertillon thus seems to have understood the improvement in discrimination that is to be obtained by combining different types of measurement from different parts of the body.

Jia and Nixon (1995) present a modern discussion of work that depends on such orthogonal (i.e. uncorrelated) data sets for improving the discrimination of automatic face recognition systems. Cephalometric analysis used in orthodontics involves the identification of anatomical points on a lateral radiograph of the head and the manual measurement of angles and distances. For surface measurement, datum points may simply be drawn on the face by hand (Kobayashi *et al.*, 1990) or may be generated by structured light techniques such as Moiré patterns (Kawai *et al.*, 1990) or projected grids (Fricker, 1985).

Stereophotogrammetry provides a way of extracting three-dimensional measurements from images and this has been used in facial analysis over a long period of time (Beard and Burke, 1967; Von Thomann and Rivett, 1982). The basis of this method is a stereoscopic pair of images taken under carefully controlled conditions and with cameras whose focal length, field of view and location have been calibrated (Newton, 1980). The two photographs are examined in a stereoplotter (e.g. Zeiss Jena Stecometer), and points that can be identified in both pictures can have their co-ordinates extracted by triangulation. Stereophotogrammetry provides precise measurements (±0.15 mm for clearly defined points, ±0.25 mm for points on the facial surface; Von Thomann and Rivett, 1982), but data extraction is slow (Von Thomann

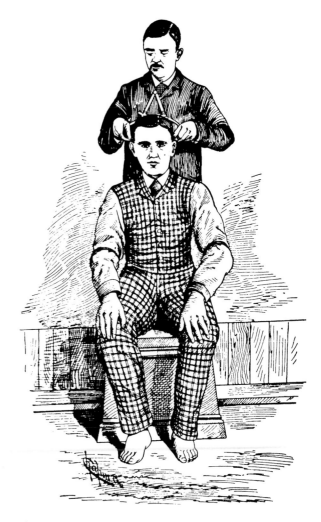

Fig. 13.2 In the English translation (Muller, 1977), Bertillon's method requires seven pages for the description of the taking of just the length and width of the head. Details of the face were recorded as a 'word picture'

reports about 2 hours per face for an expert technician). A significant problem is that the slowly changing smooth surfaces in a face do not provide many uniquely identifiable points for measurement. Structured light methods project a grid of points on to the face, thus overcoming the difficulties that stereophotogrammetry has with smooth surfaces lacking easily identifiable points.

Moiré diffraction has been used extensively in the quantification of shape, particularly for the planning and evaluation of surgery (Altobelli, 1994; Kawai *et al.*, 1990), and specialized equipment is available commercially (e.g. the Fujinon Moiré camera Model FM3013 mentioned by Kawai). The method employs a fine grating ruled on a transparent sheet through which the object to be analysed is illuminated by a point source. When viewed (and photographed) through the grating, the shadows of the lines produce an interference pattern with the lines themselves, and as the positions of the shadows are a function of the surface topology, the interference fringes contain quantitative information about the surface. As the angle between the surface and the plane of the image increases, the fringes become more closely spaced, and this limits the method to the measurement of faces with relatively flat contours.

Results from current research in computer vision (Shashua, 1994; Quan, 1995; Subbarao and Choi, 1995; Ulupinar and Nevatia, 1995; Weinshall and Tomasi, 1995) indicate that it is possible to recover the three-dimensional shape of objects from sequences of images. In particular, Azarbayejani and Pentland (1995) describe a system that recovers motion, shape and the focal length of the lens from a sequence of images. They compare the performance of this system with that of a Polhemus three-dimensional digitizer when identifying and tracking points on the surface of a face, and the results show that their system is at least as accurate as the digitizer. The errors in tracking are still of the order of 1 cm, but the results indicate that such methods can, with some further development, provide a way of extracting useful information from a sequence of uncalibrated images (e.g. security camera pictures).

THREE-DIMENSIONAL SURFACE SCANNING AND DIGITIZING

As a face is a three-dimensional object, it is likely that the most detailed measurements will come from systems that record measurements directly from the surface of the face; these include three-dimensional digitizers and laser scanners.

Three-dimensional surface digitizers employ such techniques as magnetic field measurement (Polhemus, Colchester, Vermont, USA), sound-ranging (Science Accessories Corp., Stratford, CT, USA) and the recording of the position of mechanical linkages (systems known as 'co-ordinate measuring machines' in mechanical engineering) (Browne and Sharp, Providence, RI, USA) (Thomas, 1988). All these systems offer good resolution and accuracy (in the range 0.1–1 mm), but they rely on manual probing of the surface to be measured. This will result in some deformation of the surface and is slow if any significant number of data points is to be acquired. These methods are much more suited to the measurement of individual anatomical points on skulls than to the tracing of continuous contours on the soft tissue of living subjects in whom movement, or a change of expression, may occur.

The most accurate and comprehensive measurements of faces have so far come from laser scanning machines. Moss *et al.* (1987) have described a unit built at University College, London, in which the subject is seated in a dental chair that is rotated under computer control. A pair of vertical lines of laser light are projected onto the face, and the profiles generated where the beams intersect the face are recorded using a television camera. Readings are taken every 3 degrees over most of the head and at 1 degree intervals around the nose where more detail is required. The scanning takes about 30 s and the final representation is accurate to 0.5 mm. The application of a commercial laser scanning machine (Cyberware, Monterey, CA, USA) to facial measurement has been described in detail by Altobelli (1994). The Cyberware unit is very similar to the one described above, the differences being that the subject remains still while the scanner rotates around them and there is only one line of light (Fig. 13.3).

Both these systems require the subject's head to be securely located for the duration of the scanning; they are thus only suitable for applications in which subjects are highly motivated and capable of co-operation. The very young, the old and infirm, and the unwilling all present obstacles to the use of these

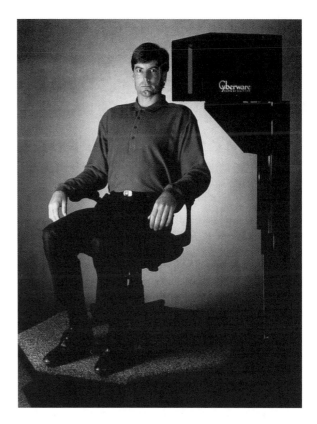

Fig. 13.3 A Cyberware digitizer and motion platform in use for scanning a face

systems, thus limiting their application in the identification of criminals.

CO-ORDINATE SYSTEMS

Once a set of data points has been created by any of the above methods, the points must be projected into a co-ordinate system related to the anatomy of the head. The location of the origin of this co-ordinate system is problematical. Altobelli (1994) suggests the use of the soft-tissue nasion when the measurements are to be used in surgical planning, but for purposes involving rotations of the head or for growth measurements, an anatomically well-defined and stable point close to the rotational centre of the head is needed. The difficulty with this is that such a point (the most anterior point on the foramen magnum, for example) will only be available radiographically. The provision of an anatomically relevant horizontal reference can also present difficulties. Some systems attempt to bring the subject into a relaxed and reproducible stance that results in the head being in a 'natural' position (see Chapter 11). Alternatives to this are the Frankfort horizontal or a plane defined by infra-orbitale and porion. The midsagittal plane can be established by bisecting a line joining the inner canthi, although this may be inadequate if the face is highly asymmetrical. Once an origin and a set of reference points and planes have been identified, three-dimensional co-ordinate geometry can be used to rotate and translate the measured co-ordinates into the anatomically defined system. (Scale is presumed to have been established by calibration of the measuring system.) For any given application, the choice of co-ordinate system and origin will depend on the nature of the application and on the data acquisition methods available.

Representations and models

A description of a face may be made at several levels of complexity. It may be simply a surface representation (an image in two dimensions, or a sculpture if it is in three). It may be a collection of images of parts of the face, a list of two- or three-dimensional co-ordinates or landmarks that can describe the basic proportions of a head. The description might also include an analytical model of the materials, structures and mechanisms comprising and controlling the face. Images consist of an array of grey-scale or colour values that have meaning only when viewed by a human observer. They contain no inherent information about the object portrayed. A geometrical or mechanical model, on the other hand, includes the physical and material characteristics of the anatomical parts of a head and can thus represent structural and functional information. The various forms of geometric and physical models are therefore a higher-level representation and contain considerably more information than do images or point-sets. The degree to which these forms of representation correspond to process of face recognition in the human brain will not be discussed here. However, it should be recognized that it is those human recognition processes that any method of identification is seeking to stimulate, so methods that best meet this requirement are the ones most likely to result in successful identifications.

The elements of an object description can be classified by the amount of information each such element carries. This classification might start with points (which are arbitrary positions in three-dimensional space) and landmarks (a point with some biological meaning, defined later). A classification could be extended to include distances, lines, angles, surfaces (two- and three-dimensional) and volumes as well as volumes that have physical properties ascribed to them (e.g. the elements in a three-dimensional finite-element model).

FACIAL MODELS BASED ON POINT DATA

Sets of points, line lengths and angles can describe the basic proportions of a face and are useful in models of growth and for anthropological comparisons (Farkas and Munro, 1987; Farkas and Posnick, 1992; Farkas, 1994). They cannot, however, describe the appearance of the face in a form recognizable by humans. Landmarks carry some additional information. Bookstein (1990) defined a landmark as follows:

> a landmark is a location that has a biological meaning as well as a geometric location in two or three dimensions. . . . The biological term for this correspondence is homology, and so landmarks are often called 'homologous points'. The most useful landmarks are . . . single points identifiable by local properties of tissue in their vicinity.

Radiographic hard tissue (cephalometric) points on the skull have the best chance of being accurately and reproducibly defined. Tooth cusps, the auditory meatii and nasion, for example, can all be identified clearly. Soft tissue points – such as the tip of the nose, 'the most anterior point of the chin' (pogonion) – are, as Bookstein points out (1978), often 'extremal' landmarks. They are defined by the geometry, rather than the biology, of the structure. Descriptions of their locations are therefore dependent on the co-ordinate system chosen for measurement, and the problem of defining an origin (or centre of rotation) has been previously discussed.

On the surface of the face, in fact, clearly defined landmarks are uncommon, and the problem with using landmark data for cephalometrics has been discussed in detail by Moyers and Bookstein (1979). Even on the skull, there may be difficulties: Baumrind and Frantz (1971) discuss errors in head film measurements and conclude that these 'stem in part from antecedent errors in landmark identification'. Moss *et al.* (1992) discuss the problems mentioned above and go on to present a method for the description of facial profiles based on the analysis of curvature. The landmarks used in this work were defined as 'mathematically derived landmarks that are particular extremal points on the outlines (i.e. points of maximum and minimum curvature)'. These authors also make the important point that, in the study of growth, it is necessary to 'consider not only the relative movement of landmarks, but also the changes in shape of the segments between the landmarks'. Some of the properties of descriptions of such segments are discussed in the next section.

OUTLINES

Measurements of point locations, lines and the angles between them evolved to describe geometrical objects and were never intended to include elements for the description of complex, irregular forms (Lestrel, 1989). Points, landmarks and lines can be linked together to form outlines of forms (for example, the profile of a face). A point's only property is its location; outlines have the additional properties of shape and size. Very simple shapes can be described completely by a shape name and a set of qualifiers (dimensions, colour and texture, for example): 'a red circle of radius two', 'a blue square of side four', 'a grey rectangle...' etc. Thus a description (in these cases, the name) of the shape and some qualifying information are combined to describe the *form* of the object. Looked at in another way, the *shape* of an object is what is left after all information regarding location, orientation, size and colour has been removed from its description. For example, the use of sets of anthropometric data to describe a face (particularly where distances are standardized to some fixed dimension such as the intercanthal distance), and the normalization of Fourier shape coefficients (Kuhl and Giardina, 1982) to provide a template by which a shape can be recognized, are typical of this separation of shape information from the rest of an object model. Simple descriptions such as those given above for geometric objects are not available for the shape of a face or head, and to represent these, richer and more detailed methods are needed.

Fourier shape analysis has been used by many workers for the description of biological outlines (Lu, 1965; O'Higgins and Williams, 1987; Kapur *et al.*, 1990; Vanco *et al.*, 1995). It has been shown to be useful for the quantification both of shape and of shape change. The output from this method is a set of numbers (coefficients) whose size depends directly on the amount of detail that is required. Typically, 30 or fewer coefficients will provide a highly accurate representation of a shape such as a facial profile (Fig. 13.4). In the case of some of the lower-order coefficients, it may be possible to ascribe anatomical meaning to their values (Fig. 13.5) (Sheridan *et al.*, 1997). Further study is required to determine the value of Fourier analysis for the identification of individual faces, but the technique seems promising.

IMAGES OF THE FACE

The current state of the art in identification often relies on an image of a face as the basic form of information. The use of such two-dimensional representations has proved very successful but has some inherent problems that limit their usefulness and which have to be taken into account when evaluating identifications obtained using such methods.

Video superimposition systems (see Chapter 12), used for the matching of skulls to photographs of living people, employ electronic techniques to manipulate video images and thus use these images as representations of a face and skull (Iscan and Helmer, 1993). There is, however, no underlying model of a face to control the modifications made to the images in these systems. Therefore, there are no internal constraints imposed on the changes of scale, viewing angle and perspective that are used to try to achieve a match. These modifications are carried out interactively by human operators who base their judgement of what is reasonable on their personal understanding of faces and photography. Fixed reference points are essential to provide some control over what is otherwise a freehand method with many degrees of freedom. These references are best provided by the teeth, and thus photographs of smiling subjects are preferable, or even essential, for this method to give valid results.

Systems used for constructing pictures of offenders and missing persons (e.g. Identikit, Photofit and FACE) all use frontal views of the face. These systems divide the face into the units that people use when describing a face (hair, eyes, nose, mouth and chin). Their purpose is to produce approximate representations of subjects that can be distributed within the police and to the media in the hope of the subject being recognized. The computer-based FACE system allows the controlled distortion ('morphing') of indi-

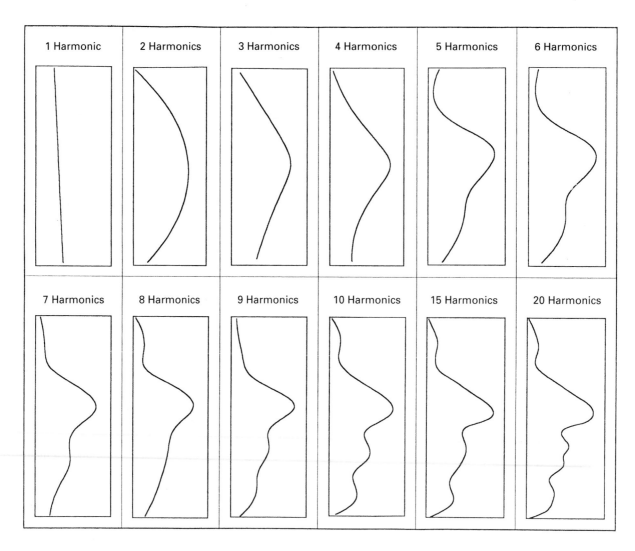

Fig. 13.4   The reconstruction of a facial profile from a set of Fourier shape descriptors. By the time 20 harmonics are in use, most of the detail in the profile is reproduced. Using 30 harmonics will give a near-perfect reproduction. Reproduced from Sheridan *et al.* (1997) with permission of the *Australian Orthodontic Journal*

vidual components, which greatly broadens the range of faces that can be represented. This process is only valid if it is assumed that a face can be depicted as two-dimensional. For many profiles, this is approximately correct, as in many faces the eyes, nose and tip of the chin do not lie far from a common plane.

If the task is to identify a person (or compare identities) from photographs, the 'flat face' assumption is weaker. Security camera pictures, for example, rarely show offenders full face or from the same viewpoint relative to the head. For comparisons between photos to have any validity, standardization of camera position and angle, as well as head position, must be attempted (Bruce *et al.*, 1992).

The rotation and scaling of pictures of faces has

two geometric sources of error. First, it requires assumptions of symmetry to fill in previously hidden surfaces. Second, if it does not take into account their three-dimensional nature, some distortion will occur. With current technology, these problems are not likely to be solved by changes in imaging methods, so systems for recognition need to be very robust or to have multiple views of each person in their databases (Beymer, 1993). Bruce *et al.* (1992) comment that 'changing the shape of such features as the nose or jaw may be achieved more naturally using a 3-D representation'. For many purposes, three-dimensional systems will be of increasing importance, particularly with the rapid increase in the affordability of computer graphics systems.

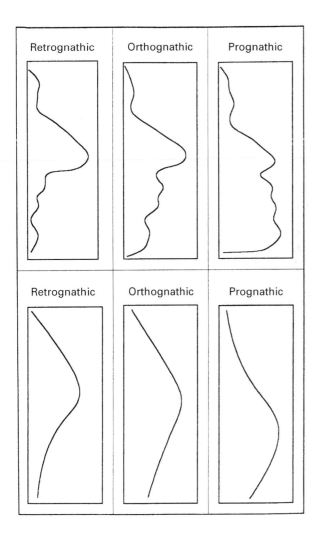

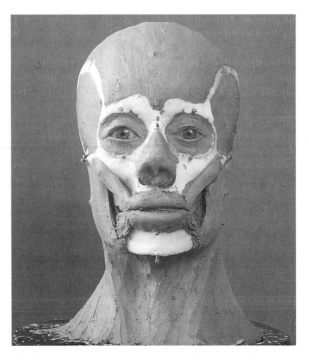

Fig. 13.6 A partially complete facial reconstruction in clay. Such work can take up to 10 days and requires the sculptor to be specially trained and to have extensive anatomical knowledge. Photo courtesy of Mr R Taylor, School of Dental Science, University of Melbourne

Fig. 13.5 Facial profiles with minimum (upper left), median (upper centre) and maximum (upper right) values of the third shape harmonic. Below are the corresponding reconstructions using the first three harmonics. Reproduced from Sheridan *et al.* (1997) with permission of the *Australian Orthodontic Journal*

THREE-DIMENSIONAL MODELS

Until it became possible to render an image of a three-dimensional numerical using computer graphics, the only three-dimensional representation of a face was that produced by a sculptor or forensic artist. Such sculpted renderings can be no more accurate than the skill and anatomical knowledge of the artist permits (Fig. 13.6); they are static, and they cannot easily be duplicated. Despite these limitations, many successful identifications of missing people have been made based on a facial reconstruction over a skull. At the time of writing, the author

knows of no quantitative system for creating such a rendering, although attempts have been made to do this (Evenhouse *et al.*, 1992). However, whenever a three-dimensional model of a face is required for identification purposes, that model is created by an artist using anatomical knowledge. Work from other areas may be applicable for identification, some of which is described below along with some general observations on the characteristics of three-dimensional models of the face.

In general, a three-dimensional model can be either a surface representation (i.e. a hollow shell with no internal structure but only size, shape, texture and colour) or a solid model, which offers the possibility of representing internal structure and mechanical properties. A model may be static or deformable; i.e. it may be simply a quantitative numerical sculpture or it may be able to reproduce changes in expression, the appearance of speech and the effects of gravity.

Three-dimensional finite element models are made up of solid 'bricks', usually tetrahedral or hexahedral in form. Physical properties, such as mass, density and elastic moduli, can be assigned to these bricks, and these properties can be made non-linear and thus able to model biological materials. A model consists of a large number of bricks of appropriate size and shape combined to approximate the object being analysed, the sizes being chosen to allow the modelling of the smallest meaningful structure desired. There is no explicit quantification of shape (compare the Fourier description of an outline, which does carry absolute shape information); these models can only directly describe shape *changes* (Lestrel, 1989). Sets of bricks representing separate layers of material (for example bone, muscle tissue, fat and skin) can be combined and the nature of the interface between them (rigidly attached or varying degrees of sliding) defined. To build such a model in sufficient detail to be recognizable as an individual would be very challenging with current technology and not necessarily very useful. The appearance would change under differing poses (due to gravity), but the models as described are essentially static: they cannot reproduce the action of muscles and changes in expression.

Explicit representations of facial anatomy (bone, muscle, fat and skin) have been used to create systems that can behave very realistically and can produce lifelike expressions. These have been constructed by Waters and Terzopoulos (1990), Waters (1992) and Lee *et al.* (1995). These models have representations of bone, three types of muscle (linear, sphincter and sheet structures) and skin (divided into dermis and epidermis). The muscle models have varying 'spring constants' that describe the relationship between tension and length, and they also have size and orientation. The facial tissue is modelled as a lattice of springs that will deform realistically under gravity and into which the outer ends of muscles are attached. Thus the effects of both changes in pose (the effects on the face being due to gravity) and the effects of muscle contraction can be reproduced. So far, this work has not attempted to recreate recognizable images of real people, but the potential to do this appears to be present. A lifelike and expressive face was created using 960 polygons and 6500 spring elements. Just how much more complex the model would have to be to imitate an individual successfully is unknown. However, this area appears to deserve further investigation. Recognition of a face depends on more than just shape (other possible characteristics include wrinkles and lines, colour and texture, characteristic expression and hairstyle), so quantitative descriptions that model only shape may well be inadequate for identification purposes.

Further possible computer methods for the representation of deformable solid objects are discussed in a review by Hersh (1990). Some of these, particularly 'space-filling blobs' and constructive solid geometry (CSG), may offer useful ideas for the realistic modelling of facial shape in the near future.

Conclusion

When reviewing mathematical modelling of the head and face, Lestrel (1989) stated, 'It is apparent that a generalised model for the characterisation of complex morphological forms remains to be developed.' This statement may well always remain true, as each application makes differing demands on the methodology and technology employed, and a truly general method may not exist. The representation of a face that is appropriate for any given purpose has to be matched to the requirements of that purpose. In O'Higgins and Williams (1987), the authors state: 'the way in which a shape is measured and the benefit of such measurements is highly dependent upon the questions that are being asked about it.' Differing methods are needed for generating a picture of an offender from a witness description, for use in studies of recognition, for facial reconstruction over a skull and so on. We can look back to the list of purposes in the introduction and at some of the possible applications for which methods are required.

The necessary precision and accuracy must be considered for any of the possible applications. These are fundamental considerations in the design of any measurement system or mathematical model. Beymer (1993) achieved good results with very simple low-resolution models – in two dimensions, and for computer recognition purposes. If the representation were to be used for facial reconstruction, a large number of data points and a level of resolution better than 1 mm would be required. At present, no complete quantitative system for such reconstruction is known to the author.

Representations may be either two- or three-dimensional, the choice being determined by the nature of the application, the type of data available and the level of complexity that can be justified. Three dimensions are essential for surgical and orthodontic planning (Linney, 1992) and are inherent in facial reconstruction. For offender identification, two-dimensional drawings or composite images have proved adequate, although advances in computer software and capabilities may make a reappraisal of this approach worthwhile. In terms of surface versus volume rendering, surgery simulation and facial reconstruction require internal anatomical information whereas identification and psychological research do not. Realistic animation may need a *model* of the anatomy, but this does not need to be an accurate representation of an individual.

In the case of the ageing of faces, the representation is required to model growth and perhaps other changes. It may be necessary to link points on a surface that describes a face with actual anatomical points and to have a set of standards for the growth of differing facial types (Langenbach *et al.*, 1995). Correspondences between anatomical points also form the basis of identification by photosuperimposition although, in this case, the points are embedded in images of the face and skull being compared. Anthropometric measurements form the basis of models of growth, and these are an essential part of any attempt to forecast the changes in appearance of childrens' faces with age. Changes in skin colour and texture, hairstyle and soft tissue thickness also need to be taken into account to complete the prediction of changes of appearance with age.

Some methods allow the facial model to generate varying expressions under control of an operator (Waters and Terzopoulos, 1990). Other models are dynamic, i.e. they are able to produce a time sequence of images in which the face is changing expression or pose. Some of the purposes to which facial models are put require such dynamic performance: image compression for video conferencing, animation and some psychological research projects being examples. Although these dynamic capabilities are more relevant to recognition studies and computer animation than they are to identification, these other fields of study may well provide the techniques that will be adopted in the next generation of identification software. Current systems for producing facial images from witness descriptions do not incorporate variable expressions as such but do allow an artist to modify the face considerably. In the future, such systems might allow a police criminal identification operator to ask a witness to choose a type of facial expression ('laughing', 'frightened', etc.) and have the face being created adopt that expression automatically.

THE NEED FOR IMPROVED QUANTITATIVE THREE-DIMENSIONAL METHODS

A recognizable, animated model of a face, perhaps based on methods similar to those of Waters and Terzopoulos, as described above, could provide a very powerful tool for the identification of individuals in many circumstances. The problems with defining a face (mentioned earlier) are overcome if a fully three-dimensional model of the head is used, but at the expense of more complex data acquisition methods. The possibilities of computer-based facial reconstruction were canvassed by Bruce *et al.* (1992), and at least two attempts have been made (or are in progress) to create tools to assist artists in producing adequate models (Evenhouse *et al.*, 1992; Langenbach *et al.*, 1995).

References

Altobelli DE. 1994: Computer-assisted acquisition of facial surface topography. In Farkas LG. (ed.) *Anthropometry of the head and face*. New York: Raven Press, 219–33.

Azarbayejani A, Pentland AP. 1995: Recursive estimation of motion, structure, and focal length. *IEEE Transactions on Pattern Analysis and Machine Intelligence* **17**(6), 562–75.

Baumrind S, Frantz RC. 1971: The reliability of head film measurements. Part 2: Conventional angular and linear measures. *American Journal of Orthodontics* **60**(5), 505–17.

Beard LFH, Burke PH. 1967: Evolution of a system of stereophotogrammetry for the study of facial morphology. *Medical and Biological Illustration* **17**, 20–5.

Beymer DJ. 1993: *Face recognition under varying pose*. Boston, MA: Massachusetts Institute of Technology, Artificial Intelligence Laboratory.

Bookstein FL. 1978: *The measurement of biological shape and shape change*. Berlin: Springer-Verlag.

Bookstein FL. 1990: *Visualizing biological shape differences*. First conference on visualization in biomedical computing, May 22–25, 1990, Atlanta, GA. IEEE Computer Society.

Bruce V, Burton M, Doyle T *et al.* 1992: Faces as surfaces. In Bruce V, Burton M. (eds) *Processing images of faces*. Norwood, NJ: Ablex.

Evenhouse R, Rasmussen M, Sadler L *et al.* 1992: Computer-aided forensic facial reconstruction. *Journal of Biocommunication* **19**(2), 22–8.

Farkas LG. 1994: *Anthropometry of the head and face*. New York: Raven Press.

Farkas LG, Munro IR. 1987: *Anthropometric facial proportions in medicine*. Springfield, IL: Charles C. Thomas.

Farkas LG, Posnick JC. 1992: Growth and development of regional units in the head and face based on anthropometric measurements. *Cleft Palate-Craniofacial Journal* **29**(4), 301–29.

Ferrario VF, Sforza C, Miani A, Poggio CE, Schmitz J. 1992: Harmonic analysis and clustering of facial profiles. *International Journal of Adult Orthodontics and Orthognathic Surgery* **7**(3), 171–9.

Fricker JP. 1985: Projected grid facial photography. *Australian Dental Journal* **30**(6), 414–7.

Hersh JS. 1990: *A survey of modelling representations and their application to biomedical visualization and simulation*. First conference on visualization in biomedical computing, May 22–25, 1990, Atlanta, GA. IEEE Computer Society.

Iscan MY, Helmer RP. 1993: *Forensic analysis of the skull*. New York: Wiley-Liss.

Jia X, Nixon MS. 1995: Extending the feature vector for automatic face recognition. *IEEE Transactions on Pattern Analysis and Machine Intelligence* **17**(12), 1167–76.

Kapur KK, Lestrel PE, Garrett NR, Chauncey HH. 1990: The use of Fourier analysis to determine age-related changes in the facial profile. *International Journal of Prosthodontics* **3**(3), 266–73.

Kawai T, Natsume N, Shibata H, Yamamoto T. 1990: Three-dimensional analysis of facial morphology using moire stripes. Part I: Method. *International Journal of Oral and Maxillofacial Surgery* **19**(6), 359–62.

Kobayashi T, Ueda K, Honma K, Sasakura H, Hanada K, Nakajima T. 1990: Three-dimensional analysis of facial morphology before and after orthognathic surgery. *Journal of Cranio-Maxillo-Facial Surgery* **18**(2), 68–73.

Kuhl FP, Giardina CR. 1982: Elliptic features of a closed contour. *Computer Graphics and Image Processing* **18**, 236–58.

Langenbach G, Forsey D, Cahoon P, Sweet D, Leroy H, Hannam A. 1995: *Facial reconstruction for the identification of growing children.* Sixth annual meeting of the International Association for Craniofacial Identification, Boca Raton, FL.

Larrabee W. 1986: A finite element model of skin deformation. Part 1: Biomechanics of skin and soft tissue. *Laryngoscope* **96**, 399–419.

Lee Y, Terzopoulos D, Waters K. 1995: *Realistic modelling for facial animation.* SIGGRAPH 95. Los Angeles, CA: ACM.

Lestrel P. 1989: Some approaches toward the modelling of the craniofacial complex. *Journal of Craniofacial Genetics and Developmental Biology* **9**, 77–91.

Linney AD. 1992: The use of 3-D computer graphics for the simulation and prediction of facial surgery. In Bruce V, Burton M. (eds) *Processing images of faces.* Norwood, NJ: Ablex, 149–78.

Lu KH. 1965: Harmonic analysis of the human face. *Biometrics* Jun, 491–505.

Moss JP, Linney AD, Grindrod SR, Arridge SR, Clifton JS. 1987: Three-dimensional visualization of the face and skull using computerized tomography and laser scanning techniques. *European Journal of Orthodontics* **9**, 247–53.

Moss JP, Campos JC, Linney AD. 1992: The analysis of profiles using curvature analysis. *European Journal of Orthodontics* **14**(6), 457–61.

Moyers RE, Bookstein FL. 1979: The inappropriateness of conventional cephalometrics. *American Journal of Orthodontics* **75**(6), 599–617.

Muller G. 1977: *Alphonse Bertillon's instructions for taking descriptions for the identification of criminals and others by the means of anthropometric indications.* New York: AMS Press.

Newton I. 1980: Medical photogrammetry. In Atkinson KB. (ed.) *Developments in close range photogrametry.* London: Applied Science Publishers, 117–48.

O'Higgins P, Williams NW. 1987: An investigation into the use of Fourier coefficients in characterizing cranial shape in primates. *Journal of Zoology* (London) **211**, 409–30.

Quan L. 1995: Invariants of six points and projective reconstruction from three uncalibrated images. *IEEE Transactions on Pattern Analysis and Machine Intelligence* **17**(1), 34–46.

Shashua A. 1994: Projective structures from uncalibrated images: structure from motion and recognition. *IEEE Transactions on Pattern Analysis and Machine Intelligence* **16**(8), 778–90.

Sheridan C, Clement J, Thomas CDL. 1995: A Fourier shape analysis study of sexual dimorphism of facial profile in adolescents and children. *Australian Dental Journal* **40**(4), 264.

Sheridan CS, Thomas CDL *et al.* 1997: Quantification of ethnic differences in facial profile. *Australian Orthodontic Journal* **14**(4), 218–24.

Subbarao M, Choi T. 1995: Accurate recovery of three-dimensional shape from image focus. *IEEE Transactions on Pattern Analysis and Machine Intelligence* **17**(3), 266–74.

Thomas D. 1988: A 3-dimensional digitiser using spherical co-ordinates. *Australian Dental Journal* **33**(2), 138–43.

Ulupinar F, Nevatia R. 1995: Shape from contour: straight homogenous generalized cylinders and constant cross-section generalized cylinders. *IEEE Transactions on Pattern Analysis and Machine Intelligence* **17**(2), 120–35.

Vanco C, Kasai K, Seergi R, Richards LC, Townsend GC. 1995: Genetic and environmental influences on facial profile. *Australian Dental Journal* **40**(2), 104–9.

Von Thomann J, Rivett LJ. 1982: Applications of photogrammetry to orthodontics. *Australian Orthodontic Journal* **7**(4), 162–7.

Waters K. 1992: Modelling three-dimensional facial expressions. In Bruce V, Burton M. (eds) *Processing images of faces.* Norwood, NJ: Ablex, 202–27.

Waters K, Terzopoulos D. 1990: *A physical model of facial tissue and muscle articulation.* Proceedings of the first conference on visualization in biomedical computing, May 22–25, 1990, Atlanta, GA. IEEE Computer Society.

Weinshall D, Tomasi C. 1995: Linear and incremental acquisition of invariant shape models from image sequences. *IEEE Transactions on Pattern Analysis and Machine Intelligence* **17**(5), 512–7.

Places on the Internet where facial analysis or face recognition are discussed include:

- Face recognition home page: http://www.cs.rug.nl/~peterkr/FACE/face.html
- Facial animation home page: http://mambo.ucsc.edu/psl/fan.html
- The Sheffield Facial Reconstruction Project: http://www.shef.ac.uk/~assem/evison.html

CHAPTER 14

Facial reconstruction and approximation

RG TAYLOR, C ANGEL

Introduction	177	Three-dimensional facial reconstruction	181
Preliminary collection of data	177	Duplication of the reconstruction	184
Duplication of the skull	178	Conclusion	185

Introduction

Three-dimensional reconstruction of the face from a skull may be carried out to assist in the identification of human remains but is only used when more reliable methods have failed or are impossible. As a technique used for identification, it has definite limitations, but it still has a valuable role in forensic identification. The three-dimensional reconstruction image may later be altered, via computer software or other means, enabling further characterization and adjustment in a more efficient and rapid manner than with traditional three-dimensional reconstruction methods.

Variations of many aspects of the reconstruction method described in this chapter are possible (Caldwell, 1986; Krogman and Iscan, 1986), but a successful reconstruction can only be carried out if the person is familiar with the normal human anatomy of the skull and attached soft tissues, dental occlusion, sculpting and split-mould techniques of duplication. The steps involved in a reconstruction may include collection of preliminary data, duplication of the skull, reconstruction of the soft tissues and duplication of the reconstruction.

Preliminary collection of data

Although the skull is the basis of the reconstruction, other valuable physical remains may be available. Occasionally, reconstruction of only part of the skull soft tissues is required, and close inspection of the soft tissue remaining by the person carrying out the reconstruction is obviously then vital. Jewellery found with the deceased, such as earrings and necklaces, may be incorporated in to the final reconstruction, as may hats, glasses or other accessories. The finding of hair with the human remains is obviously invaluable in choosing hair colour and style in the reconstruction. Details of race, sex, age and build may be obtained by a thorough examination of skeletal remains, teeth, clothing and jewellery (see Chapters 2, 5 and 6). This information is usually provided by other specialists such as police, forensic pathologists, anthropologists and odontologists, either directly or in the form of written reports, and should be avidly sought for every reconstruction.

Close examination of the skull may reveal details that affect the final reconstruction. Clearly, if the facial skeleton is incomplete or not intact, a preliminary reconstruction of the bony skeleton will be required (see Chapter 5). Occasionally, bony pathology will be present, which may influence the soft tissue reconstruction and lead to asymmetry. More commonly, the prominence of certain bony landmarks, such as the supraorbital ridges and zygomas, will affect the general appearance of the eyes. The ruggedness of muscle attachments, profile of the jaws and bony face, and symmetry of the nasal bones may all give clues to the gross appearance. The dentition and/or dentures should be closely examined as they give clues to articulation of the mandible with the maxilla. It is possible that loss of the vertical dimension of the face owing to excessive wear of the occlusal surfaces, abnormal posturing of the mandible and soft tissue support of the lips may have occurred.

Duplication of the skull

Although the reconstruction may be carried out directly on the skull, as advised by Caldwell (1986), it is often preferable to duplicate the skull and carry out the reconstruction on a plaster model. Advantages of using a duplicate include minimizing damage to the skull and having the skull available as a reference during the reconstruction. It may even be essential if the skull is available only for a short time or if multiple reconstructions of the single skull are to be made.

Uncommonly, some of the soft tissues covering the skull remain intact but not those of the face. In such cases the skull with its attached soft tissue is duplicated. However, usually only the bony skull and minimal or no other soft tissue remains are present. In this cases, the skull is cleaned and the remaining soft tissue removed. If the skull is incomplete, damaged or fragmented, these defects need to be repaired, for example with wax (Fig. 14.1a). The degree of accuracy with which this can be done varies with the site of the damage and decreases with increasing size of the defect.

Re-articulation of the mandible is relatively simple if natural or artificial teeth are present. The mandible is positioned so that the teeth are in centric occlusion and the mandibular condyles in the glenoid fossae of the temporal bone. The mandible is then held in place by the judicious use of wax (Fig. 14.1b). In an edentulous person in whom no dentures are found, average measurements are used to establish the vertical dimension between the mandible and maxilla, and occlusal wax rims similar to those used in the construction of dentures are used. A similar technique is used when there are an insufficient number of teeth to articulate the mandible with the maxilla. The wearing of dentures can dramatically affect facial appearance and emphasizes the importance of accurate positioning of the mandible.

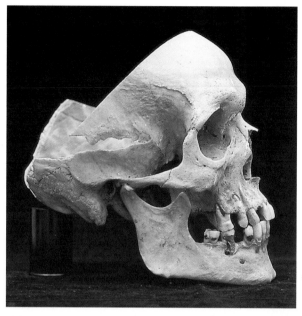

(a)

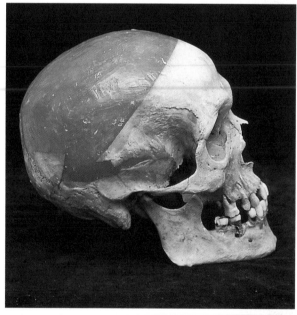

(b)

Fig. 14.1 (a) Skull dried and cleaned for duplication. (b) Repair of a substantial part of the calvarium has been required on this skull. Sizeable repairs to the facial skeleton may considerably reduce the accuracy

Prior to duplicating the skull, unnecessary undercuts, such as the foramen magnum, the external acoustic meatus, the anterior and posterior nasal openings and the zygomatic arches, are blocked out. Modelling clay is a useful material for blocking out undercuts as it is pliable, non-toxic, inert and easily washed away after duplication has been completed. The orbits are fitted with plaster or prosthetic eyes at this stage to remove the undercut of the bony orbit. Again, modelling clay is used to hold the eyes in position. The eyes are centered in a line between the midpoints of the superior and inferior orbital rims, and should be just visible when viewed from above, as advised by Gatliff and Snow (1979) (Fig. 14.2).

A split-cast technique is employed to duplicate the skull. The skull is supported by modelling clay so that the face is upright and the plane passing through the mental sulcus, body of the mandible, zygomatic arch, external acoustic meatus and parietal bones is horizontal (Fig. 14.3). A horizontal table of clay 5 cm wide is added around the entire skull and notched at regular intervals (to facilitate later accurate positioning of both halves of the completed cast). A suitable quantity of impression material (e.g. 450 g alginate powder) is mixed and applied to the skull, initially by rubbing it on to the surface by hand and then by pouring it over the skull. The impression material needs to be strong, flexible and slow-setting. Once set, thin plastic film is applied to the outside of the impression material (to act as a separating medium). An outer plaster supporting layer is then poured. Before the plaster is set, a shallow groove is made in

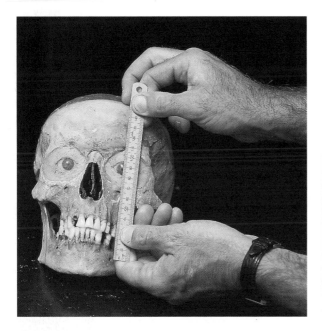

Fig. 14.2 The prosthetic eye is positioned midway between the superior and inferior orbital margins on the skull prior to duplication

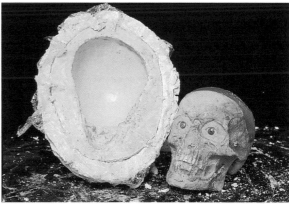

(a)

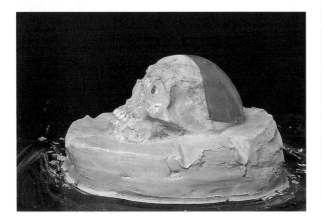

Fig. 14.3 The initial step in the production of the split-cast mould involves embedding the skull in modelling clay. A table of clay 5 cm wide is built around the skull and notched at regular intervals. (This will result in accurate joining of the two halves of the completed cast)

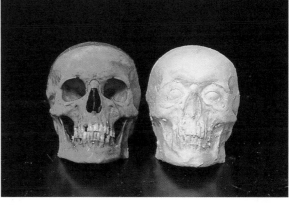

(b)

Fig. 14.4 (a) The skull being devested. The completed split cast is carefully separated to avoid tearing the impression material. (b) The original skull should be compared with the duplicate model. Used carefully, several models can be made from the single split cast

Table 14.1 Soft tissue thicknesses

Depth sites	Welcker (1883) Germans	His (1895) Germans		Kollman and Buchly (1898) Swiss		Suzuki (1948) Japanese		Rhine and Campbell (1980) American blacks		O'Grady et al. (1990) Male		Female Thin		Female Well nourished	
		M	F	M	F	M	F	M	F	AV	SD	AV	SD	AV	SD
Occipital	6.8														
Middle of parietal	5.3														
Upper forehead		4.06	4.16	3.07	3.02										
Hairline															
Middle forehead	4.3					3.0	2.0	4.75	4.5	4.6	1.4	2.5	1.1	3.6	1.1
Glabella		5.10	4.75	4.29	3.90	3.8	3.2	6.25	6.25	6.6	2.0	4.8	1.2	6.0	1.5
Nasion/nasal root	5.9	5.55	5.0	4.31	4.1	4.1	3.4	6.00	5.75	6.8	1.2	4.9	1.0	5.8	2.2
Mid nasal bone	3.3	3.37	3.0	3.13	2.57					3.3	1.3	2.7	1.1	2.8	0.6
Tip of nasal bone	2.2			2.12	2.07	2.2	1.6	3.75	3.75	3.9	1.6	2.5	0.8	3.8	1.9
Mid philtrum		11.49	9.75	11.65	10.1			12.25	11.25	12.9	4.1	8.9	2.1	12.3	2.8
Akanthion															
Upper lip margin Prosthion	11.0	9.51	8.26	9.46	8.1			14.0	13.0	11.0	3.0	7.3	2.7	8.3	2.5
Mental sulcus	10.6	10.26	9.75	9.84	10.95	10.5	8.5	12.0	12.0	11.9	2.9	10.4	1.3	13.2	2.6
Mental eminence	8.5	11.43	10.75	9.02	9.37	6.2	5.3	12.25	12.25	9.1	2.3	5.4	1.0	8.9	2.9
Beneath chin		6.18	6.5	5.98	5.88	4.8	2.8	8.0	7.75	9.4	3.3	5.3	1.3	7.5	2.1
Mid supraorbital		5.89	5.5	5.41	5.15	4.5	3.6	4.75	4.50	8.0	1.6	5.4	1.3	7.4	1.3
Mid suborbital		5.08	5.25	3.51	3.65	3.7	3.0	7.5	8.5	11.6	4.4	5.6	1.9	9.6	3.1
Lateral orbit						5.4	4.7	13.0	14.25	13.0	5.0	7.7	1.9	11.7	3.4
Mid zygomatic arch				4.33	5.32	4.4	2.9	8.75	9.25	10.3	3.7	6.3	2.3	10.0	2.3
Supra glenoid/base of zygomatic arch		6.07	6.75	7.42	7.1			11.75	12.0	13.3	4.4	7.6	3.8	11.4	3.9
In front of masseter		8.65	8.1	7.76	6.16					13.5	4.8	9.0	3.2	12.7	4.6
Mid ramus		18.05	17.05	17.01	14.83					24.3	6.2	14.3	2.7	22.9	4.2
Gonion		12.21	11.5	8.72	7.56	6.8	4.0	14.25	14.25	15.5	7.1	8.3	2.2	14.6	4.9

AV = Average; SD = Standard Deviation; M = Male; F = Female.
Modified and compiled from Caldwell (1981), Krogman and Iscan (1986) and O'Grady et al. (1990).

it to facilitate tying of both halves of the mould together at later stages. When the plaster has set, the supporting clay is removed and the second half of the mould constructed in a manner similar to that of the first half. The two halves of the mould are then carefully removed from the skull (Fig. 14.4a). A suitable quantity of plaster is mixed and manually rubbed over the inner aspect of each half of the mould. These are then filled. Both halves are repositioned together accurately (using location notches) and tied together (using string in scribed groove), and the plaster is allowed to set. The duplicate plaster skull is then carefully uncovered and checked for accuracy; further duplicates can then be made if required (Fig. 14.4b). For convenience and to minimize the risk of damage, the duplicate plaster skull is mounted on a revolving workstand with a metal bracket long enough to allow space to reconstruct the neck. A hole is drilled in the region of the foramen magnum to a distance of about 4 cm, and the metal bracket is inserted and fixed in place with a new mix of plaster. When the plaster has set, the exposed portion of the metal bracket is fixed to the turntable with the duplicate skull's centreline vertical and Frankfort plane horizontal.

Three-dimensional facial reconstruction

The basis of the soft tissue reconstruction is the use of average soft tissue thicknesses for given anatomical landmarks (Table 14.1). Unfortunately, the amount of data that has been published on soft tissue thicknesses related to the skull is quite limited. The limitations include relatively small numbers of subjects in all studies, few comparisons of soft tissue thicknesses in different races (Lebedinskaya *et al.* (1993) being a recent exception but a by no means definitive study) and few studies detailing sex and age differences. Comparison of the studies is difficult because of the varying methods of measurement, the varying points at which measurements are taken, the different racial groups studied and the differing status of the subjects (e.g. alive versus dead, fixed versus unfixed tissues). Additional problems are encountered with the ear and nose, which have a cartilaginous frame rather than direct bony support. A considerable amount of individual variation is possible in these structures as well as in the hairstyle, length and colour, and their reconstruction

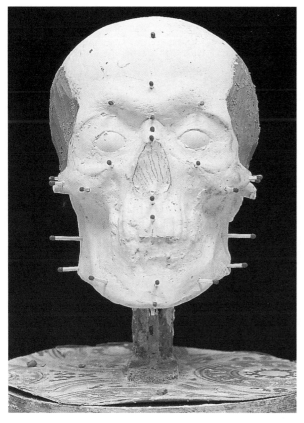 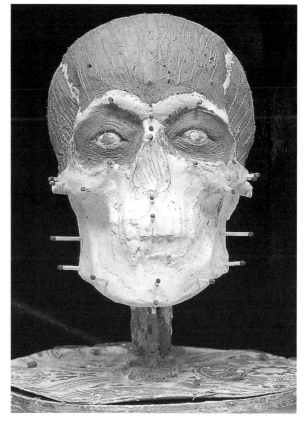

Fig. 14.5(a) (b)

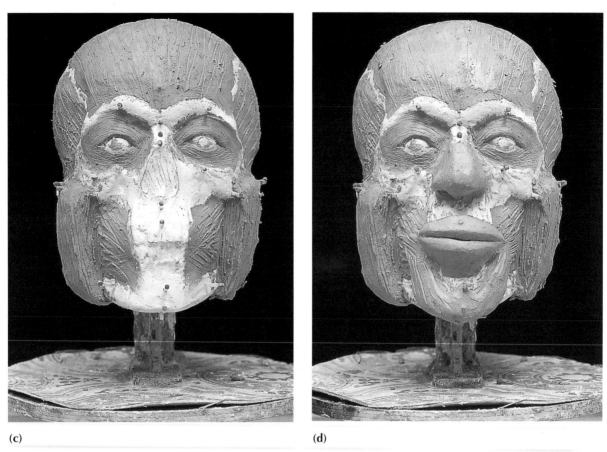

(c)   **(d)**

Fig. 14.5 (a)–(d) These figures show the transition from duplicate skull with soft tissue thickness markers to reconstruction of the underlying muscles, nose and lips

is probably the most variable and least accurate.

Another significant problem is that the number of reconstructions of childrens' faces reported in the literature is minimal. The soft tissue thicknesses in Table 14.1 are based on those of adults, and their value in reconstructions of a child's face is questionable. Hodson *et al.* (1985) measured soft tissue thicknesses in a small number of children using an ultrasound technique and found that tissue thickness tended to decrease with age in children. Differences between adult and child tissue thicknesses were clearly demonstrated by Gerasimov (1971). With the advent of magnetic resonance imaging and ultrasound, more objective and reproducible measurement of soft tissue thicknesses on large numbers of subjects may be possible and would clearly be desirable. However, the importance of the accuracy of soft tissue thicknesses may be overestimated given that, ultimately, a two-dimensional image of the three-dimensional reconstruction is generally used for identification purposes.

The anatomical landmarks from Table 14.1 are

marked on the duplicate skull using wooden or plastic markers. These are cut to the average soft tissue thickness for a given point and glued to the skull. Coloured plastic or the coloured ends of safety matches are useful for this purpose as the coloured ends are visible through a thin layer of clay. Reconstructions building the soft tissue thickness in bulk without regard to the underlying soft tissue anatomy have been performed (e.g. Gatliff and Snow, 1979), but in this chapter, a technique in which muscles are built up in an anatomical manner is described. The temporalis, masseter, buccinator and occipito-frontalis are initially built up, followed by orbicularis oris and orbicularis oculi. The soft tissues of the neck are built up in bulk (size is greatly helped if a shirt with a collar is found on the body), although the bulge of the sternocleidomastoid muscles and the manubrial notch are usually highlighted. At this stage, it is often useful to reconstruct the nose and lips before forming the other muscles.

The lips are approximately as wide as the inter-pupillary distance (Caldwell, 1986), but considerable variation of form occurs with age, sex, race, occlusion and loss of vertical dimension. In young adults, the lip tends not to cover the upper incisors entirely, but it may in older age, when considerable tooth attrition or inadequate dentures are present. Class II division 2 occlusions are associated with a short upper lip and deep mental sulcus, whereas class III occlusions are associated with protrusion of the lower lip. The philtrum of the lip is affected by the length of the lip, the lip support given by the teeth and the shape of the base of the nose. The philtrum is usually placed in the midline of the face, but this may not correspond to the midline of the teeth (Fig. 14.5).

The nose is difficult to reconstruct because of the limited underlying bone and the wide individual variation possible. The profile of the nose is arbitrarily determined by projecting two lines from the skull midline, as suggested by Gerasimov (1971). The first is a continuation of the inclination of the nasal bones, and the second is a horizontal line from the anterior nasal spine. On average, Gatliff (1984) found the width of the nose to be 1.67 times that of the anterior nasal aperture, but Schultz (1918) found that racial and individual variations were considerable. The nose is positioned in the midline unless obvious bony asymmetry is present.

The muscles of facial expression are then added, followed by completion of the completion of the soft tissue around the eyes. The eyelids normally cover part of the iris and extend from 2 mm lateral to the medial orbital rim to 4 mm medial to the lateral orbital rim (Caldwell, 1986). The orientation of the palpebral fissure varies between races; for example, Asians typically have a palpebral fissure that passes inferiorly from the lateral to the medial aspect. At this stage, the tissues are built up to within 1 mm of the soft tissue thickness markers and the ears are then reconstructed. The latter are arbitrarily positioned so that the ear canal is positioned at the external acoustic meatus and set obliquely with a 15 degree posterior inclination. Caldwell (1986) noted that virtually all authors experienced in facial reconstruction found ears 'complicated' to reproduce. Finally, fleshing of the face is carried out to the tips of the depth markers, and characterization may be added if indicated. For example, an aged appearance is simulated by the addition of wrinkles and the accentuation of skin folds. Similarly, further racial characterization may also be carried out if indicated (Fig. 14.6).

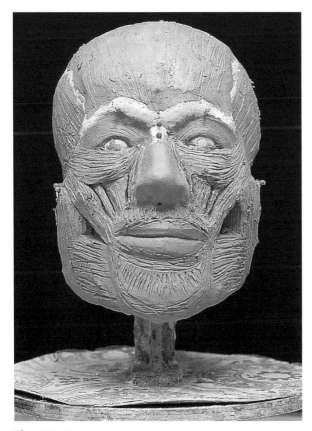

Fig. 14.6(a)

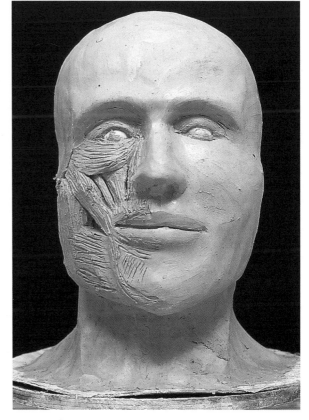

Fig. 14.6(b)

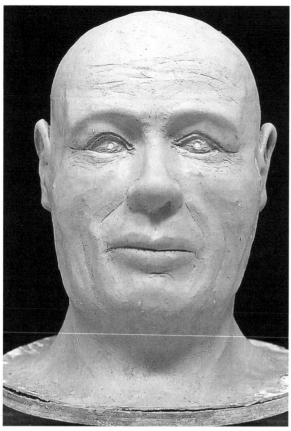

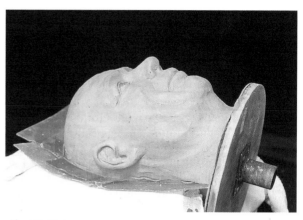

Fig. 14.7(a)

Fig. 14.6(c)

Fig. 14.6 (a)–(c) Completion of the reconstruction involves simulation of the skin (fleshing out), placement of the ears and final characterization of the face

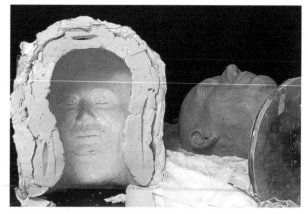

Fig. 14.7(b)

Duplication of the reconstruction

Duplication of the clay reconstruction is also advisable as a plaster model is considerably more durable than a clay model. The clay reconstruction is duplicated using a split-mould technique similar to that used to duplicate the original skull. The only significant difference is that the clay reconstruction is supported by towels, and sheets of wax are used to form the 5 cm table around the head (Fig. 14.7). On the plaster reconstruction additional identifying material may be added, for example hair, jewellery and spectacles if these were found with the body. Alternatively, a two-dimensional image of the reconstruction may be carried out and additional alterations made with the use of computer software. This is often a more efficient method of finishing the reconstruction (Fig. 14.8).

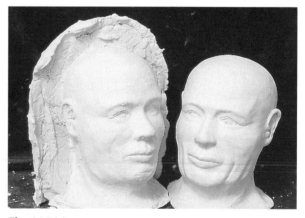

Fig. 14.7(c)

Fig. 14.7 (a) Duplication of the reconstruction is similar to duplication of the original skull. However, the reconstruction is supported by towels, and a wax table is built around to support the first half of the split mould. (b) Impression of the clay reconstruction. (c) Plaster casts of the clay reconstruction

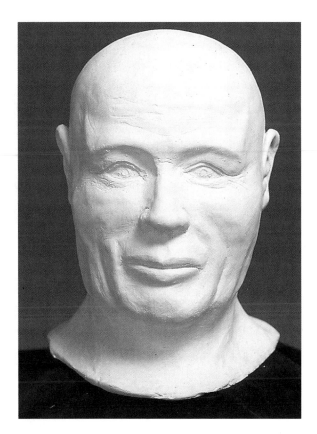

Fig. 14.8 Complete three-dimensional plaster model

Conclusion

A technique of three-dimensional reconstruction of the face carried out on a duplicate plaster skull using average soft tissue thicknesses is described. Unfortunately, the data on soft tissue thickness are limited and hardly ideal, but this is perhaps not as crucial as might be expected given that a two-dimensional image is ultimately used for identification purposes. Of more concern is their limited usefulness in children and the accuracy in reconstruction of the lips, eyes, hair, nose and ears. Alteration of these latter structures is time consuming on three-dimensional reconstructions and more efficiently carried out on two-dimensional images using computer software. Bearing the above limitations in mind, three-dimensional reconstructions are clearly only used when other methods have failed. The reconstruction will at best produce an image with features similar to the ante mortem appearance of the deceased and, if pub-licized appropriately, may aid in obtaining a successful identification.

References

Caldwell MC. 1981: The relationship of the human skull and its application in forensic anthropology. MA thesis, Arizona State University.

Caldwell MC. 1986: New questions and some answers on the facial reproduction techniques. In Reichs KJ. (ed.) *Forensic osteology: advances in the identification of human remains.* Springfield, IL: Charles C. Thomas, 229–55.

Gatliff BP. 1984: Facial sculpture on the skull for identification. *American Journal of Forensic Pathology* **5**, 327–33.

Gatliff BP, Snow CC. 1979: From skull to visage. *Journal of Biocommunication* **6**, 27–30.

Gerasimov, MM. 1971: *The face finder.* London: Hutchinson.

His W. 1895: Anatomische Forschungen ueber Johann Sebastian Bach's Gebeine und Antlitz nebst Bemerkungen ueber Dessen Bilder. In Adhandlungen der Mathematisch-Physikalischen Klasse der Konigl. *Sashsischen Gesellschaft der Wissenschaften* **22**, 379–420.

Hodson G, Lieberman LS, Wright P. 1985: In vivo measurements of facial tissue thicknesses in American Caucasoid children. *Journal of Forensic Sciences* **30**, 1100–12.

Kollman J, Buchly W. 1898: Die Persistenz der Rassen und die Reconstruction der Physiognomie prahistorischer Schadel. *Archiv für Anthropologie* **25**, 329–59.

Krogman WM, Iscan MY. 1986: *The human skeleton in forensic medicine.* Springfield, IL: Charles C. Thomas.

Lebedinskaya GV, Balueva TS, Veselovskaya EV. 1993: Principles of facial reconstruction. In Iscan MY, Helmer RP. (eds) *Forensic analysis of the skull.* New York: Wiley-Liss, 183–98.

O'Grady JF, Taylor RG, Clement JG. 1990: Facial tissue thickness: a study of cadavers in Melbourne. Poster presented at the International Association of Forensic Science Scientific Symposium, Adelaide, South Australia, October 1990.

Rhine JS, Campbell HR. 1980: Thickness of facial tissues in American Blacks. *Journal of Forensic Sciences* **25**, 847–58.

Schultz AH. 1918: Relation of the external nose to the bony nose and nasal cartilages in whites and negroes. *American Journal of Physical Anthropology* **1**, 329–38.

Suzuki K. 1948: On the thickness of the soft parts of the Japanese face. *Journal of the Anthropological Society of Nippon* **60**, 7–11.

Welcker H. 1883: *Schiller's Schadel und Todenmaske, nebst Mittheilungen uber Schadel und Todtenmaske Kant's Braunschweig.* Fr. Vieweg und Sohn, 1–160.

CHAPTER 15

Computer modelling of facial form

A LINNEY, AM COOMBES

Introduction	187	Summary	198
Recording the facial surface in three dimensions	187	Conclusion	198
Visualization of three-dimensional data sets	189		
Identification applications of three-dimensional facial surface recordings	190		

Introduction

Apart perhaps from monozygotic twins, each one of us has a unique face determined by a mixture of genetic and environmental influences. The face ought therefore to be a good means of identifying an individual. To do this 'beyond reasonable doubt', however, has proved to be a difficult task. Two kinds of evidence on identification are commonly heard in court in cases involving either surveillance photography or surveillance videotaping. These are recognition by an individual who is familiar with the subject, and identification by comparison of sets of measurements on the surveillance images with a homologous set taken from images of the suspect. In both identification by recognition using only visual and mental faculties and in identification by the use of quantifiable facial traits, there is still much room for error. An important measure of error in this situation is the relative number of false-positive identifications. In terms of human recognition, it is easy to believe that some form of training in visual recognition would reduce the number of false-positive identifications. However, in spite of experiments designed to test this

idea, improvements in performance have not been satisfactorily demonstrated (Shapiro and Penrod, 1986). It is also impossible to estimate the chances of being wrong in any particular situation of individual recognition. Furthermore, it is difficult to envisage any development in human training that could improve this situation. In the case of using quantifiable traits, however, it is always possible that new technology will improve this means of identification. This method is also always amenable to the calculation of the probabilities of false-positive identification in individual cases, provided that sufficient relevant data have been collected.

Recording the facial surface in three dimensions

To date, the work on identification both by human recognition and by metric analysis has been based on two-dimensional images such as photographs and video frames. Faces have been considered as seen from only a limited number of viewpoints (Bledsoe,

1964, 1966; Samal and Iyengar, 1992; Bruce, 1988). Methods of facial analysis using three-dimensional recordings or images of the face have been developed largely for medical and surgical purposes, for which special systems of recording the facial surface have been developed. One such device is the optical scanner designed and constructed by the Department of Medical Physics and Bioengineering at University College, London. This device conveniently produces an accurate three-dimensional recording of the surface of a subject's face directly as digital information stored on a computer system. A brief description of this system is given here, but the system has been described in detail elsewhere (Moss *et al.*, 1989). The layout of the system is illustrated in Fig. 15.1. The technique is to record on-line the shape of a line of light projected onto the face (Fig. 15.2) and viewed obliquely via collecting mirrors by a Charge Coupled Device (CCD) video camera. Two collecting mirrors, one either side of the face are used to avoid loss of information due to obscuration by prominent features, particularly the nose. The distortion of the line as it appears on the face is determined by the facial form. Simple geometric analysis based on the surveying principle of triangulation allows the shape of the distorted line to be transformed into a set of three-dimensional co-ordinates of points along the line illuminating the facial surface. By rotating the subject, the whole of the facial surface is scanned. More than 50 000 co-ordinate measurements are made on the facial surface in approximately 7 seconds, with an accuracy of the order of 0.5 mm.

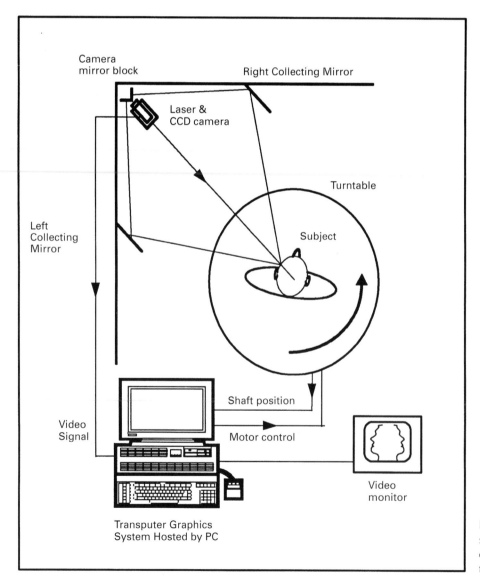

Fig. 15.1 Layout of the system for producing three-dimensional recordings of the facial surface

Distorted light line
reflecting facial form

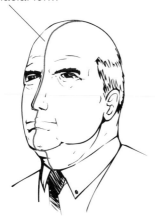

Fig. 15.2 Illustration showing a light line projected onto the face, which appears distorted by the facial shape when viewed obliquely

Visualization of three-dimensional data sets

The data collected on the face by optical scanning comprise the spatial co-ordinates of a very large number of points on its surface. In this form, the data are not immediately very useful, and methods are needed to present them in a meaningful way. Visualization of the data as a facial form is one of the most appropriate methods. Along with this viewing facility, tools must be provided to affect a mathematical analysis or to make comparisons that yield numerical indices of similarity. As the data are not collected in a random fashion but are structured into lines, a faceted representation of the facial surface is easily generated. The surface now consists of many thousands of small triangles and, in this form, may be displayed on a video screen as a smooth surface using a number of well-established graphics techniques (Foley *et al.*, 1990). To create realistic surface images with a good three-dimensional 'feel' to them, Gouraud interpolation (Gouraud, 1971) is used for surface rendering. An example of three-dimensional facial surface data rendered on a video screen in this way is shown in Fig. 15.3.

Along with the software that has been written to display the facial surface, programmes have also been written which allow the face to be analysed in a number of ways. For example, distances may be measured interactively by marking points on the face using a mouse-driven cursor. Figure 15.4 shows that the shapes of sections of the face may be extracted. For

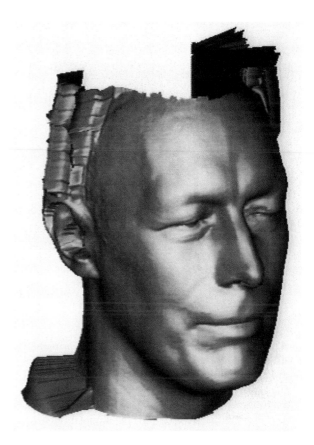

Fig. 15.3 An example of three-dimensional facial surface data rendered as a facial image on a video screen

the identification applications that we consider in this chapter, the important facts are that the display system allows the face to be viewed at any magnification and from any direction, and be illuminated in a variety of ways. Perspective can also be correctly represented in the image. Thus it is possible to take any number of photographs from a robbery or still prints from a video sequence and match these in viewpoint and illumination with a suspect's face recorded in three dimensions by the optical scanner. The comparison then made will be free of the effects of viewpoint differences and, to some extent, lighting differences. These effects often severely limit comparisons based only on two-dimensional material. Moreover, since the visualized facial surface may be rotated to any viewpoint, the stability of various measurements against changes in viewpoint may be quantified.

In the past two decades, a considerable amount of effort has been devoted to developing systems to record anatomical surfaces with accuracy. Newer optical scanners are providing facial surface colour in addition to shape (Incremona, 1995), and this will clearly be of added benefit in any comparison, the images generated being photo-realistic in this case.

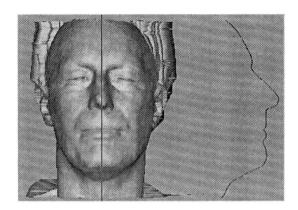

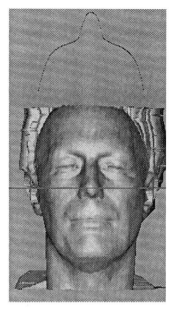

Fig. 15.4 Interactive extraction of shapes of sections of the face (as a profile through the level indicated)

Thus, using three-dimensional recording technology and suitable visualization by means of computer graphics, it is possible to overcome some of the most difficult problems in interpreting two-dimensional surveillance material. In the case of a crime recorded photographically or on video, the facial image of a suspect may be matched in viewpoint and, to an extent, illumination to a large sequence of images in the recording. This maximizes the probability of correct identification and minimizing false positive identification. With suitable software, all of this may be demonstrated interactively on a computer screen in a legal conference or courtroom setting.

Identification applications of three-dimensional facial surface recordings

We now consider several identification applications that could benefit from the use of three-dimensional recordings of the facial surface. For each application, we also suggest the kinds of technique that might be used to carry out the identification based on our experience, and some experiments for which we present the results.

APPLICATION TO CONTROLLED ENTRY

For one possible application – controlling entry to buildings and restricted areas – three-dimensional recordings of the facial surface offer great poten-

tial. Here, the task is to identify the person under inspection as one belonging to a limited group of individuals who are allowed entry. In this case, three-dimensional facial recordings will be available of all of the members of the privileged group. Two problems exist. The first is to devise a method for recording the face rapidly as an individual seeks entry. The second is to devise methods of making a rapid and reliable comparison with all prerecorded faces of the group. We do not intend to discuss here the possible designs for the physical set-up of the entry recording system, but it should be possible to devise a relatively simple structured light system. For example, these data might be collected by projection of multiple laser lines onto the entry-seeker's face viewed obliquely by one or more CCD cameras, similar to the systems of Nixon (1985) or Halioua and Liu (1989). Since so much information of a high quality would then be available, it should be possible to produce a unique description of every individual face in quantitative morphological terms that could be used for comparison.

The constraints on the position of the subject's head are important, and these should naturally be as few as possible. It would be inappropriate to demand, for example, that the head be placed in a very precise position in the entry inspection space, or in a very specific orientation. Ideally, the subject would be requested to stop and look ahead momentarily on seeking entry. This has important implications for the requirements of the methods and algorithms for making the comparisons with the facial database. Two approaches have been examined for such a comparison. The first requires the registration of the two facial surfaces to be compared. That is to say, the surfaces must be transformed into a co-ordinate system in which the corresponding features of each are located, as far as possible, at the same three-dimensional co-ordinates. The second method considered is based on surface shape analysis and produces a description of the surface that is independent of its position and orientation.

Registration method

The registration of two facial surfaces depends on the identification of corresponding facial features, or rather single points on features usually referred to in this context as 'homologous landmarks'. Assuming that no scaling or perspective correction is required, at least three such non-colinear landmarks must be identified to achieve registration. However, it is important to note that, generally speaking, the greater the number of points, the more accurate the registration. Once a set of homologous points is identified, the registration can proceed automatically using a registration algorithm for three-dimensional data such as that described by Fright and Linney (1993). This algorithm works by iteratively estimating the transformation required to minimize the sum of the squares of the distances between homologous points on each surface, producing a 'least squares' registration. Although a measure of the match in shape of the two surfaces is now given by this sum of squares of distances, the degree of match is computed only for the chosen landmarks. To compare more of the surface, an axis is chosen behind the surfaces, and the radial distances of the surfaces from this axis at corresponding points are determined at regular intervals over the entire region of overlap of the surfaces. The sum of the squares of the differences in distance of each surface along each radial direction may now be used as an index of the surface match. Regions of the face that are the least affected by facial expression are given greater weight. Some regions that are highly mobile may, of course, be excluded from the comparison altogether.

Figure 15.5 shows two face scans of the same individual taken at different times before registration. Figure 15.6 shows the two face scans registered to each other using nine selected landmark points. Figure 15.7 shows the registered face scans of two different individuals. In this case, using as few as nine landmarks, the sum of the distances squared between homologous landmark pairs is already approximately a factor of ten greater for registered scans of different faces than that for the same individual's face recorded at different times. To visualise a complete comparison of two registered facial surfaces, differences of distances of points on the facial surfaces taken radially from an approximately vertical axis approximately through the centre of the head are computed.

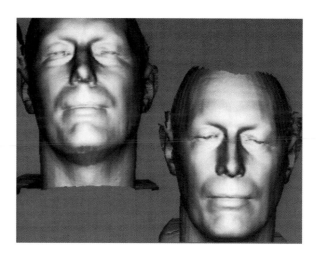

Fig. 15.5   Two face scans of the same individual taken at different times before registration

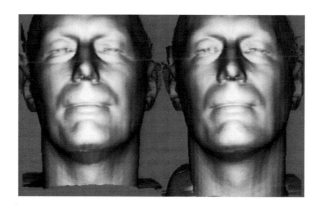

Fig. 15.6   Two face scans from Fig. 15.5 registered to each other using nine selected landmark points

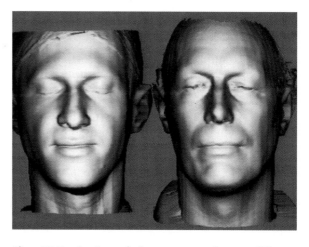

Fig. 15.7   Registered face scans of two different individuals using nine landmarks

These distances may then be represented by dividing them into ranges and displaying distance ranges on a colour scale. Figure 15.8 shows a visual representation of such a comparison for the same individual's face recorded at different times. Figure 15.9 shows the same display for the faces of different individuals. The small differences seen in the comparison of scans of the single individual's face recorded at different times reflect a combination of the accuracy of the scanning system and possible differences in facial expression between the two scans. Differences between different individuals, as illustrated by Fig. 15.9, are, in comparison, quite marked.

Shape analysis method

In discussing the registration technique, we have not discussed how the landmarks are to be determined. Facilities exist for the manual selection of landmarks using horizontal and vertical profiles through the data to assist the operator. However, this is costly in terms of time and therefore not appropriate for a rapid door-entry system. What is needed is a way of automatically selecting landmarks for use by the automatic registration algorithm. In seeking such an algorithm, we have developed a method that would allow landmarks to be automatically determined and even to avoid the necessity of registration of the facial surfaces at all.

This method arises from the differential geometry of the surface that allows surface shape to be characterized. At any point on a surface, there are two kinds of curvature that describe the shape of the surface. These are known as the Gaussian curvature and the mean curvature, which may be derived from the maximum and minimum principal curvature values at each point on the surface. Lipschultz (1969) gives a good review of the mathematical theory of differential geometry, while Yokoya and Levine (1989) and Besl and Jain (1986) present the appropriate algorithms governing its application to numerical data defining surfaces. These curvature measures are rooted to the surface and are independent of the position and orientation of the surface in space. For our problem of comparing facial surfaces, this means that they have the important property of being independent of viewpoint. Besl and Jain (1988) found that, by utilizing the values of the Gaussian and mean curvatures, they could classify each surface point as belonging to an area having one of eight 'fundamental' shapes: peak, pit, ridge, valley, saddle ridge, saddle valley, flat and minimal. These are illustrated in Fig. 15.10. Clusters of data points with the same shape classification form distinct patches, or regions, of that shape on the surface. A surface could thus be segmented into regions, each having a distinct shape.

We have applied this idea to the human face,

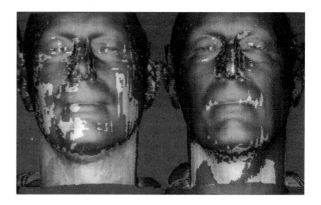

Fig. 15.8 Visual representation of the comparison of the same individual's face recorded at different times

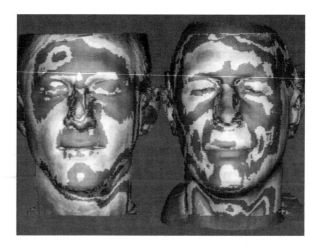

Fig. 15.9 Visual representation of the comparison for the registered facial scans of two different individuals

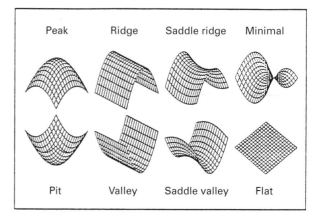

Fig. 15.10 Fundamental surface types: peak, pit, ridge, valley, saddle ridge, saddle valley, flat and minimal

implementing algorithms to calculate the Gaussian and mean curvatures from the facial surface data collected from the optical surface scanner (Coombes, 1993). The surface data are segmented into patches of each fundamental shape. The distributions and characteristics of these shape patches are independent of the viewpoint from which the face is seen and are likely to be as unique as the face itself. Using pseudo-colours to represent each fundamental shape, the face can be visualized via computer graphics as a patchwork of these shapes. It appears that the segmentation into shape patches matches the human interpretation of facial features.

The 'faceprints' of two individuals produced in this way are shown in Fig. 15.11. These now reflect the three-dimensional structures of the faces and are therefore likely to be very individual in character. Although no experiments have so far been carried out on a larger population to establish their degree of individuality.

We have demonstrated that the faceprints are repeatable for different data sets collected for the same individual (Coombes, 1993). Thus, for a controlled entry system application, comparison could be made between the faceprint of an individual and the stored faceprints of the allowed population. Some methods have already been developed for comparison of these faceprints, but further automation is needed to provide a practical system. Artificial intelligence methods seem to offer great promise in this respect (Yager, 1984a, b; Zadeh, 1988).

Limitations of using 'faceprints' for controlled entry

Since facial expression distorts facial shape, and thus the mathematical representation, a neutral expression would need to be adopted by the entry-seeker. Because the data collected are vulnerable to error caused by light scattering and this affects the accuracy of the shape description, spectacles would need to be removed. Facial hair could similarly disrupt performance.

APPLICATION TO IDENTIFICATION FROM SURVEILLANCE RECORDINGS

In situations in which a crime has been recorded by photographic or video means, three-dimensional data will be available for the suspect, that is provided that the law permits them to be obtained and the suspect is prepared to co-operate.

To date, the surveillance material has mostly been compared with photographs of the suspect's face taken from a number of viewpoints. In preparing evidence for the prosecution, it is often difficult to obtain photographs of the suspect from viewpoints that are sufficiently close to those from which the criminal is alleged to have been seen. This arises because the suspect will not allow specially posed photographs to be taken. Consequentially, comparisons are very limited and largely confined to discussion of the relative proportions of the face. However, if one is presenting defence evidence, it is often possible to take as many photographs of the suspect as one likes within, of course, the limits of time and cost. We have also sometimes been able to collect three-dimensional data using the optical surface scanner subject only to the suspect being at liberty to visit our laboratory. In Figure 15.12, a three-dimensional scan is shown which is brought into alignment with the viewpoint from which a photograph has been taken. Projection lines, taken from

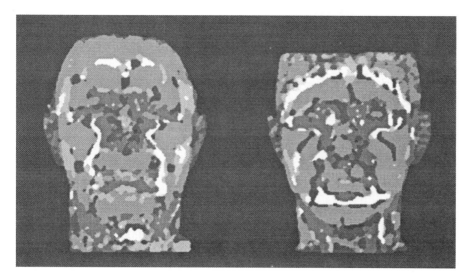

Fig. 15.11 The 'faceprints' of two individuals based on the pattern of fundamental surface-type patches

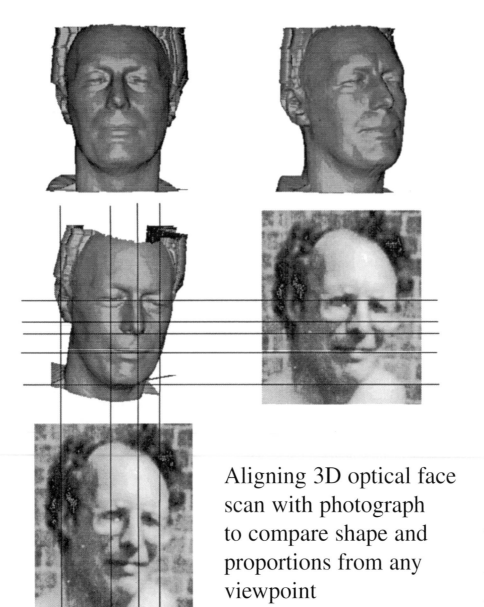

Aligning 3D optical face scan with photograph to compare shape and proportions from any viewpoint

Fig. 15.12 A three-dimensional scan is shown which is brought into alignment with the viewpoint from which a photograph has been taken. The projected lines allow a comparison of the facial proportions

the scan to the photograph, allow the images to be scaled to the same size and for it to be demonstrated that facial proportions on the photograph and the scan are the same. It may also be seen that the direction of illumination has been simulated, showing that the surface illumination pattern on the forehead may be matched. Since this pattern depends on the shape of the forehead, this represents further evidence of the identity of the individuals compared.

In our experience, the average crime surveillance recording provides a reasonable number of images of the criminal for comparison with the suspect's face. Methods of comparison generally revolve around the

measurement of the relative facial proportions (i.e. configuration of facial features) and the shapes of these features. In particular, the appearance of the shape of the criminal's face seen against a background can normally be compared for a range of viewpoints, thus offering information on the three-dimensional shape of the face. Since facial outline images in surveillance recordings are frequently found to be sharper than the internal features of the face, owing to poor image contrast, this comparison often proves to be especially important.

The advantage of having a three-dimensional facial data set of the suspect is that it allows comparisons to be made with the criminal from any viewpoint. Small, quantifiable adjustments can be made in the position of the head that allow us to say more precisely how accurate the comparison is. Moreover, the reliability of the comparison can be demonstrated visually to the court, using the suspect's own head to show the effect of discrepancies in rotational alignments or head inclination and, given the right equipment, an interactive demonstration is possible. An example of the method applied to an actual surveillance recording of a robbery is shown in Fig. 15.13. Because of the ability to change, in small steps, the viewpoint from which the three-dimensional scan is seen, it was demonstrated to the court in this case that it was not possible to match the face of the robber to that of the suspect from any viewpoint. At the same time, it was easily possible to produce a match between the three-dimensional scan and the suspect's own photograph. The suspect was found not guilty.

COMPARISONS WITH DATABASES

A number of methods for the objective identification of faces have been proposed by researchers who have, to different degrees, applied current technology. Some systems have aimed at identifying features to be compared, while others leave this to an operator but provide for parameters of the comparison to be recorded. These parameters or features are then used in an algorithm that determines the degree of match between features and the probability that this degree of match can be relied upon for positive identification.

To make the step from accuracy of the comparison to reliability of the identification and an estimation of the probability of false positives, a database of facial features for a sample of the relevant human population is essential. This database may consist of measurements showing the position of features against some baseline. The database may include measurements of shapes of facial features classified against a scheme wide enough to encompass the various general permutations of features and sensitive enough to discriminate effectively, or against a combination of both. The population sample must be of the correct ethnic group, sex and probably age to validate the identification. From this database, the chance of a random feature match, and hence the chances of a false-positive identification, can be estimated (Hildendorf and Irving 1978, Mardia *et al.*, 1996).

A computer system known as VIAS (video identity assessment system) has recently been developed in the UK. This contains the elements necessary to carry out this procedure, including on-screen feature measurement and classification using a sample data-

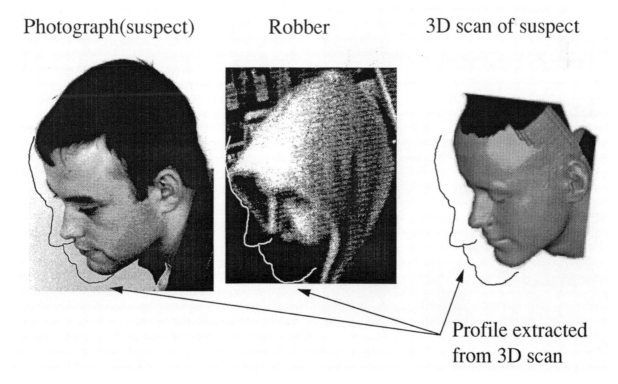

Photograph(suspect)   Robber   3D scan of suspect

Profile extracted from 3D scan

Fig. 15.13 An example of the method applied to an actual surveillance recording of a robbery used in evidence

base of one representative population (white males). Examples of interactive comparison screens are shown in Fig. 15.14. For each face, 29 measurements and the classification of 43 features are possible, provided that facial images depicted from certain viewpoints are available for both the suspect and the criminal. The requirement of closely similar viewpoints is a limiting factor for this system, although investigation has shown that a number of the measurements and classifications are not so sensitive to small viewpoint differences that the method is invalidated. The creation of a complete database of three-dimensional scans would remove this limitation, and work is currently being undertaken to do this. In the meantime, however, it is still possible to use a smaller sample of three-dimensional scans to investigate the sensitivity of various measurement and

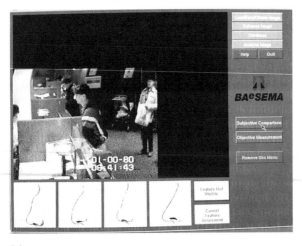

(a)

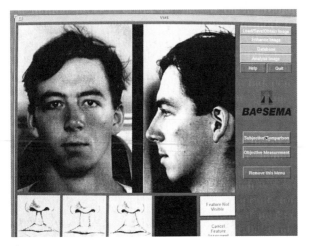

(b)

Fig. 15.14 Screens used for interactive classification and assessment using a sample database of one representative population (white males)

feature comparisons to viewpoint. Figure 15.15, for example, illustrates the insensitivity of one facial angle to head rotation, as demonstrated using a three-dimensional surface scan. The angle in question for this individual appears almost constant up to a rotation of 15 degrees from the lateral view of the head towards the observer. In addition, methods for making corrections for viewpoint differences have been proposed that are found to work under many conditions (Kamel *et al.*, 1994).

The database allows the estimation of (1) the frequency of a particular combination of feature classifications and facial measurements, and (2) the chances of any match being found across these features. There is also a possibility of providing guidance on which measurements and feature classifications will produce the best result in terms of individual identification. Figure 15.16 shows the fraction of a young white population in our database matching a set of features as a function of the number of features used.

Both classifications and measurements are made interactively via the main VIAS presentation screen. The measurements are continuous values, but the classifications are discrete. The classifications are therefore coded with a unique numerical code to enable a search of the databases to be made for a match of the entire coded pattern for a face under investigation. For the measurements, the measured data for the investigated face are represented as a range, which, it is suggested, should correspond to the $P < 0.01$ confidence interval about the mean. This is based on the ten measurements that have been made during the interactive session. Subjects in the database with measurements falling into the ranges defined in the above manner will be treated as 'matching'. This output will be an estimate of the frequency of occurrence of the feature combination in the population. This allows an estimation to be made of the probability of a false-positive identification. The probability (P) that at least one other face will provide a match in a population (N) may be calculated using the formula:

$$P = 1 - (1 - f)N$$

where f is the matching fraction found in the database population (Koehler, 1993).

The database provides the possibility of answering the question 'What fraction of the population would match in terms of a given set of features and measurements?' With the number of possible pairs that can be formed with the current database, this can be estimated with a good degree of precision. Figure 15.16 shows how the number of matching pairs typically varies with number of features compared. It is not yet clear how this estimation can be used in evidence, as some reasoning still has to be made to

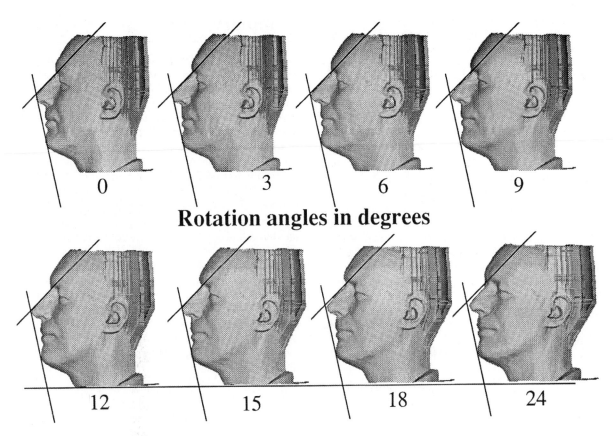

Rotation angles in degrees

Fig. 15.15 Using three-dimensional scans to show that a profile angle for this individual appears almost constant up to a rotation of 15 degrees towards the observer from the lateral view of the head

establish how this information would relate to the confidence one might place in the identification of a given individual. A tentative suggestion is this. One would be able to say that the suspect and the surveillance subject match in the following set of features and measurements, the probability of a pair of individuals in the population showing this degree of match in the same set of features being so many per 1000. Therefore, the probability of a match of this sort being found between two individuals selected at random from the population is low/high (a value can be given). The objection by defence might be that their client has not been randomly selected but has been selected deliberately because he resembles the surveillance subject. We are not sure, however, that this invalidates the presentation of such probabilities for the consideration of a jury, since it might then be argued that the probability should be interpreted as a measure of the difficulty one might have in finding a person who would match. If this is shown to be very difficult, the significance of having found such an individual (against whom there is likely to be other circumstantial evidence) will be high.

By testing various combinations of features, it should eventually be possible to determine the most

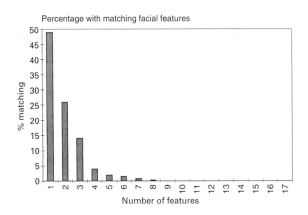

Fig. 15.16 The fraction of a young white population matching a set of features as a function of the number of features used

important features and measurements for arriving at a 'positive identification' with the lowest rate of false positives. Initially, it must be assumed that the measurements that have the greatest spread in the database and which have the least dependence (as measured by correlation coefficients) on other measures will provide the best discrimination. In the case of the classified features, the best features will, similarly, be those with the highest number of classes and the lowest degree of association with others.

RECONSTRUCTING THE FACES OF FOUND SKULLS

Three-dimensional facial scans have also proved useful in reconstructing the faces belonging to found skulls to assist in their identification. The method has also been applied to cases in which parts of the face are missing, rendering it unidentifiable. The same methods have been applied to the reconstruction of the faces of historical figures using their skulls. (A reconstruction of a Viking was undertaken by the Jorvik Viking Museum in York, UK and is on display there; the face of Alexander the Great has also been attempted.)

Traditionally, a medical artist has been employed to build up the face using clay. In the first stage, the clay representing the soft tissues is built up over the skull to a given depth at a number of landmark points, about 40 points usually being used. At each point, the depth of the clay above the skull is given in tables compiled from many measurements taken from cadavers by forensic scientists. Allowance is made for the build, age and sex of the individual. These can often be estimated from the skeletal and other remains. After the clay is applied, the artist blends the surface, interpreting it as he or she sees fit. The process is demanding and it takes a number of days to complete one face.

The availability of three-dimensional data derived from a selection of faces has led to a computerized version of this technique being developed (Vanezis *et al.*, 1989). In this version, the face of an individual of approximately the same age, sex and build is taken and overlaid on to a three-dimensional optical scan of the skull to the required depths at each landmark point. Interpolation between the landmarks takes place, adjusting the facial surface to produce a smooth variation between them. The resulting face seems to follow the skull structure well. However, the nose given tends to be that of the initial individual. This is because there is no bony tissue to guide the shape of the tip of the nose. It would be advantageous to implement a software algorithm for altering the nose shape across at least the more common types in order to make full use of the capability offered by this technology.

The advantages of this computerized version are that is it much quicker and that a number of possible faces can be produced. This can be done either by using a different initial face or by adjustment of soft tissue depths at landmarks. This may well help to jog someone's memory of the face and contribute to a police investigation.

Summary

A method is described for capturing a large number of ordered three-dimensional co-ordinates on the facial surface using an optical surface scanner. These data recordings are then displayed to show the facial surface of the subject as it would be seen from any selected viewpoint and under different lighting conditions, using a notional point source and diffuse light illumination model. The use of this form of recording and presentation of the face for identification is discussed, and examples are given of the methods already practically explored. The methodology facilitates the investigation of the appearance of an individual's face from different viewpoints and allows comparisons to be made with a face viewed or recorded for security purposes on video or in security camera photographs from particular viewpoints. This is advantageous for the forensic investigation of the identity of the criminal. Three-dimensional facial data may also be used to build graphics images of plausible faces over found skulls.

It is concluded that methods of this kind using three-dimensional information offer promise in several identification scenarios. These may include access to restricted areas, in facial identification from photographic or video material collected by surveillance cameras and in the search of larger databases for potential suspects.

Conclusion

Systems for recording the facial surface in three dimensions are becoming more widely available. Combined with a computer graphics system for visualizing the data collected as a facial form, this technology represents a powerful resource for the identification of individuals by means of facial shape and configuration comparisons. Preliminary investigations indicate that it should be possible to increase the probability of correctly identifying a criminal recorded by a surveillance system from a group of suspects. Furthermore, it should be possible accurately to assess the reliability of this identification in terms of the probability of false positives. Three-dimensional databases of faces are currently being collected, which will be of great use in assessing identification techniques based on photo and video comparisons. With a suitable data collection system, the technology also has considerable potential for controlled entry. It has been shown that analysis of the facial data for comparison with the features of a limited group with entry privileges could be made automatically. Finally, it has been shown that three-dimensional data on the facial surface can be used to reconstruct plausible faces over found skulls in a flexible and convenient manner.

The extent to which the sample population database can be utilized depends on the quality of the surveillance (criminal) and comparison (suspect) material as well as on their correspondence in terms of viewpoint. Until now, the two-dimensional nature of the comparison material and reference database has restricted the usefulness of facial comparisons. However, the arrival of machines for the quick and easy acquisition of three-dimensional data and their commonplace use could soon mean that three-dimensional databases of faces will become available. These will enable comparisons to be made with any available surveillance material and will also remove the question of viewpoint similarity. They will further provide an index of the reliability of identification. The enormous amount of information contained in the surface shape of the face will dramatically increase the possibility of unambiguously asserting the identity of an individual and of computing a precise determination of the probability of false-positive identification.

Acknowledgements

We would like to thank BAeSEMA Ltd and the Police Foundation for their help in developing VIAS which is now being marketed by Forensic Technology Ltd. Thanks to the Medical Graphics and Imaging Group at UCL for their complementary work and to Simon Hughes for allowing us to use images of him in this chapter.

References

Besl PJ, Jain RC. 1986: Invariant surface characteristics for 3D object recognition in range images. *Comp. Vision, Graphics and Image Processing* **33**, 33–80.
Besl PJ, Jain RC. 1988: Segmentation through variable-order surface fitting, *IEEE-PAMI* **10**, 167–92.
Bledsoe WW. 1964: *The model method in facial recognition.* Report #PRI:15. Palo Alto, CA: Panoramic Research.
Bledsoe WW. 1966: *Man-machine facial recognition.* Report #PRI:22. Palo Alto, CA: Panoramic Research.
Bruce V. 1988: *Remembering faces.* Amsterdam: North-Holland.

Coombes AM. 1993: Shape classification: towards a mathematical description of the face, PhD thesis, University of London.
Foley DF, van Dam A, Feiner SK, Hughes JF. 1990: *Computer graphics, principles and practice.* New York: Addison-Wesley.
Fright WR, Linney AD. 1993: Registration of 3-D head surfaces using multiple landmarks. *IEEE Transactions on Medical Imaging* **12**, 515–20.
Gouraud H. 1971: Continuous shading of curved surfaces. *IEEE Transactions on Computers* **C-20**(6) 623–8.
Halioua M, Liu H-C. 1989: Optical three-dimensional sensing by phase measuring profilometry. *Optics and Lasers in Engineering* **11**, 185–215.
Hildendorf EL, Irving BA. 1978: False positive identification. *Medicine, Science and the Law* **18**(4), 255–62.
Incremona A. 1995: Whole body imaging for visualisation and animation; new alternatives. *Advanced Imaging* **10**(7), 56.
Kamel MS, Shen HC, Wong AKC, Hong TM, Campeanu I. 1994: Face recognition using perspective invariant features. *Pattern Recognition Letters* (15), 877–83.
Koehler JJ. 1993: Error and exaggeration in the presentation of DNA evidence at Trial. *Jurimetrics Journal* **34**, 21–9.
Lipschutz MM. 1969: *Differential geometry.* New York: McGraw-Hill.
Mardia KV, Coombes A, Kirkbride J, Linney A, Bowie JL. 1996: On statistical problems with face identification from photographs. *Journal of Applied Statistics* **23**(6), 655–75.
Moss JP, Linney AD, Grindrod SR, Mosse CA. 1989: A laser scanning system for the measurement of facial surface morphology. *Optics and Lasers in Engineering* **10**, 179–90.
Nixon M. 1985: Eye spacing measurement for facial recognition. *Proceedings SPIE* **575**, 279–85.
Samal A, Iyengar PA. 1992: Automatic recognition and analysis of human faces and facial expressions: a survey. *Pattern Recognition* **25**(1), 65–77.
Shapiro PN, Penrod S. 1986: Meta-analysis of facial identification studies. *Psychological Bulletin* **100**(2), 139–56.
Vanezis P, Blowes RW, Linney AD, Tan AC, Richards R, Neave R. 1989: Application of 3D computer graphics for facial reconstruction and comparison with sculpting techniques. *Forensic Science International* **42**, 69–84.
Yager RR. 1984a: Linguistic representation of default values in frames, *IEEE-Transactions on Systems. Man and Cybernetics* **14**(4), 630–4.
Yager RR. 1984b: Approximate reasoning as a basis for rule-based expert systems. *IEEE-Transactions on Systems. Man and Cybernetics* **14**(4), 636–43.
Yokoya N, Levine MD. 1989: Range image segmentation based on differential geometry: a hybrid approach, *IEEE-PAMI* **11**(6), 643–9.
Zadeh LA. 1988: Fuzzy logic. *Computer* **21**(4), 83–92.

PART 3

The changing face

CHAPTER 16

Growth of children's faces

SA FEIK, JE GLOVER

The problem of missing children	203	Soft tissues	211
Growth and maturation	204	Gender differences in the face	212
Cranium	206	Individual variation	214
Cranial base	206	Correlations between biological ageing methods	219
Face	207	Facial types	219
Facial growth	209	Growth prediction	220
Dentition	210		

The problem of missing children

In Victoria, Australia, a state of approximately 4 million people, some 7500 people on average go missing every year. Of the 7603 reports of missing persons in the period July 1993 to June 1994, 49.6% were female and 51.4% were male; those aged 16 years or under comprised 62.3% (Kapardis, 1995). Recent Victoria Police data indicate that although 85% of all missing persons are relocated within 1 week of their disappearance, 1% take longer than 1 year to relocate and 1% are never relocated, either dead or alive (Victoria Police Missing Persons Unit, 1995).

The Victorian authorities accept the following definition of a runaway teenager: 'any young person under the age of 17 years, who is missing and gone overnight, without parents' permission to be away from home' (Vincent, 1990). Regardless of the strategies adopted by parents, guardians or providers of residential care, there are large numbers of runaway teenagers from homes and absconders from institutions. This is an international phenomenon (Haselden, 1991; Victoria Police Missing Persons Unit, 1991). The overall Australian statistics relating to missing persons (low incidence, high early recovery rate and low numbers of long-term unsolved cases) might suggest that the problems associated with long-term missing persons are not significant. However, agencies such as 'Parents of Missing Children', 'Families and Friends of Missing Persons' and the 'Salvation Army' report that the anguish of those who cannot locate relatives who disappeared mysteriously, especially young children, is continuous and does not fade with time. The emotional toll impinges on all aspects of life and frequently renders an affected individual incapable of leading a normal life. Media reports of further missing person cases or the discovery of an unidentified corpse renew their distress. Neither the passage of time, the birth of other children nor the pursuit of other interests entirely eases the emotional trauma. Until the missing person is located, whatever the outcome, these people remain significantly affected by their loss (Jones, 1988; Safe, 1995).

In Australia there was sufficient concern about the incidence and prevalence of homelessness amongst children and young people for the Human Rights and Equal Opportunity Commission to launch, in 1987, a national inquiry into homelessness as it affected those persons. This inquiry investigated many data sources from around the country but concluded, after 2 years of inquiry, that 'it is impossible to state precisely how many homeless children and young people there are in Australia ... there are at least 20 000 to 25 000 homeless children and young people across the country ... the likely figure is actually 50 000 to 70 000 children and young people who are homeless or at serious risk'. (Human Rights and Equal Opportunity Commission, 1989).

International statistics relating to missing persons are hard to obtain, principally as a result of the differing levels of organization responsible for monitoring the problem and the operational differences in police forces around the world. In the UK, for example, there are 43 independent police forces of differing sizes and capabilities within England and Wales alone. Each has a regional responsibility for the location of missing persons, but it was not until very recently that a national missing persons bureau was established. Registration of an individual as a missing person depends upon widely accepted criteria including length of absence (usually greater than 28 days) and perceived vulnerability at the time of the disappearance.

Similar problems are also found in the USA where, despite the diversity of regional and local law enforcement agencies, the Federal Bureau of Investigation (FBI) has a central co-ordination responsibility for missing persons. Since the passage of the 1982 Missing Children's Act by Congress, there has been a steady increase in the number of missing persons reported to the police. The total increase since 1982 is 528% (154 341 entries in 1982 versus 964 264 entries in 1995), but the 1995 increase of 1.5% is the smallest annual increment since 1982. Further Congressional legislation in 1990 (the National Child Search Assistance Act) mandated the immediate reporting of every missing child to the FBI National Crime Information Centre (NCIC). These reports have increased by 45.2% since 1990. In 1995 there were 804 151 juvenile missing persons cases recorded as well as 95 497 endangered cases in which the missing individual (adult or child) was perceived to be missing under circumstances such that their physical safety was endangered (National Centre for Missing and Exploited Children, 1996).

Given that so many of the long-term missing persons are young, the changes associated with their normal physical maturation from adolescence to adulthood make visual identification by others difficult. Any available photographs of these persons are naturally somewhat outdated, and the time elapsed since their last photograph or sighting ensures that existing records can be misleading. A small proportion of missing children or teenagers die prematurely as a consequence of their disappearance. A need therefore exists to update old records to facilitate subsequent identification; this can only be done from a knowledge of age changes as they affect the individual's appearance.

Growth and maturation

Children, whether under a family's watchful gaze or otherwise, inevitably grow and change – it is the nature of the beast, so to speak. We all unthinkingly know and expect this, yet for the various authorities and experts involved in the identification of children who have gone missing, this can present a considerable challenge. A child goes missing, and with the passage of time, it may be an adolescent or even an adult whom the police have to find. From knowledge of the missing child's current appearance (e.g. an existing photo), can we predict what the teenager or adult may look like? This is not an easy task as a description of a person's appearance simply in number terms, for example proportional sizes of various parts of the face, which may be within the realms of predictability, does not do justice to the complex process of growth and is a poor substitute for visual experience (Israel, 1978). However, a start has to be made somewhere. An introduction to some of the concepts governing growth may serve as a useful prelude to a description of the characteristics of a baby's face and the changes that occur in the face as the infant grows into a child, an adolescent and finally an adult.

Falkner and Tanner (1978), in the preface to their book *Human growth*, succinctly define 'growth' as 'the study of change in an organism not yet mature'. This definition includes 'development', which the British Medical Dictionary states as being 'the series of changes by which an individual embryo becomes a mature organism'; thus not only quantitative but also qualitative changes are involved. Growth and development together refer not only to anatomical and physiological changes but also to 'the emergence of psychological attributes, ideas and understanding as well as the acquisition of motor and sensory skills' (Sinclair, 1989). Although the anatomical and physiological changes are the most important in determining a person's appearance, other factors also contribute subtly to the identification of living, growing persons. The above definitions are still incomplete in that growth continues throughout life and does not cease at maturity; it is a continuous process extending from fertilization until death.

Growth involves a series of changes rather than simply an enlargement of existing structures. It may involve removal of material – for example, as the head enlarges, some bony tissue is removed to maintain an appropriate skull curvature – or it may produce a reduction in size, for example regression of lymphoid tissue beyond adolescence. It may also involve substitution, such as replacement of the deciduous dentition by the permanent one or replacement of cartilage by bone at some growth centres. The process of growth also results in alterations in form. The most obvious are the secondary sex changes that distinguish girls from boys at puberty, but less obvious ones, such as changes in the shape of the nose and chin, also occur. Differentiation of tissues to enable more complex functions to be performed is also a feature of growth.

Finally, a distinction has to be made between growth of the whole, for example the head, and growth of its parts – orbits, nose, etc. Different parts grow at varying rates at different times, and not all cease growing at the same time. The growth of one part may be controlled by the activity of another at a different stage of development, as seen in the influence of hormones on other body systems. Since the parts are interconnected, growth of one part necessitates translation of another, so the relative positions of structures change with age. This process of differential growth of parts means that the proportions of the body change as the child grows and matures (Sinclair, 1989). The head provides a striking example of this in that the greatest difference between the appearance of the newborn and the adult is in proportionality (Israel, 1978). The skull is a complex structure comprising 22 bones, each with its own individual growth pattern, which may differ in rate and direction of growth. The observed changes in shape from infancy to maturity are the result of integrated activity; growth of each bone affects adjacent bones and others further away, necessitating a balanced readjustment. Thus studying the skull on a regional basis may be misleading but is hard to avoid when describing the process.

The head consists of the neurocranium (calvarium plus cranial base), whose main function is to house and protect the brain, and the viscerocranium (nasofacial complex), concerned with the mechanisms for respiration, mastication and speech (Sullivan, 1978). The very different functional requirements are reflected in the greatly differing growth patterns of the two regions. The calvarium displays a so-called neural pattern of growth, associated with the very

rapid growth of the central nervous system in the early stages of childhood, while the face as a whole follows a curve closer to that of the S-shaped somatic curve of general body growth (Fig. 16.1).

A few comparisons between a baby's and an adult's head illustrate the importance of this differential growth rate on proportionality and hence appearance. The head of an infant constitutes one quarter of its total body length, whereas that of an adult constitutes approximately one eighth of its stature. Thus, with growth, the head undergoes a relative decrease in relation to the total body (Baer, 1977). A similar situation pertains in the head itself in that the volume of the skull in the neonate is eight times that of the face, while in the adult skull volume is only double that of the face (Fig. 16.2). Differences in the rate and timing of growth in head length (in the anteroposterior plane) versus width also occur, and produce changes in cranial form. The cranial or cephalic index (breadth as a percentage of length) is used to express this proportionality (Hajnis, 1987), and the terms dolicocephaly (long-headedness), mesocephaly and brachycephaly (short- or round-headedness) are commonly used to describe cranial form. Because of the asynchronous development of head length (87.1%) relative to head width (83.8%), at 1 year of age the infant has a dolicocephalic skull with a mean cephalic index of 75.9. With age, the index increases, and head width is 77.8% of length by 18 years (Farkas *et al.*, 1992a).

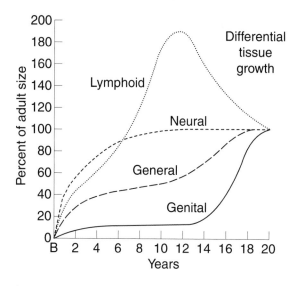

Fig. 16.1 Growth of systems and organs: Scammon's curves. The percentages of adult weight attained are plotted against the age in years. Reprinted from Baer (1977) with permission. Original illustration from Harris JA *et al.* (1930) *The measurement of man*, University of Minnesota Press, Minneapolis University of Minnesota

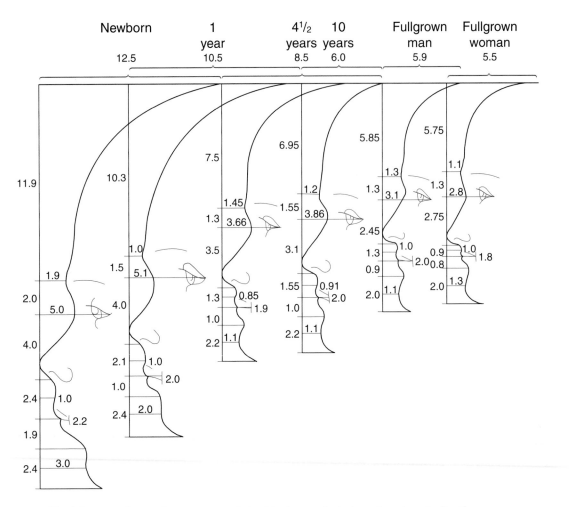

Facial proportions change a great deal between babyhood and maturity: the nose becomes proportionally much larger and the forehead proportionally smaller

Fig. 16.2 Change in facial proportion with age. Reprinted from Liggett (1974) (after Krukenberg, *Der Gesichtsausdrück des Menchen*) with permission

Cranium

Brain growth, which dictates cranial expansion, means that the brain attains nearly 50% of its total weight by 1 year of age, 75% by 3 years, 90% by 7 years and is essentially complete by 10–12 years (Israel, 1978). Growth of bone in the sutures in the vault of the skull is therefore very rapid at first. Greater sutural apposition occurs peripherally than centrally as cerebral growth exceeds brain stem growth. The inner table of the vault bones ceases growth when the cerebrum stops growing, but the outer table continues to grow for a longer period (Enlow, 1990). This leads to increased thickening of the skull. After the first few years, many sutures interlock, and from this time on, sutural adaptation to

bony displacement is limited, ceasing altogether at around the time of puberty. The infant has prominent frontal and parietal eminences. However, the forehead of the baby is narrow relative to both head and face width as seen in the adult (Farkas *et al.*,1992a). As the child grows, the frontal sinus in the forehead develops by excavation of the frontal bone while bone is concurrently deposited on the surface, forming the brow ridges, which become more pronounced beyond adolescence, particularly in males.

Cranial base

Although the cranial base separating the calvarium from the face is not visible when looking at a child's face, it greatly influences facial growth. The cranial base is commonly divided into two sections: anterior and posterior to the pituitary fossa. The anterior segment follows a neural growth pattern, and apart from continuing deposition on the frontal bone as mentioned above, is relatively stable beyond 8 years of age (Stamrud, 1959). This area is therefore frequently used as a reference for evaluating the growth of other areas of the face. The nasofacial complex is attached to the anterior cranial base by a series of sutures orientated in such a way that growth results in a downward and forward movement of the face relative to the base of the skull. The posterior segment contains the spheno-occipital synchondrosis, a cartilage growth area, displaying a somatic growth pattern. This structure is considered by some to be the pivotal point of craniofacial growth as both cranial and facial sutures radiate from it, thus creating a close interrelationship between the calvarium, the cranial base and the face (Ranly, 1988). Growth here not only contributes to growth in the length of the skull but also results in the mandible being pushed forward. The synchondrosis ossifies in late adolescence or early adulthood.

ORBITAL REGION

The infant orbits are large, because of the early development of the eyes, and the orbital rims appear vertical, gaining anterior obliquity in adulthood (Enlow, 1990). The intercanthal distance, i.e. the distance between the inner corners of the eyes, is 84.1% complete by 1 year and attains full development relatively early (8 years in females and 11 years in males). In, contrast, biocular width, i.e. the distance between the outer corners of the eyes, shows small but continuous changes until adolescence (Farkas *et al.*, 1992b). The relationship between these two measurements, expressed as the intercanthal index, reaches its mature value around puberty. It greatly influences visual judgement of the relative proportions of structures in the eye region (Hreczko *et al.*, 1990).

Face

While calvarial expansion is largely dictated by the growth of the nervous system, facial growth is more closely associated with the functional requirements of respiration, mastication and speech. Hence the development of structures such as the nasopharynx, muscles of mastication, tongue and teeth influences facial growth.

For descriptive purposes, the face is frequently divided into an upper and a lower section. The upper

consists of the orbits and their contents (covered above), the nasomaxillary complex, including the maxillary sinuses, and the upper alveolar process and teeth. The primary bone is the maxilla, with contributions from a number of others. The lower face comprises the mandible with its associated alveolar process, teeth and soft tissues.

Farkas and Posnick (1992) undertook a comprehensive study of the growth patterns of the head and face in approximately 1500 North American Caucasians between 1 and 18 years of age. By measuring the distances between a number of surface landmarks (Fig. 16.3) at various ages and comparing these with the sizes attained at maturity (taken to be 18 years), they were able to determine the levels of development reached by different regions of the face (Farkas *et al.*, 1992c) at specific ages and to illustrate the changes in proportionality. A brief summary of their findings will be presented to show the overall pattern of development before describing how facial growth occurs.

Face height

By 1 year of age, face height shows a moderate level of development (mean 67.8% in both sexes). By 5 years, this increases to 83% of eventual adult size. The growth increment between 5 and 18 years of age (54.1% of the total) is significantly greater than that between 1 and 5 years (45.9%). Two periods of rapid growth (defined as growth per cent per annum of 6% or more) occur in the early years, and in males only, a second smaller spurt is seen in adolescence (14–15 years). Maturation is reached at age 15 in males and 13 in females.

Upper face height

At 1 year and 5 years old, the developmental level of upper face height is comparable to that of total face height. Similarly, more than half the total growth increment (1–18 years) occurs between 5 and 18 years of age. Of the total growth increment, approximately 32% in males and 44% in females is attained during the rapid growth phase between 1 and 4 years. Mature size is reached 1 year earlier than for total face height.

Lower face height

Mandibular height at 1 year approaches 67% of its adult value, and by 5 years nearly 88% (the latter being approximately 6% higher than upper face height). In contrast to the regions described above, the total growth increment between 1 and 5 years is significantly greater (63.1%) than that after 5 years. Two rapid growth phases, occurring between 1–2 and

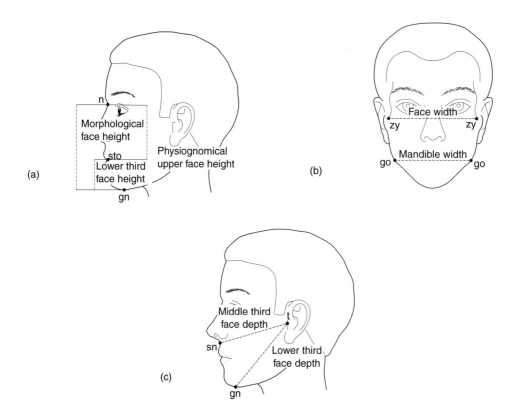

Fig. 16.3 (a) Schematic drawing showing the three vertical height distances. The height of the face (morphological face height: n–gn) is measured between the the nasion point (n) of the nasal root and the chin point (gnathion: gn). The upper face height (physiognomical upper face height: n–sto) is the projective distance between the nasion point (n) and the stomion (sto) landmark in the middle of the labial fissure between gently closed lips. The mandible (lower third face) height (sto–gn) is measured between the stomion (sto) point of the labial fissure and the gnathion (gn) landmark of the chin. (b) Schematic drawing showing the horizontal measurements of the face. The width of the face (bizygion diameter or upper face width: zy–zy) is the projective distance between the most lateral points of the zygomatic arches right and left (zygion: zy). The width of the mandible (bigonian diameter or lower face width: go–go) is measured between the right and left gonion landmarks (go), localized at the angles of the mandible. (Reprinted with permission from Farkas LG, Kolar JC, Munro IR. Craniofacial disproportions in Apert's syndrome: an anthropometric study. *Cleft Palate J*, 1985, **22**, 256.) (c) Schematic drawing showing the depth measurements of the face in the maxillary and mandibular regions. Middle face depth (maxillary depth: t–sn) is the projective distance between the tragion landmark of the ear (t) and the subnasale point (sn), localized at the midpoint of the columella base. Lower third face depth (mandibular depth: t–gn) is the projective distance between the ear's tragion landmark (t) and the chin point (gnathion: gn). Reprinted from Farkas *et al.* (1992c) with permission

3–4 years, account for approximately 53% in males and 58% in females of total lower face height. Maturation levels are attained at 15 years in males and 12 years in females.

Upper face width (bizygomatic diameter)

The developmental level of upper face width at 1 year old is somewhat greater (72%) than face height (67%), but by 5 years, the levels are comparable. Similarly, greater growth in width is seen between 5 and 18 than between 1 and 5 years. Rapid growth

occurs between 3 and 4 years of age, and maturation is reached at the same age as face height.

Lower face width (bigonion diameter)

Mandibular width attains a high level of development relatively early, approaching 80.2% by 1 year and 92% by 5 years, considerably more growth occurring between 1 and 5 years than after this time. In males, three periods of rapid growth are scattered between the ages of 3 and 13 years; in females, rapid growth is evident between 6 and 7 years. Age of maturation is relatively early: 13 in males and 12 in females.

Maxillary depth

Face depth has progressed to a greater developmental level than face width at 1 year (76.6%) and 5 years (85.5%) of age, and similarly, greater growth is seen between 5 and 18 years than between 1 and 5 years. Apart from a period of rapid growth in males between 3 and 4 years of age, only gradual growth is observed, maturation levels being reached at 14 in males and 13 in females.

Mandibular depth

The depth of mandible shows slightly lower values at 1 year (74.2%) and 5 years (84.7%) of age than maxillary depth. Otherwise, the growth pattern is similar except that no periods of rapid growth are seen. Mature size is reached 1 year later than maxillary depth in males but at the same age in females.

Summary of morphometric findings

By 1 year of age, the width and depth measurements of the face attain a greater developmental level than does the height. The latter subsequently shows the greatest relative growth increments until maturity. Only mandibular height and width show greater growth increments between 1 and 5 years than between 5 and 18 years. All the other dimensions measured show greater increments in the latter period, exhibiting gradual growth after 5 years. The face matures between 12 and 15 years in males and 2 years earlier in females.

Facial growth

The nasofacial complex grows by a combination of two processes: displacement and drift. Displacement is the bodily relocation of a bone by movement of adjacent structures pushing against it, while drift results in movement of bone in space by apposition on one surface and concurrent removal from the other.

UPPER FACE

Displacement predominates here till about age 7 or 8, and by this means, the maxilla is pushed downwards and forwards. The primary cause of this displacement appears still to be controversial. The nasal septum has a role, but it is obviously not the only influencing factor as, in its absence, the nose does not grow but maxillary development is relatively normal. After 7 or 8 years of age, the anterior cranial base stabilizes, the ossified nasal cartilage fuses with the underlying bone, the vomer, behind the septal cartilage, and drift largely takes over. Very rapid growth during the first 3 or so years is followed by considerable slowing (Fig. 16.4). At birth, the nostrils (floor of nose) are at approximately the same level as the eyes (lower margin of orbits). With growth, this distance steadily increases until well into adolescence, proportionally more so than for other areas of the face. This vertical increase occurs through enlargement of the nasal cavity by removal of bone from the internal surfaces and deposition superficially on the palate. Air sinuses develop by a similar process of resorption of bone internally. The largest of these, the maxillary sinus or antrum, grows in spurts coinciding with the eruption of the molars associated with it (Sinclair, 1989). As the maxilla is pushed forward, it grows posteriorly at the tuberosity with little apposition occurring anteriorly. Room is thus created for the developing permanent molars: the tuberosity contains the first molar at 3 years, the second molar at 6 years and the third molar at 12 years (Sullivan, 1978).

LOWER FACE

The lower face looks diminutive in the infant. At birth, the mandible is in two halves, which fuse by the end of the first year, so any further growth in width is by the process of drift. Fill-in growth occurs in the cartilage of the condyle as the mandible is displaced downwards and forwards by the growth of other structures. The ramus grows proportionally more than the body, and the angle where these meet decreases progressively with growth, from around 140 degrees in the infant to 120 degrees in the adult. The face therefore looks more 'upright' with age, particularly after adolescence, when many of these facial changes occur (Sinclair, 1989). The mandible increases in length by progressive distal relocation of the ramus; as bone is removed from the anterior aspect, creating room for the developing molars, new bone is deposited posteriorly. Deposition of bone on the chin point and its removal near the tooth roots means that the teeth progressively move upright to prevent root exposure and therefore the chin becomes more prominent. The profile becomes less retruded as the child grows, so the mandible must grow more than the maxilla. It also enlarges very considerably in height to allow for the descent of the upper face, the growth of the alveolar processes and the eruption of the teeth (Fig. 16.5).

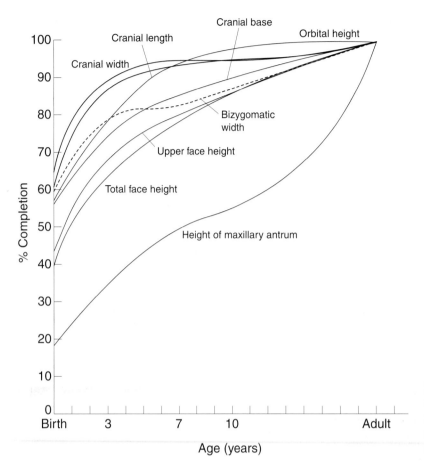

Fig. 16.4 Cranial and facial measurements (males). The changing dimensions of the craniofacial complex. Reprinted from Ranly (1980) with permission

Dentition

At birth, the infant appears toothless, with a space anteriorly between the arches that is filled by the tongue as the infant swallows. The shape of the dental arches is established with the eruption of the primary dentition. The first teeth – the lower central incisors – appear at around 6–7 months of age, and the primary or deciduous dentition is usually complete by 30 months of age. It comprises 20 teeth: a central and a lateral incisor, a canine and two molars in each quadrant. The deciduous anterior teeth are smaller, whiter and more vertically positioned, and usually have gaps between them in both arches, thus distinguishing them from the permanent teeth. Little change is evident in the dentition between 2.5 and 6 years of age, when the first permanent teeth begin to erupt. The first of these is usually the lower, then the upper, first molar, which erupts behind the last deciduous tooth, followed closely by the lower central incisors. The mixed dentition phase is the period when the child has erupted primary and secondary teeth in the mouth together. This phase usually lasts from about 6 to 12 years, and during this time, much change is evident as the primary teeth exfoliate and are replaced by permanent ones. At around 9 years old, when children have eight permanent incisors erupted anteriorly but still have deciduous teeth posteriorly, they typically go through a transitional stage often referred to as the 'ugly duckling stage'; the upper central incisors appear large and have a gap between them, while the lateral incisors appear crooked and the corresponding lower incisors, appear, if anything, slightly crowded. The child normally grows out of this stage; the spaces close and the teeth straighten up as the maxillary canines (the eye teeth) emerge around the age of 11–12. The deciduous molars are replaced by permanent premolars between 10 and 12 years old. Little increase in arch width is seen beyond 8 years (Sillman, 1964), but the arches increase considerably in length to make room for the eruption of the second molars at around 12 years and the third molars, usually between 17 and 21 years.

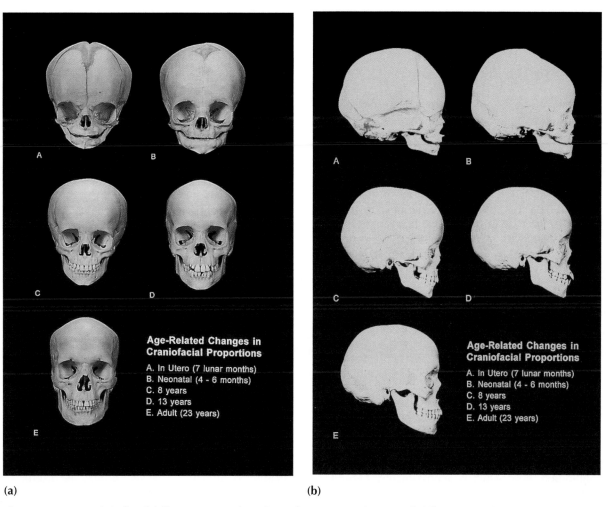

Fig. 16.5 Series of skulls of different ages with scaling effects removed to reveal differences in shape and proportion. (a) Frontal view. (b) Corresponding lateral views of the same specimens shown in (a)

Soft tissues

Soft tissues are important when considering a child's changing appearance as that is what people see. An infant is incapable of making fine muscular movements; hence, there is little subtlety in facial expression. As the child grows, a greater range of emotions can be expressed, and by adolescence, with increasingly complex feelings being portrayed, they are often all too expressive. In late adolescence and early adulthood, transient changes of expression and colour impart richness to the face. The colouring of the face is also more subtle: 'some artists maintain that the portraiture of the teens and twenties needs a lighter and more skilful brush, a much more delicately varied palette' (Liggett, 1974). As a balance is struck between sensibility and control, the most varied and interesting facial expressions may be seen.

Relatively few studies have been dedicated to an analysis of the soft tissues of the face, and there seems to be a divergence of opinion on a number of issues; however, some generalizations can be made. The outline of the soft tissue profile does not correspond well with the underlying skeletal framework because of the variable soft tissue thickness over different parts of the facial skeleton (Peck and Peck, 1970). There is sexual dimorphism in the amount and timing of soft tissue development, which tends to lag behind skeletal development, especially in males. A good example of this is seen in the increased anterior projection of the nose, which continues after skeletal growth ceases. In females, a large proportion of soft tissue development has been attained by age 12, while in males, there is continued growth until age 17; hence their soft tissue dimensions are greater for many parameters. The shapes and the positional relations of the nose, lips and chin remain relatively constant throughout the developmental period for both sexes (Genecov *et al.*, 1990).

NASOLABIAL REGION

The baby's nose is different from that of an adult in that it looks smaller and wider and is nearly always concave, with a sunken bridge (Liggett, 1974). In a study similar to that mentioned above, Farkas *et al.* reported on the growth of the nasolabial region (1992d) and the ear (1992e). They showed that, at 1 year of age, the developmental level of nose height (from the nasion at the root of the nose to the sub-nasale at the base of the columella) reaches a mean of 59% and, with considerable early rapid growth, the level reached by 5 years is approximately 80%. A significantly larger growth increment occurs beyond 5 years (largely between 5 and 8 years) than between 1 and 5 years. Males differ from females in displaying a spurt in nose height around puberty and by showing continuing growth for a longer period (Prahl-Andersen *et al.*, 1995). The width of the nose (distance between the alae) is more highly developed at 1 year old than is the height (79.5% versus 59%), and it increases to approximately 87% by 5 years. The total growth increment after 5 years is therefore small. Over 95% of final nose height and width is reached by 14–15 years in males and 12 years in females. The apparent early imbalance between nose height and width is remedied with growth, and at maturation, nose width is approximately two-thirds of nose height.

The skin portion of the upper lip (base of the columella to the upper vermilion line) and the total upper lip height (i.e. including the vermilion portion) achieve approximately 81% of eventual adult size by 1 year of age and approximately 93% by 5 years. The height of the vermilion portion is not as well developed (63.7% at 1 year increasing to 87.4% at 5 years). Maturation of total upper lip height is observed at 11 years old in males and 5 years in females. Because of this difference in developmental times of lip and nose height, the upper lip in a young child looks too high; with age, this discrepancy is corrected, and in a well-balanced adult face, the upper lip height equals approximately 43% of nose height (Farkas *et al.* 1992d). The nasolabial angle becomes smaller with growth, and the difference in this angle between the sexes decreases after 9 years of age (Prahl-Andersen *et al.*, 1995). However, according to Genecov *et al.* (1990), it is unlikely that the change in the nasolabial angle with growth is more than a few degrees, and the angular characteristics of the nasal complex essentially remain virtually unchanged.

CHIN

The thickness of the soft tissues on the chin increases with growth. In girls, growth velocity decreases beyond 9 years of age whereas boys show a growth spurt around puberty (Prahl-Andersen *et al.*, 1995).

EAR

Ear width develops rapidly in early childhood, reaching approximately 93% of its final size by 1 year in both sexes, only a few millimetres less than the adult value. Mature dimensions are attained at 7 and 6 years of age in males and females respectively. A lower developmental level of ear length at 1 (76.4%) and 5 years (86.6%) accounts for the greater growth observed between 5 and 18 years and the later maturation of ear length at 13 in males and 12 in females. The discrepancy between width and length development means that the ear is relatively wide in early childhood, and preservation of proportionality between ear length and face height up to age 18 can be achieved only by normal growth increments in both features.

Gender differences in the face

A number of differences relating to growth have been mentioned already; however, it may be useful to point out some of the features affecting appearance that distinguish males and females. The following observations are generalizations, and there is obviously a range and considerable overlap between the sexes. In females, there is greater retention of juvenile features. Female faces are usually smaller in overall size, being about four-fifths the size of those of the male. The jaw and the brow ridges are less pronounced. The nose is proportionally smaller, wider and more concave, with a bridge that is more depressed, more akin to that of a baby. The mouth, similarly, is proportionally smaller, the upper lip shorter and the lipline higher in females (Prahl-Andersen *et al.*, 1995). Finer, smoother skin and a thicker layer of fatty tissue covering the facial muscles lead to a perception of decreased facial movement, which is associated with femininity (Fig. 16.6). This smooth, unruffled appearance is often enhanced by cosmetics, which are also used to accentuate the eye region. Females have larger eyes and, when young, stronger eyebrows, longer eyelashes, darker irises and sometimes natural eye shading so that the eye region looks darker than in the male (Liggett, 1974). The effects of cosmetics can

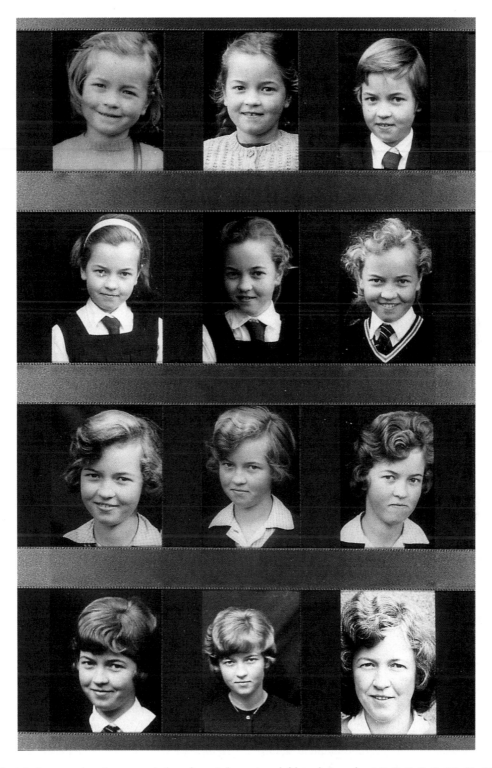

Fig. 16.6 Serial photographs of a person's face from infancy to adulthood. Female at 5, 6, 7, 8, 9, 10, 11, 12, 13, 14, 15 and 35 years of age (from top left to bottom right in rows)

alter the appearance of a face and enhance its femininity, potentially affecting ease of identification of teenage girls (Fig. 16.7).

Individual variation

BIOLOGICAL AGE

The information given above may be misleading in that specific events are said to occur at certain chronological ages. The values, however, are for the so-called 'average' child, and individual children, who display different developmental rates, may not conform to this growth pattern, hence attaining certain landmarks at different ages from those specified. The concept of a biological age, as opposed to a chronological age, needs to be introduced: 'Biological age represents an aggregate or composite of many discrete developmental factors' (Baer, 1977). It is not feasible to assess all the systems in the body so, most commonly, certain key indicators of development are used. Each measure is different, and to enable direct comparisons to be made between them, raw scores must be converted into a single system. This is usually expressed in terms of age equivalents, i.e. the average age at which a particular level of development is attained. For example, a 6-year-old boy may have a bone maturation level of the average 7-year-old; he is then said to have a bone age of 7, and in skeletal development he is 1 year in advance of his chronological age. A number of physical and mental traits can be expressed in terms of age equivalents, and by comparing these, one can determine whether a child is advanced in some areas and slow in others. A single biological age can be arrived at by assessing and averaging the developmental ages of all the bodily systems measured; this then represents a composite picture of the child's level of development. Lay people, for example the police, are often unaware that children's development may not be uniform: maturation levels can differ within and between individuals.

Another way of expressing a child's developmental level or maturity is on a percentage basis from 0 to 100. This can be done because, unlike for example with stature, which is not uniform in adulthood, all children reach the same end point, i.e. a fully mature adult with the same bone maturity, the same number of permanent teeth (excluding pathological aberrations) and the same secondary sex characteristics. To define and measure maturity, either the timing of the occurrence of single events or, preferably, a series of events that always occurs in the same sequence is needed. Noting the attainment of a developmental 'milestone', such as the emergence of the first permanent molar, can indicate the distance the individual has travelled along the road to full maturity (Tanner, 1975).

Six so-called 'indices of maturity' have been developed to assess a child's maturation level: bone age (synonymous with skeletal age, radiological age or anatomical age), dental age, sexual age, neural age, mental age and physiological age. Which body systems are assessed is determined by the child's age and by the particular area of interest, be it the child's physical or mental development. The former is usually of greater importance in the forensic area, and the indices determining bone age, dental age and occasionally sexual age are most widely used and will therefore be discussed more fully below.

BONE AGE

The determination of this index relies on the premise that each bone passes through a sequence of recognizable stages during its development until it reaches a reasonably constant final shape. These stages can be defined and recorded radiographically. When bones ossify, they are rendered radio-opaque, so the times of appearance of certain stages of development, such as the primary and secondary centres of ossification, and the progressive enlargement and change in shape of an epiphysis (secondary centre of ossification at the end of a bone) or a short bone can be observed. For example, each long bone begins with a primary centre of ossification and then changes in shape and size until ultimate fusion of primary and secondary centres (i.e. the shaft with the epiphysis, on obliteration of the cartilage growth plate). Although the sequence of changes is more or less the same for a given bone, individual timing may differ greatly in early, average and late-maturing children. The reproducibility of the sequence enables comparison between individuals. Hand–wrist radiographs are most commonly used to assess skeletal maturation. This is based on the premise that the developmental level of the bones in this area is indicative of that in the skeleton in general, which may not always be the case. The hand and wrist region has a large number of centres of ossification and can be easily radiographed with minimal radiation exposure to the rest of the body. The assessment of skeletal maturation from radiographs is based on the recognition of maturity indicators, i.e. the stages of development previously mentioned that are visible radiographically and can be used to determine the maturity level of a bone.

A number of systems have been developed to assess skeletal maturation. Greulich and Pyle constructed an atlas of skeletal development at different ages. An updated version (Pyle *et al.*, 1971) is still in

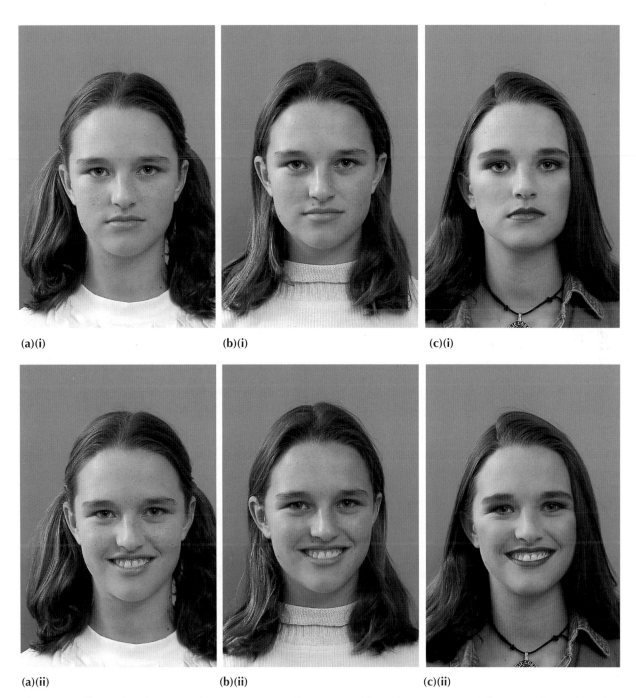

(a)(i) (b)(i) (c)(i)

(a)(ii) (b)(ii) (c)(ii)

Fig. 16.7 Effects of make-up on the apparent age of a person: girl aged 13 years. (a) Make-up used to reduce the apparent age of this teenager. The prominence of the cheeks has been reduced, the lips de-emphasized and the freckles enhanced. Apparent age – 10 years? (b) The teenage subject unaltered. Real age – 13 years. (c) Make-up used to make the subject look older. The contours of the face have been exaggerated, the cheeks enhanced and the eyes and eyelashes emphasized. Pigmentation of the lips has been augmented and the jawline 'strengthened'. The freckles have been covered. Apparent age – 18 years?

use today. The atlas method has the advantage that it is quick and easy to use. A given child's radiograph is compared with the standard films in the atlas and the 'closest match' obtained; the child is then said to have a bone age corresponding to this. Ideally, individual bones are then compared as there is considerable genetic variation in the order of appearance of centres of ossification, and delay in the appearance of a given centre does not necessarily mean that overall skeletal maturation is retarded. Difficulty may be encountered in extrapolating from one stage to the next. Another disadvantage is that the standards were derived from upper middle-class North American children who tended to be skeletally advanced; children from different socio-economic levels and ethnic origins may not conform to this. There are also problems with using 'age' in a system measuring maturity: a 'skeletal year', unlike a chronological year, is not constant at all stages of development.

Systems using bone-specific techniques were developed in an attempt to overcome some of these problems. Tanner and his co-workers (1962) developed a system based on assigning numerical scores to bones depending on their level of maturity. Eight or nine stages are recognized for each bone; the bones are weighted and the scores assigned accordingly. Three different methods may be used – TW2, RUS and Carpal – using 20, 13 and 7 bones respectively (Tanner *et al.*, 1983). Scoring the radius, ulna and finger bones (digits I, III and V), i.e. the RUS method, seems to be sufficiently reliable for clinical use and is the method most commonly used. The result can be recorded as a percentage of final maturation or as a 'bone age', which is taken as the age on a constructed centile chart at which the 50th centile score corresponds to the actual score of the given child. The newest system, the FELS method, was developed by Roche *et al.* (1988) and uses 98 maturity indicators. The recorded grades are entered into a computer that provides the bone age and the standard error, the only method that provides an estimate of error.

The ability to assess skeletal maturation has led to the development of more accurate methods of height prediction. Bayley and Pinneau (1952) constructed tables that were designed for use with the Greulich and Pyle atlas, which assesses skeletal maturation. Using the appropriate table, i.e. accelerated, average or retarded, and knowing the child's current stature, his or her predicted final height can be determined much more precisely than if the pattern of development is not known. However, the Bayley and Pinneau method only provides a semiquantitative allowance for bone age and covers the age range beginning at 8 years. Tanner *et al.* (1983) developed a number of equations in which height increments, RUS increments and, in the case of girls, menarcheal status could be included to improve the predictive power. The accuracy of prediction varies depending on the particular equation used, the difference between predicted height and attained height being as great as 8 cm in some instances. A particularly large adolescent growth spurt may occur, and this is always wholly unpredictable.

DENTAL AGE

As with the skeletal system, the dental system may be used to assess a child's developmental level. In cases in which a child's chronological age is unknown, and birth records are unavailable, dental age can sometimes be used to approximate chronological age as teeth are less prone to environmental changes than are most other body systems. This also applies under adverse conditions such as chronic malnutrition, where growth is stunted and bone maturation delayed, but dental development proceeds relatively normally. Initially, dental development was determined by the number of teeth present in the mouth at each chronological age. An example of its early use for age determination was the Factory Act in nineteenth-century Britain, in which the eruption of the second molar at around 12 years of age was used to indicate that a child was old enough for factory employment (Sinclair, 1989). Cattell (1928) was the first to assign a dental age based on the number of teeth that had appeared in the mouth.

However, there are some difficulties with using tooth emergence or eruption as a criterion for determining dental age, not least of which is the lack of agreement on definitions of emergence and eruption. Assessment of the number of teeth present may be useful on a population basis but may be quite inaccurate for the individual child. This may be attributable to local factors affecting the dentition such as infection, crowding, early loss of the overlying deciduous teeth, etc., all of which can affect the timing of eruption. The other great limitation on the use of this method is that the periods during which it can be applied are restricted. Between approximately 2.5 years, when the primary dentition has erupted, and 6 years, when the permanent teeth begin to emerge, there is no change in the number of teeth present. Similarly, after the eruption of the second molars at around 12 years, little change is evident in the mouth. The third molars, the wisdom teeth, are usually ignored as their presence and appearance are highly variable, and they are frequently missing.

For the above reasons, a better system of age estimation was sought. Gleiser and Hunt (1955) first put forward the idea that an assessment of tooth calcification, rather than emergence, may be more useful. 'Dental formation or calcification, which is a continuous developmental process, should be considered as a better measure of physical maturity than a short-lived and environmentally dependent phenomenon such as dental emergence' (Demirjian, 1978). The time over which somatic maturation can be monitored is considerable since the dental system has two overlapping periods of development for the two sets of teeth: the primary dentition period extends from the third month of intrauterine life to the third postnatal year, the secondary dentition (excluding the wisdom teeth) from 6 months to 14–15 years of age. Teeth, like bones, go through a set sequence of stages until they are fully mature, and these developmental stages can be followed radiographically. Utilizing this concept, many workers (Garn *et al.,* 1958; Nolla, 1960; Moorees *et al.,* 1963; Liliequist and Lundberg, 1971) have, over time, developed rating systems looking at different teeth, or combinations of a number of teeth, to assess a child's dental maturity. Amongst others, these systems all suffer from the disadvantage that absolute values for the lengths of teeth, crowns or roots have been used in describing the various stages, and there is considerable variation in tooth length between individuals.

To eliminate some of these problems, Demirjian *et al.* (1973) devised a system based on the same principle as the skeletal age assessment of Tanner *et al.* (1975), described above. Using a panoramic radiograph of all the teeth, seven left mandibular teeth (from central incisor to second molar) are assessed. Weighted scores are assigned to each of eight stages from calcification of the cusp (0 for no calcification) to closure of the apex. Letters rather than numbers are used, as with the bone scoring system, as the stages are not equidistant. A maturity score of between 0 and 100 is obtained. Scores and percentile standards are calculated separately for boys and girls because, as with skeletal maturation, girls tend to be more advanced in the development of their permanent dentition than boys. The standard sample originally consisted of approximately 1400 boys and girls of French-Canadian origin. This was subsequently enlarged to over 2000 children of each sex, and centile charts are now available for children aged 3 to 17 years (Demirjian and Goldstein, 1976). As with the bone scoring system, the maturity score can be converted to a dental age by using the 50th centile score. Because panoramic radiographs are not always readily available, or the first molar may have been extracted, two additional systems based on scoring only four teeth have been developed. Equal biological weights for each tooth are used in the three systems, and the correlation between them is quite high at most ages. As with skeletal maturation, there are some population differences, and these need to be considered when comparing children from different environments with the French-Canadian standards.

SEXUAL AGE

The development of an individual's secondary sex characteristics during puberty can also be used to provide further information on the child's progress towards maturity. However, the sequence and timing of the particular events that occur during this period vary considerably from one person to the next (unlike the relatively fixed sequences of development in bones and teeth), and knowing when one of these events occurs gives us little information of when the others may occur. Also, the time of commencement of these changes gives little indication of the rate of progress, so that those who start early do not necessarily reach sexual maturity first; some children complete puberty in 2 years, others in close to 5 (Sinclair, 1989).

Noting the time of first appearance of a particular feature or the attainment of a certain stage of organ development can be used to provide an estimate of an individual's sexual age. Charts such as those shown in Fig. 16.8 for the average American boy and girl show the range of ages during which each event occurs and can be used to compare an individual's developmental pattern with that of a standard group. In boys, the first sign of puberty is the further development of the infant testes. The testicular volume can be measured by palpation and comparison with a device called an orchidometer. The average volume of an adult testicle is about 20 mL, and when a volume of 6 mL is attained, the boy can be considered to have begun puberty (Sinclair, 1989). No precise scale for measuring the development of the external genitalia (penis and scrotum) has been devised, but Tanner (1962) divided the process into five stages that could be described and differentiated from each other, stage 1 being prepubertal and stage 5 indicating the end point of adolescent growth.

A similar system is used to classify the appearance of pubic hair. The mean age for the first appearance of pubic hair in European boys is just below age 12 (Marshall and Tanner, 1970). Axillary hair usually first appears more than a year after the onset of pubic hair growth (Neyzi *et al.,* 1975). Facial hair, which is first seen at the corners of the upper lip, is later still, at a mean age of just over 14.5 years. Hair then spreads across the upper lip and onto the upper part of the cheek and the midline area below the lower lip. This is on average not before the age of 16.5 years. Complete development of both genitalia and pubic hair normally precedes hair growth on the chin (Tanner, 1962). Breaking of the voice, which accompanies rapid growth of the larynx, is not heard until about the termination of penile growth and usually occurs close to the time of maximum growth velocity in height. Once a boy has a male voice, he can be assumed to have attained or passed his peak height velocity (Hägg and Taranger, 1982). Thus in boys, the externally visible signs of puberty such as the growth spurt, facial hair and male voice do not occur until relatively late when they are nearly sexually mature.

This differs from the situation in girls, in whom the visible signs of puberty occur earlier. Breast enlarge-

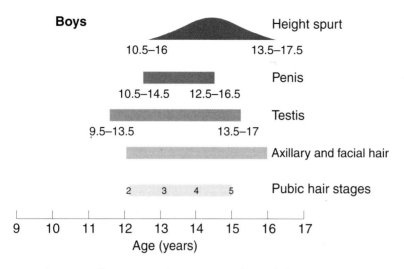

Sequence of events at puberty in boys

(a)

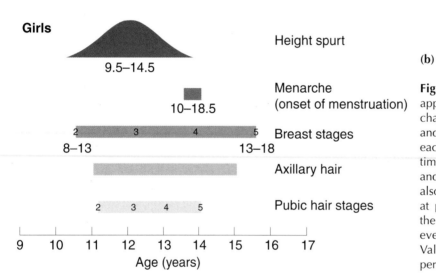

(b)

Fig. 16.8 (a) Sequence of appearance of the secondary sex characteristics for an average boy, and the range of ages during which each event occurs. The amount of time generally required for the penis and testes to complete their growth is also shown. (b) Sequence of events at puberty for an average girl, and the range of ages during which each event occurs. Reproduced from Valadian and Porter (1977) with permission

ment, which precedes peak height velocity, is the first visible sign of puberty. Both breast development and pubic hair appearance have been divided into five stages for descriptive purposes and to facilitate the estimation of sexual age. Breast development is fairly variable: it may begin as early as 8 years of age in some girls and, in late developers, may not be complete until age 19 or later. Most girls, however, have commenced before their thirteenth birthday. The first appearance of pubic hair usually occurs at a mean age of just over 11 (van Wieringen *et al.*, 1971). Axillary hair development normally occurs once breast development is well underway, but in some normal girls it may precede it.

The timing of the occurrence of menarche (onset of menstruation) has been most widely studied as precise data can be obtained for this event. It occurs fairly late in puberty, invariably after peak height velocity has been reached, and corresponds to the period of maximal deceleration in height. Differences between populations in age at menarche are due to genetic and environmental factors. There has also been a secular change. During the twentieth century, menarche has occurred progressively earlier in many parts of the world, but in some Western countries, this trend is no longer apparent and the age of menarche appears to have stabilized. Modern European population means lie between 12.9 and 13.4 years, with the exception of Italians, who reach menarche earlier (around 12.5–12.6 years) (Marshall, 1978). In Australia and New Zealand, the median is similar to that of the UK, i.e. 13.0 years (Jones *et al.*, 1973).

Correlations between biological ageing methods

In studies using dental emergence criteria, greater correlations were found between dental age and chronological age than between dental emergence and bone age, age at peak height velocity or age at menarche (Lamons and Gray, 1958; Meredith, 1959; Nanda, 1960; Bjork and Helm, 1967). Similar conclusions were drawn from studies using tooth calcification criteria (Hotz, 1959; Green, 1961; Demirjian, 1978). Lewis and Garn (1960), on finding less variability in dental development than skeletal development, suggested that the former is a better criterion of biological maturation than is ossification and that dental maturation could be used to determine chronological age. It is generally agreed that there is no close relationship between the growth of the face, which follows the general somatic pattern, and dental development: the skeletal and dental systems are substantially independent.

Facial types

As already mentioned, head shape can be described as dolichocephalic, brachycephalic or the intermediate form, mesocephalic. The facial complex is attached to the cranial floor, which acts as a template for establishing many of the characteristics of the face. The dolichocephalic head form tends to be associated with long, narrow protrusive faces, termed leptoprosopic. Conversely, the brachycephalic head form frequently establishes a face that is short, broad and less protrusive, also known as euryprosopic (Fig. 16.9). In different population groups, one or the other type tends to predominate. However, as with all biological variables, a distribution range from one extreme to the other is seen in each group. In northern and southern continental Europe, as well as the UK, Scandinavia, northern Africa and some Near and Middle Eastern countries, the dolichocephalic head form is more common, whereas brachycephaly tends to predominate in central Europe (Alpine head form) and the Far East (Oriental). Another, quite distinctive head form, called the dinaric, is found at the geographic interface between the dolicho- and brachycephalic regions. This admixture produces not a mesocephalic skull but one that is technically brachycephalic because the posterior portion of the skull has been flattened; however, the face itself appears more dolichocephalic (Enlow, 1990).

Since the association of a particular face type with head form does not always hold true, a facial index has been developed to classify the face more accurately. Cole (1963) defined the facial index to be 'the length of the face from the root of the nose to the bottom of the chin, expressed as a percentage of the greatest breadth across the cheek bone' (this differs from the cephalic index, which is breadth divided by length). The values for the facial indices given by Cole are: broad <85, medium 85–88, and narrow >88. In more recent orthodontic literature, these facial types are usually referred to as brachyfacial (broad), mesofacial (medium) and dolichofacial (narrow). The facial types differ in such characteristics as the slope of the forehead, nose shape, set of the eyes, prominence of cheekbones, facial profile and position of mandible, and therefore occlusion.

Dolichofacial individuals tend to have vertically longer and more protrusive noses, sometimes aquiline in contour, with a downturned tip. The bridge and root of the nose are higher, and the nasal profile follows the line of the sloping forehead, which is characterized by a pronounced glabella and upper orbital rims. Because the nasal region and the supraorbital ridges are protrusive, the cheekbones appear less prominent and the eyes more deep set. The midface is long to provide adequate airway capacity, but correspondingly narrow; therefore, the palate and maxillary arch conform to this. The direction of mandibular growth tends to be downward and backward, so the chin and lower lip appear retrusive and the profile convex. Individuals with this facial type often have a tendency towards an open bite (the upper and lower teeth do not overlap) and crowded arches. This may be accompanied by mouth-breathing and a high lip line, resulting in a gummy smile. This is obviously an extreme example, and dolichofacial individuals may have a normal occlusion through compensatory adjustments in various facial components.

Brachyfacial characteristics are obviously the obverse of those listed above. The nose is shorter, straighter or often concave, and with a more rounded tip. The nasal bridge is lower, breaking from a more bulbous and upright forehead. The brow ridges are not as pronounced, but the eyes tend to bulge more. The wider, flatter face makes the cheekbones appear more prominent. Both facial types have an approximately equivalent airway capacity so the midface in the euryprosopic face is shorter but broader, as are the palate and maxillary arch. The lower jaw and chin are more protrusive and the profile straight or even concave. The mandible tends to rotate up and forwards with growth, which may result in a deep bite and an everted lower lip. The fully developed dental arches show a squaring of their shape without crowding of teeth.

From the descriptions given earlier, it can be seen that many of the features characteristically ascribed to a brachyfacial individual also apply to a baby or female face. In fact, before puberty, the faces of boys and girls are comparable, and it is often easy to mistake one gender for the other. Only at adolescence do the facial differences between the sexes become marked, and since girls' faces grow very slowly beyond about 13 years of age, their appearance as young adults is not as greatly altered as is that of males.

Ricketts and his orthodontic colleagues (1979) described a number of angles that could be measured on lateral head radiographs to determine an individual's facial type. On the basis of these angles, facial patterns were defined. 'Mesofacial' describes an average facial pattern with a normal maxillo-mandibular relationship, a harmonious musculature and a pleasant soft tissue profile; if a malocclusion exists, it is usually classified as class I. 'Brachyfacial' is associated with a horizontal growth pattern, and if a malocclusion is present, it is typically a class II division 2, i.e. there is a deep bite and the front teeth are more upright. 'Dolichofacial' implies a vertical growth pattern, and the malocclusion frequently associated with this facial type is class II division 1, in which the lower arch is distal relative to the upper, and the front teeth are more proclined – the typical 'buck teeth' appearance.

Few studies, particularly longitudinal ones, have been carried out on the stability of facial types with growth. However, from the information available, it appears that the concept of logarithmic growth holds true, i.e. there is a change in size but not in shape and direction, at least on a population basis. Moss (1964), in a cross-sectional study, reported that, during growth, upper and lower face height maintain their relative proportionality of total face height. Similarly, Ricketts (1981) showed that the growth direction of the mandible did not change with age. Bishara and Jakobsen (1985) concluded that there is a strong tendency to maintain the original facial type with age since 77% of their longitudinal sample were categorized as having the same facial type at 5 and at 25.5 years. Moreover, comparison of the growth curves of the different parameters (they measured 48) showed that the curves consistently demonstrated parallelism regardless of the facial type, i.e. relativities were maintained. Differences between the three facial types, particularly in the vertical relationships, were more pronounced at adulthood compared with childhood. This would perhaps make identification of a missing child who subsequently displays markedly dolichofacial tendencies more difficult, as greater change can be expected. In addition, there is a large variation in the amount of growth and in the size and relationships of the various facial components within each facial type. These factors ensure that predicting the growth of an individual child, particularly one whose growth pattern is unknown, is not an easy matter.

Growth prediction

At present, attempts at 'predicting' what a missing child will look like some years hence are purely subjective, based on an individual police artist's concepts of how the child's appearance will change. Modifications made to existing photos to simulate growth changes are largely dependent on the particular artist's skills, intuition and observational capacity, and therefore the success of the venture is likely to be very variable. Can science as well as art be employed in this process to produce a better outcome?

'The simplest method of prediction assumes that growth will take place as a linear expansion along the long axis of the structures being examined and that its amount is quantified as averaged growth increments added progressively through time' (Macri and Athanasiou, 1995). Growth prediction presented as above may sound relatively straightforward, but it is, however, fraught with difficulties. Some of these are (1) the wide range of morphological differences between individuals, (2) the varying rates and directions during the growth period, (3) the varying influence of modifying environmental factors, (4) variation in the timing of the different areas of active growth, and (5) a lack of correlation between the size of facial structures at an early age and the ultimate adult size (Ari-Viro and Wisth, 1983). Other difficulties, as perceived by Rakosi (1982), are the variable growth rates in regional growth sites; for example, the mean annual rate of increase in the base of the maxilla between 8 and 14 years of age is approximately 0.8 mm while that of the mandibular base is 1.9 mm. These are simply means derived from a specific population, and no allowance is made for individual differences in biological age or growth pattern. Function may also affect the final form attained; for example, the tautness of the lower lip may prevent compensatory proclination of the lower incisors in individuals with a retruded mandible. The major limitation of the method outlined above, therefore, is that individual variability is not taken into account.

In the area of growth prediction, the greatest amount of work has been done in the field of cephalometry, i.e. the analysis of standardized radiographs of the head and part of the neck; this method has now largely replaced classical anthropometric measurement methods. Even though cephalometry may not be directly applicable to the problem in hand, i.e. predicting what a child will look like, as radiographs of missing children will be available only in rare instances, much has been learned about craniofacial skeletal morphology and the similarities and differences between and within different population groups through the use of this method. Studies

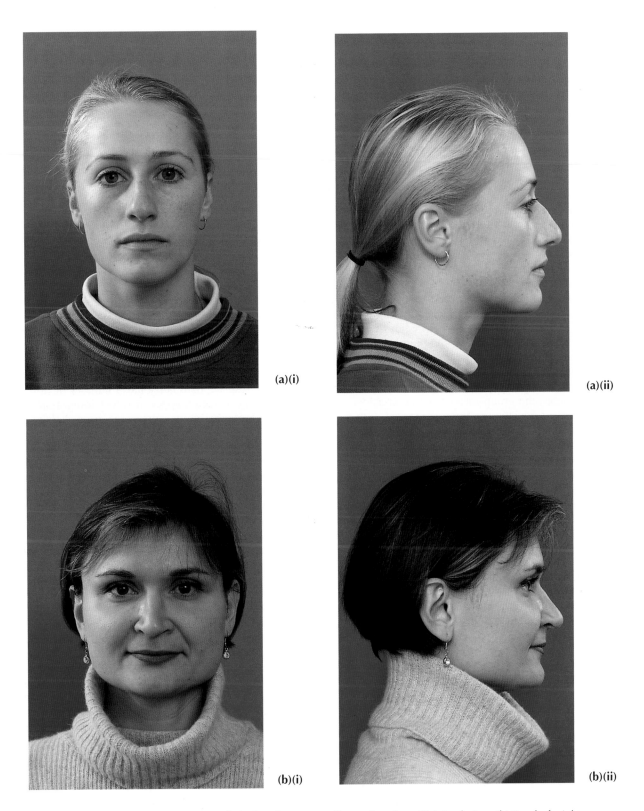

Fig. 16.9 Different facial types. (a) Dolichofacial teenager: (i) anterior view, (ii) lateral view. (b) Brachyfacial teenager: (i) anterior view. (ii) lateral view

of general trends and the variability of craniofacial growth through time have been conducted using radiographs taken at multiple time points on a longitudinal basis. From these, standards for growth patterns characterizing various growth types have been developed (Riolo *et al.*, 1974; Broadbent *et al.*, 1975; Popovich and Thompson, 1977). Using such data, attempts have also been made to develop algorithms for the prediction of craniofacial growth, and some computer-based methods have been commercialized (Ricketts *et al.*, 1979).

The current controversy about growth prediction may be more a matter of interpretation in that the ability to predict growth on a group basis is mistaken for the ability to predict growth of the individual. The generation of statistical predictors using cephalometry is partly determined by topographical correlations, and biologically meaningful correlations are poor; hence a large part of the total variation in individual cases is unexplained. Because of individual variation in growth, it is easier to predict the mean value of any parameter than it is to predict the value for any single individual in the group from which the mean is drawn. In predicting change in the individual, not only the group mean but also the individual's deviation from the group mean must be considered. If the standard deviation is small compared with the mean, i.e. there is relatively little individual variation in particular parameters, the use of the mean in individual cases may be satisfactory. An additional problem in the case of the individual is the error with which the particular individual is measured. This is usually a larger problem than with groups, where error is randomized, and may be greater than the average measured change. On a group basis, growth prediction can be very precise, and the precision increases as the group size is augmented. However, when mean values derived from earlier studies are used, consideration must be given to how well the previously acquired means approximate the true means of the population under study. Questions relating to the measurement techniques used, regional or cultural differences and secular trends need to be addressed. The more similar the groups are, and the less variation there is in the effect that is to be predicted, the better is the predictive power.

As mentioned earlier, a 'pattern extension' method is traditionally used to predict growth by adding mean annual increments during a given time period. This ignores individual differences in growth increments, variations in biological age and the timing of the adolescent growth spurt, by adding the same amount to each child. Therefore, growth prediction in individual cases is currently not good enough to be clinically useful in orthodontics.

Attempts have been made to improve on this method. Buschang *et al.* (1990), using a longitudinal database, employed a multilevel prediction procedure with a requirement for an earlier follow-up before the required time of prediction, i.e. the individual child's previous growth pattern was considered. Parental and/or sibling data were used in a couple of studies (Saunders *et al.*, 1980; Suzuki and Takahama, 1991) and appear to enhance the predictive power. Another method of growth prediction has focused on proportional relationships amongst facial landmarks within a rectilinear co-ordinate system using a mesh diagram (Moorees *et al.*, 1991). Despite the fact that the facial type of an individual has been shown to be relatively stable between 8 and 16 years of age, standard errors, using this method, show a range in individual response to growth that lowers the precision of prediction sought.

Cephalometry currently appears to be the only feasible method for investigating the spatial relationships between cranial structures and between dental and surface structures. Ultrasound imaging, magnetic resonance imaging (MRI) and computed tomography (CT) can also be used for this purpose, but costs are higher and resolution lower than with cephalometry at present.

Nevertheless, cephalometry has a number of limitations, many of which apply also to photogrammetry, i.e. the taking of measurements from standard photographs of the face. The absence of anatomical references whose shape and location remain constant over time, together with the lack of sufficient standardization in image acquisition and measurement procedures, makes comparisons at different time points difficult. An added complication is the inherent ambiguity in locating landmarks since they often lack well-defined outlines. Cephalograms and photographs present static two-dimensional projections of a dynamically changing three-dimensional object, so information about biological processes and three-dimensional shape is lost. Paired co-planar images are needed to obtain true three-dimensional co-ordinate data, but this is not yet standard procedure. The application of digital technology and processing may facilitate growth analysis by improving superimposition accuracy and by eliminating errors derived from intra- and interobserver variability through the use of computerized, non-subjective landmark identification (Cohen and Linney, 1986).

Thus, in summary, when attempting to predict the growth of children's faces to assist in human identification, consideration should be given to all known factors that can influence facial growth. The main factors include biological age, gender, ethnicity, facial type and growth prognosis as well as the anatomical relationships between the component parts of the face. Currently, no simple formulae can be universally applied to determine this, nor has any method been devised to make precise prediction of growth of an individual a reality. However, on a population basis, fairly precise prediction is possible. The most accurate growth prediction is likely to occur when a large reference group is used to derive standard values and when this reference group is similar to the individual or population under investigation. The urgency of the social problem of missing children has stimulated enormous research in this area. At present, prediction of the way in which a particular child's face will age still relies largely on subjective artistic impressions. However, as our anatomical knowledge and understanding improves, the use of scientific and computer modelling techniques should lead to improved results in predicting the growth of faces.

References

Ari-Viro A, Wisth PJ. 1983: An evaluation of the method of structural growth prediction. *European Journal of Orthodontics* **5**, 199–207.

Baer MJ. 1977: *Growth and maturation. An introduction to physical development.* Cambridge, MA: Howard A. Doyle.

Bayley N, Pinneau SR. 1952: Tables for predicting adult height from skeletal age: revised for use with the Greulich–Pyle hand standards. *Journal of Pediatrics* **40**, 423–41.

Bishara SE, Jakobsen JR. 1985: Longitudinal changes in three normal facial types. *American Journal of Orthodontics* **88**, 466–502.

Bjork A, Helm S. 1967: Prediction of the age of maximum pubertal growth in body height. *Angle Orthodontist* **37**, 134–43.

British Medical Dictionary. Revised edition. London: Claxton, 1963.

Broadbent BH Sr, Broadbent BH Jr, Golden WH. 1975: *Bolton standards of dentofacial development and growth.* St Louis: C.V. Mosby.

Buschang PH, Tanguay R, LaPalme L, Demirjian A. 1990: Mandibular growth prediction: mean growth increments versus mathematical models. *European Journal of Orthodontics* **12**, 290–6.

Cattell P. 1928: *Dentition as a measure of maturity.* Cambridge, MA: Harvard University Press.

Cohen AM, Linney AD. 1986: A low cost system for computer-based cephalometric analysis. *British Journal of Orthodontics* **13**, 105–8.

Cole S. 1963: *Races of man.* London: British Museum.

Demirjian A. 1978: Dentition. In Falkner F, Tanner JM. (eds) *Human growth.* Vol. 2: *Postnatal growth.* New York: Plenum Press, 413–44.

Demirjian A, Goldstein H. 1976: New systems for dental maturity based on seven and four teeth. *Annals of Human Biology* **3**, 411–21.

Demirjian A, Goldstein H, Tanner JM. 1973: A new system of dental age assessment. *Human Biology* **45**, 211–27.

Enlow DH. (ed.) 1990: *Facial growth.* Philadelphia: W.B. Saunders.

Falkner F, Tanner JM. (eds) 1978: *Human growth.* Vol. 2: *Postnatal growth.* New York: Plenum Press, vii–viii.

Farkas F, Posnick JC. 1992: Growth and development of regional units in the head and face based on anthropometric measurements. *Cleft Palate-Craniofacial Journal* **29**, 301–29.

Farkas LG, Posnick JC, Hreczko TM. 1992a: Anthropometric growth study of the head. *Cleft Palate-Craniofacial Journal* **29**, 303–8.

Farkas LG, Posnick JC, Hreczko TM, Pron GE. 1992b: Growth patterns in the orbital region: a morphometric study. *Cleft Palate-Craniofacial Journal* **29**, 315–18.

Farkas LG, Posnick JC, Hreczko TM. 1992c: Growth patterns of the face: a morphometric study. *Cleft Palate-Craniofacial Journal* **29**, 308–14.

Farkas LG, Posnick JC, Hreczko TM, Pron GE. 1992d: Growth patterns of the nasolabial region: a morphometric study. *Cleft Palate-Craniofacial Journal* **29**, 318–24.

Farkas LG, Posnick JC, Hreczko TM. 1992e: Anthropometric growth study of the ear. *Cleft Palate-Craniofacial Journal* **29**, 324–7.

Garn SM, Lewis AB, Koski PK, Polacheck DL. 1958: The sex difference in tooth calcification. *Journal of Dental Research* **37**, 561–7.

Genecov JS, Sinclair PM, Dechow PC. 1990: Development of the nose and soft tissue profile. *Angle Orthodontist* **60**, 191–8.

Gleiser I, Hunt EE Jr. 1955: The permanent mandibular first molar: its calcification, eruption and decay. *American Journal of Physical Anthropology* **13**, 253–81.

Green LJ. 1961: The interrelationships among height, weight, and chronological, dental and skeletal ages. *Angle Orthodontist* **31**, 189–93.

Hägg U, Taranger J. 1982: Maturation indicators and the pubertal growth spurt. *American Journal of Orthodontics* **82**, 299–309.

Hajnis K. 1987: Categories in classical anthropometric systems. In Farkas LG, Munro IR. (eds) *Anthropometric facial proportions in medicine.* Springfield, IL: Charles C. Thomas, 9–17.

Haselden R. 1991: Lost children. *Weekend Guardian*, 4–6.

Hotz R. 1959: The relation of dental calcification to chronological and skeletal age. *Transactions of the European Orthodontic Society* **35**, 140.

Hreczko T, Farkas LG, Katic M. 1990: Clinical significance of age-related changes of the palpebral fissures between age 2 and 18 years in healthy Caucasians. *Acta Chirurgica Plastika* **32**, 194–204.

Human Rights and Equal Opportunity Commission 1989: *Our homeless children (Report of the National Enquiry into Homeless Children).* Canberra: AGPS.

Israel H. 1978: The fundamentals of cranial and facial growth. In Falkner F, Tanner JM. (eds) *Human growth*, Vol. 2: *Postnatal Growth.* New York: Plenum Press, 357–80.

Jones B. 1988: *Searching for Tony.* Richmond, Victoria: Spectrum Publishers.

Jones EL, Hemphill W, Mayers, ESA. 1973: *Height, weight, and other physical characteristics of New South Wales children.* Part I: *Children aged 5 years and over.* Sydney: New South Wales Department of Health.

Kapardis A. 1995: *Missing persons in Victoria: myths and realities.* First International Missing Persons Conference, Melbourne, Victoria, 2–5 April 1995.

Lamons FF, Gray SW. 1958: A study of the relationship between tooth eruption age, skeletal development age, and chronological age in sixty-one Atlanta children. *American Journal of Orthodontics* **44**, 687–91.

Lewis AB, Garn SM. 1960: The relationship between tooth formation and other maturational factors. *Angle Orthodontist* **30**, 70–7.

Liggett J. 1974: *The human face.* London: Constable.

Liliequist B, Lundberg M. 1971: Skeletal and tooth development. *Acta Radiologica Diagnostica* **11**, 97–112.

Macri V, Athanasiou AE. 1995: Sources of error in lateral cephalometry. In Athanasiou AE (ed.) *Orthodontic cephalometry.* London: Mosby-Wolfe, 125–40.

Marshall WA. 1978: Puberty. In Falkner F, Tanner JM (eds) *Human growth*, Vol. 2: *Postnatal growth.* New York: Plenum Press, 141–81.

Marshall WA, Tanner JM. 1970: Variation in the pattern of pubertal changes in boys. *Archives of Disease in Childhood* **45**, 13–23.

Meredith HV. 1959: Relation between the eruption of selected mandibular permanent teeth and the circumpubertal acceleration in stature. *Journal of Dentistry for Children* **26**, 75–8.

Moorees CFA, Fanning EA, Hunt EE Jr. 1963: Formation and resorption of three deciduous teeth in children. *American Journal of Physical Anthropology* **21**, 205–13.

Moorees CF, Efstratiadis SS, Kent RL Jr. 1991: The mesh diagram for analysis of facial growth. *Proceedings of the Finnish Dental Society* **87**, 33–41.

Moss ML. 1964: Vertical growth of the human face. *American Journal of Orthodontics* **50**, 359–76.

Nanda RS. 1960: Eruption of human teeth. *American Journal of Orthodontics* **46**, 363–78.

National Centre for Missing and Exploited Children Fact Sheet, 1996. Arlington, Virginia: US Dept. of Justice.

Neyzi O, Alp H, Yalcindag A, Yakacikli S, Orphon A. 1975: Sexual maturation in Turkish boys. *Annals of Human Biology* **2**, 251–9.

Nolla CM. 1960: The development of the permanent dentition. *Journal of Dentistry for Children* **27**, 254–66.

Peck H, Peck SA. 1970: A concept of facial esthetics. *Angle Orthodontist* **40**, 284–317.

Popovich F, Thompson GW. 1977: Craniofacial templates for orthodontic case analysis. *American Journal of Orthodontics* **71**, 406–20.

Prahl-Andersen B, Ligthelm-Bakker ASWMR, Wattel E, Nanda R. 1995: Adolescent growth changes in soft tissue profile. *American Journal of Orthodontics and Dentofacial Orthopaedics* **107**, 476–83.

Pyle SI, Waterhouse AM, Greulich WW. 1971: *A radiographic standard of reference for the growing hand and wrist. Prepared for the United States National Health Examination Survey.* Cleveland, Ohio: Press of Case Western Reserve University.

Rakosi T. 1982: *An atlas and manual of cephalometric radiography.* London: Wolfe.

Ranly DM. 1988: *A synopsis of craniofacial growth.* Norwalk, CT: Appleton & Lange.

Ricketts RM. 1981: Perspectives in the clinical application of cephalometrics. The first 50 years. *Angle Orthodontist* **51**, 115–50.

Ricketts RM, Bench RW, Gugino CF, Hilgers JW, Schulhof RJ. 1979: *Bioprogressive therapy.* Denver, CO: Rocky Mountain Orthodontics.

Riolo ML, Moyers RE, McNamara JA, Hunter WS. 1974: *An atlas of craniofacial growth: cephalometric standards from the University School Growth Study, the University of Michigan.* Monograph 2, Craniofacial Growth Series. Ann Arbor: University of Michigan Center for Human Growth and Development.

Roche AF, Chumlea WC, Thissen D. 1988: *Assessing the skeletal maturity of the hand-wrist: FELS method.* Springfield, IL: Charles C. Thomas.

Safe M. 1995: Missing. *Australian Magazine*, 36–41.

Saunders S, Popovich F, Thompson GW. 1980: A family study of craniofacial dimensions in the Burlington Growth Centre sample. *American Journal of Orthodontics* **78**, 394–403.

Scott JH. 1954: The growth of the human face. *Proceedings of the Royal Society of Medicine* **47**, 5.

Sillman JH. 1964: Dimensional changes of the dental arches: longitudinal study from birth to 25 years. *American Journal of Orthodontics* **39**, 729–55.

Sinclair D. 1989: *Human growth after birth* (5th edn). Oxford: Oxford University Press.

Stamrud L. 1959: External and internal cranial base: a cross-sectional study of growth and association in form. *Acta Odontologica Scandinavica* **17**, 239.

Sullivan PG. 1978: Skull, jaw, and teeth growth patterns. In Falkner F, Tanner JM. (eds) *Human growth*. Vol. 2: *Postnatal growth.* New York: Plenum Press, 381–412.

Suzuki A, Takahama Y. 1991: Parental data used to predict growth of craniofacial form. *American Journal of Orthodontics and Dentofacial Orthopaedics* **99**, 107–19.

Tanner JM. 1962: *Growth at adolescence.* Oxford: Blackwell.

Tanner JM. 1975: The measurement of maturity. *Transactions of the European Orthodontic Society* **51**, 45–60.

Tanner JM, Whitehouse RH, Healy MJR. 1962: *A new system for estimating skeletal maturity from the hand and wrist, with standards derived from a study of 2,600 healthy British children.* Parts I and II. Paris: Centre International de l'Enfance.

Tanner JM, Whitehouse RH, Marshall WA, Healy MJR, Goldstein H. 1975: *Assessment of skeletal maturity and prediction of adult height: TW2 method.* London: Academic Press.

Tanner JM, Whitehouse RH, Cameron N, Marshall WA, Healy MJR, Goldstein H. 1983: *Assessment of skeletal maturity and prediction of adult height* (2nd edn). London: Academic Press.

US Department of Justice. 1996: *National Centre for Missing and Exploited Children Fact Sheet.* Arlington, VA.

Valadian I, Porter D. 1977: *Physical growth and development from conception to maturity.* Boston: Little, Brown.

van Wieringen JC, Vebrugge HP, De Haas JH. 1971: *Growth diagrams 1965 Netherlands.* Groningen: Wolters-Noordhoff.

Victoria Police Missing Persons Unit. 1991: *Statistics.* Melbourne: Victoria Office.

Victoria Police Missing Persons Unit. 1995: *Statistics.* Melbourne: Victoria Office.

Vincent C. 1990: *Teenage runaways Australia and USA: perspective.* First National Police Conference on Missing Persons, Penrith, NSW, 11–13 September, 1990.

CHAPTER 17

Age changes to the face in adulthood

R NEAVE

Introduction	225	Milestones in ageing	227
General remarks	225	Conclusion	231
The ageing process	226		

Introduction

There is only one thing in life that we can be certain of, and that is that we will die. Given that we are privileged to live for a reasonable life span we will also age. What is not certain is just how the ageing mechanisms will affect the outward appearance of our face and at what point in our life they will start to take effect. This chapter will confine itself to the question of how the appearance of an adult face may change as a result of the ageing process. It will further attempt to outline the stages at which the primary alterations to an individual's facial features may occur. It must be borne in mind, however, that there are no absolute certainties about age changes in the face, and as with most other forces that operate upon the human body, genetic and environmental influences will be the most potent.

General remarks

In common with the majority of other biological functions, there is a recognizably predictable pattern that can be seen with age changes. The male will change slowly but steadily for most of his life, whereas the female, while changing all the time, tends to have accelerated changes after the menopause. This predictability of the broad patterns of change explains why there are stereotypic images for certain types of 'character' in most folk tales throughout the world. More importantly, knowledge of these changes enables an individual to develop a tolerably objective mental database upon which to draw when endeavouring to describe a particular type of person. Such a mental database is essential for the cartoonist and the illustrator, and one sees it being drawn upon in the theatre, particularly in dance and opera, in which the nature of a character must be instantly recognizable.

This character symbolism can be found in all cultures throughout the world. Descriptions that are frequently used, such as 'the wrinkled little man', 'she looked like a witch', 'the rosy-cheeked youth', 'he had the appearance of a seafaring man', etc., assume that the recipient of these descriptions understands the significance of their meaning. They carry with them not only a literal description of the appearance of a person but also some indication of the probable age of the character being described. We routinely associate wrinkles with age, and the 'wrinkled little man' in the mind's eye is an elderly man, probably with white hair or bald. 'Looking like a witch' is much more informative if we consider the classic European image. The classic witch is depicted as having a long hooked nose and pointed chin; thus the character being described is edentulous, wrinkled and thin, has a poor skin complexion and is again probably white haired. All these are features that one associates with great age. 'Rosy-cheeked youth' implies good health, vulnerability and possibly desirability. The 'seafaring man' is different again. The description implies a degree of maturity, strength and self-reliance gained by facing and combatting the elements and the forces of nature. In particular, it further implies the gaze of a man whose looks boldly into the distance rather than down a microscope or over the realm of a desk. Such recognizable features can frequently be seen; otherwise, such descriptions would not exist which thereby support the observation that there exist clearly recognized features that may be associated with age changes.

The ageing process

The ageing process is unpredictable in terms of the speed with which changes are likely to take place in different individuals. Some retain a youthful appearance for much of their lives and age more rapidly in later years, whereas others will have a very mature look relatively early in life. By the sixth decade, however, these differences will tend to even out, both the initially mature and the youthful now looking very similar.

The physical mechanics of changes to the face are common to all races of humankind. How and when these changes occur will be greatly influenced by the environment and lifestyle. Long exposure to strong sunlight will accelerate the onset of wrinkles and creases. Furthermore, not only does the ultraviolet light affect the skin, causing such permanent physical changes to take place, but the natural reaction of the face when exposed to bright light is to screw up the soft tissues around the eyes. This will in turn cause the rest of the face to stretch and contract, causing a network of lines and wrinkles to play on the surface of the skin. These ultimately become etched into the skin relatively early in life. Diet plays an important role in the development of the whole of the body, and in the adult, this will often be manifested in the outward appearance of the face. This is particularly so if the abrasiveness of the diet is enough to cause excessive attrition of the teeth resulting in the loss of, or damage to, teeth and gums.

The process of ageing, of appearing to be older, is largely a degenerative process. The primary changes take place in the skin, in the first instance, with loss of tissue elasticity and colour changes. Colour changes will take place in the hair in the majority of people, although the rate of pigmentation loss is unpre-

dictable, varying greatly between individuals. Some people retain a full head of hair without any colour changes from childhood to over the age of 80. In others, the hair can lose all its colour by 30. In males, hair loss is another change that is associated with subjects of over 50 but can be very advanced in subjects as young as the age of 25. The predisposition of one individual to lose his hair and of another to maintain a full head of hair into old age is largely a genetic factor, as is the loss of pigmentation. Alterations to skin colour are more noticeable in later life, although the much-admired smooth and blemish-free skin of the young is unlikely to persist much after the age of 30. In much later life, the skin develops blotches and spots of a brownish hue, similar to freckles.

Alterations that take place in the bone and the cartilage are likely to have far less dramatic effects to the facial appearance and will take place at a time much more in keeping with the biological age of a person. Bone resorption of the alveolar processes of the mandible and maxilla takes place naturally during life but is greatly accelerated following tooth loss.

Marginal growth of the cartilaginous portions of the nose and the ears is again something that is more likely to reflect the biological age than the colour of the hair. In extreme old age (80+), the cranium may become slightly more elongated. All these alterations to the bone are frequently accompanied by changes to the rest of the skeleton, resulting in a change in posture that will also modify the overall appearance of a person's face.

Any consideration of apparent age from the visual appearance of the face of an individual must therefore be looked upon as uncertain. One can appreciate just how misleading many assumed points of reference may be when we remember that many people will have some loss of hair pigmentation by the age of 55. Conversely, there are those who will retain full hair colour until well beyond the age of 75.

Most changes that occur as the face ages may be considered to be structurally superficial. However, the changes that take place to the cartilage and bone are structural. These affect both the shape and the proportions of the face. Changes in the dentition may arise from resorption of some of the bone of the mandible and maxilla. Dental problems may in turn exacerbate this bone loss. These changes will affect the appearance of both the overlying soft tissue and the facial proportions. Having reduced numbers of teeth, and eventually possibly none to support, the bones of the mandible and maxilla will become smaller. Such a reduction in size will alter the dimensions of the lower part of the face, changing the proportions of the whole face. Alterations of this sort will be less apparent if dentures are worn, although the features of the mouth and surrounding area then become rather flattened. The ultimate overall effect upon the appearance of a person is that the nose will seem more prominent. The chin will look smaller but may seem to project further forward; the distance between the nose and chin will decrease, which results in the upper part of the face seeming larger.

Such changes to the proportions are important in the process of recognition as the spatial relationship between individual features are altered. The overall proportions of a head and face are fundamental to recognition. When changed, for whatever reason, albeit age or trauma, they will have a profound effect upon the face. The caricaturist who emphasizes the most pertinent features of a subject's face frequently makes a well-known personality even more easily recognizable than he or she would be from a photograph.

The soft tissue features surrounding and including the mouth are modified as the underlying support is reduced, allowing them to fall inwards, and the muscle bulk in the lips and cheeks becomes more discrete. As these changes occur, the upper lip becomes shorter, the philtrum will become less well defined, almost lost, while the white roll will lose its definition and the visible vermilion border of the lips will be greatly reduced.

This process naturally takes place over a considerable length of time and may be more realistically associated with elderly subjects, in whom further subtle alterations will take place. A degree of bone resorption will routinely be observed in most subjects by the age of 70 even if they have retained all their dentition. This, coupled with discrete increases in the cartilaginous parts of the nose and the ear, results in what is recognized as an elderly face.

The superficial alterations that affect the face as it first matures and then progressively ages are far easier to identify in the older subject as they are clearly likely to be more extreme, heavily etched and deep seated.

Milestones in ageing (Fig. 17.1)

YOUNG ADULTHOOD

When we look at how such changes may occur over a series of 10 year periods, in both males and females, it soon becomes evident that, while many individuals will not conform, a general pattern exists that holds good for us all. By taking as the starting point individuals in early adulthood (i.e. a 20-year-old who is healthy and living in a climate that is neither intensely hot nor intensely cold), we can consider the sorts of change that might occur over the next six decades.

Initially, it would be seen that the skin is smooth and highly elastic. The elasticity in the skin confers on it the ability to fold, crease and quickly revert to its former shape without leaving any trace. It is important to note this as creasing will always be repeated at the same site; it is this repetition that will determine where creases that are more permanent will appear when they become 'set'. The young face has a roundness to it. This is particularly noticeable in females, in whom there is often more underlying fat than in the male, giving rise to the characteristically smooth appearance of their cheeks. The skin is thinner, smoother and more translucent in the female, giving it a more delicate lustre. Any coarsening or disruption of the underlying structures will naturally affect this translucency in the skin, giving rise to a less than perfect appearance, which is also perceived as being a slightly older one. By the end of the third decade, the face will normally have assumed the degree of maturity and alertness, and in most cases the general expression, that it will habitually wear throughout life. This may be gentle, fierce, worried, cheerful, etc. Such expressions do not necessarily mirror the individual's character, but it is easy to understand how a constant worry may be accompanied a constant frown, which will in turn result in a permanently lined forehead. It is not easy to analyse just which changes have occurred signifying that the face being studied is that of a mature but young face as opposed to a very young face. In many cases, it is merely superficial factors such as hairstyles, which may in the male be accompanied by the growing of a beard and/or moustache, that account for this confusion. Less obvious may be the general thinning down of the face and the loss of some of the buccal fat, giving the cheeks a less childish look. These changes will in turn most probably be accompanied by the line of the mandible being slightly more accentuated.

ADULTHOOD

By the end of the third decade, folds lines and creases are starting to become 'set'. Thus a few discrete lines can frequently be observed across the forehead, in the region of the nasiolabial crease and at the outer corners of the eyes. These changes are unlikely to be very pronounced. Nonetheless, one cannot ignore the fact that young adults may be subjected to many outside stresses, which may accelerate the appearance of the features previously seen routinely on the more mature face. Such factors will include lifestyle, episodes of trauma or accident and illnesses, all of which are likely to be experienced to some degree by many individuals.

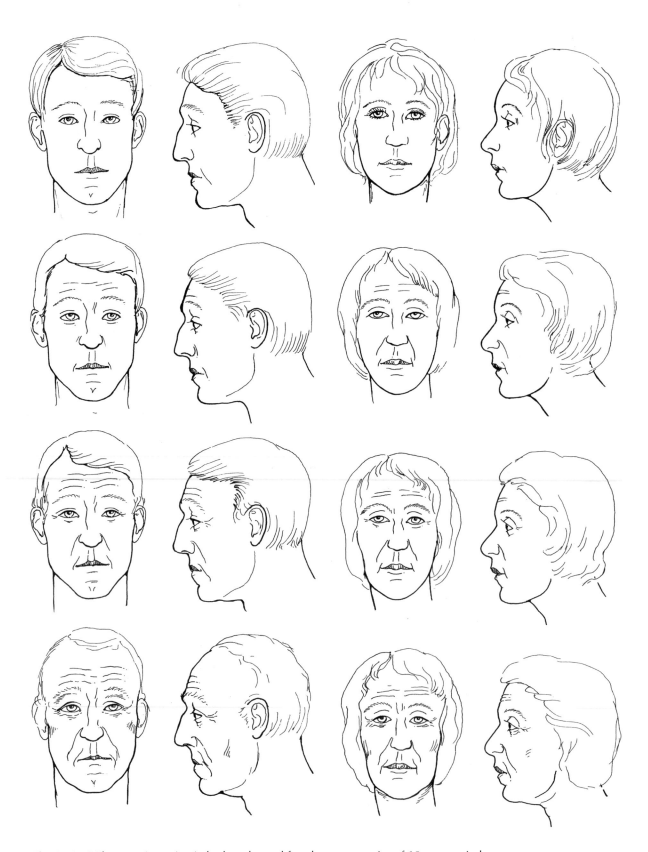

Fig. 17.1 Milestones in ageing in both males and females over a series of 10 year periods

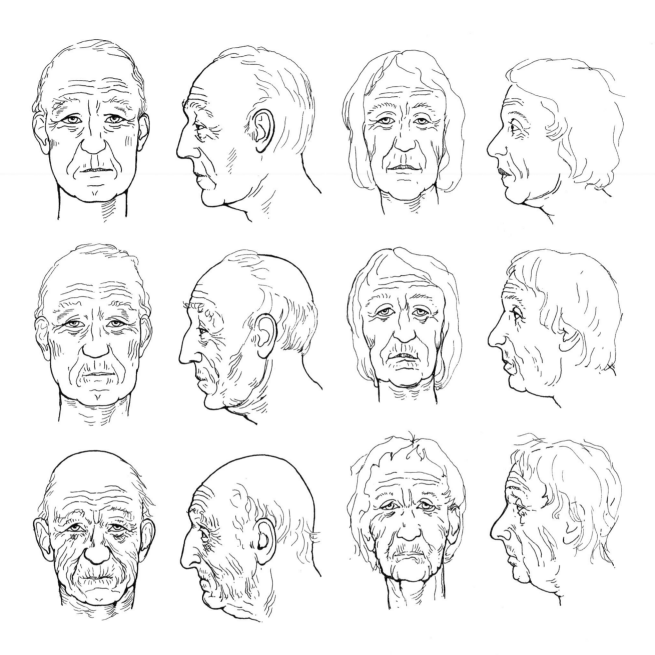

The period between the ages of 30 and 40 is often accompanied by quite noticeable modifications to an individual's appearance. The conclusion of the fourth decade will see the majority of the folds and creases that routinely appeared when the face was animated becoming 'set' into the surface of the skin. Another crease that may occur is in the region of the nasion; this will run horizontally and is the result of the action of the procerus muscle. The face is, by this stage, accumulating features that require time to form and, as such, are an indication of maturity.

Many of the facial creases that are noted as an indication of age lie in the upper one third of the face, essentially in the forehead and the tissues around the eyes. Amongst the first to appear and become permanent are those horizontal creases which cross the forehead. These may be accompanied by vertical creases arising in the region of the nasion and moving over the glabella. The creases around the eyes, often referred to as 'laughter lines', spring from the lateral canthus. Unlike forehead creases, which will remain reasonably constant once formed, the creases around the eyes tend to increase and spread with increasing age. Pouches may also start to develop under the eyes, and while these are not necessarily permanent, the lines and creases that will result are likely to remain. In subjects who have a low or very well defined palprebral crease in the upper eyelid, there is a strong likelihood of the outer canthus becoming partially obscured as this starts to droop. This feature can become very noticeable on some individuals in later life.

Another feature that can be observed routinely in both males and females is the formation of a discrete hollowing of the cheeks below the inferior border of the zygomatic bone. This increased hollowing is not evident in people with naturally hollow cheeks or very prominent cheekbones but is in many people a feature of the older face.

Of all the changes that take place with age, the most subtle is probably the change in skin texture from smooth to uneven. This change occurs earlier in the male and is often apparent around the age of 40. This change is less likely to be noticeable in the female until after the menopause and will normally be less overt, even in old age. Often, when examining photographs of poor quality in which the grain can be readily seen, the subject looks much older because the skin texture appears coarse and thus older. This can give an erroneous impression of maturity.

MIDDLE AGE

By the end of the fourth decade, it is generally possible to see whether a face will, in broad terms, either become fat or remain lean. The nasolabial creases will have formed, although there is a tendency for this to happen later in those with pronounced prognathism. It is during this period that the skin starts to become less smooth, particularly in males.

Alterations will take place in the distribution of the hair, particularly in some males. While this can be extreme in some cases, it is normally likely to be no more than a degree of recession of the hair line at the temples, possibly accompanied by some loss of pigmentation.

The period from 40 to 50 years of age can involve many profound alterations to the superficial appearance of the adult face, although the actual proportions of the face will remain unchanged. The most obvious alteration to the appearance of the face involves changes to the hair. This change includes varying degrees of depigmentation in both males and females, together with the loss of varying amounts of hair in the male. There is an added complication in the males who wear beards and moustaches in that one part may change colour while another remains unaffected. The variations in the way in which male hair can change are therefore legion, although hair loss is confined to the scalp and does not affect the lower facial hair.

As mentioned earlier, the female face tends to change more rapidly after the menopause. However, some of these changes start during this period of changing hormonal status. The former, more youthful skin will now begin to lose its elasticity more rapidly, allowing lines and wrinkles to form. These are accompanied by an unevenness to the surface of the skin. All of these are changes seen much earlier in the male. The face of both male and female will thicken slightly, and the forehead creases, along with most of the other folds and fixed lines in the skin, now become more clearly defined.

Around the eyes, there may develop numerous very subtle modifications to the surrounding tissues. In many cases, the eyebrows can become coarse and grow longer, particularly in the male. There may be loss of some of the fullness above the eye just below the supraorbital margin, accompanied by a sagging of the tissues of the lower eyelid. The lines at the outer canthus will become more prominent, the overall appearance often being that the eye loses the wide-open, expectant look that is so much a feature of the youthful face. There are seldom any notable changes to the nose in this decade, although the alae creases may become more marked in some people. In the lower portions of the face, the mouth will undergo some subtle changes, just as with the eyes, as both areas are subject to constant movement. The lips routinely become less full, losing the pouting appearance that can be observed at an earlier age in some people. Creases radiating out from the mouth running at right angles to the underlying fibres of the obicularis oris muscle sphincter may develop, principally on the upper lip, and are more noticeable in females.

A general thickening of the face during this period is frequently accompanied by a thickening of the tissues under the chin, which in turn results in the development of a submental crease. A further development in the region of the chin occurs along the lower border of the mandible, where tissue tends to 'drop' from the face just in front of the anterior border of the masseter muscle. This alters the shape of the face, particularly in its anterior aspect, as by now the effects of gravity, combined with the results of loss of tissue tone and elasticity, will start to be manifest.

By the middle of this decade, the skin begins to sag around the neck, becoming particularly noticeable in later life in slim individuals; however, this feature is not likely to become very pronounced until the middle of the next decade.

LATER MIDDLE AGE

Those who have remained largely unaffected by the more overt age changes are unlikely to remain untouched between the ages of 50 and 60. There will almost certainly be some loss of hair pigmentation in both males and females, accompanied in many cases by further recession of the hair in the males. The main changes at this time consist of a steady progression of those indicated earlier, but the increase of creases, wrinkles and coarsening of the skin surface is a significant feature. The sclera of the eye may become slightly yellow and some of the small blood vessels more prominent. The limbus of the iris can appear less well defined when the corneoscleral junction becomes clouded or slightly blurred. In some individuals, this is accompanied by the formation of a discrete white ring around the cornea, referred to as an arcus senilis. All of these changes give the eyes an older look by the end of the fifth decade.

Teeth may be lost at this stage in a person's life. Indeed, in many societies, the loss of the majority the teeth during life is not considered abnormal. Tooth loss is accompanied by a reduction in biting force, which will accelerate bone resorption at many cranial buttresses distant from the mouth. Thus there may well be some slight-to-moderate alterations of the overall proportions of a face during this period. These alterations can include the lower third of the face becoming shorter, deepening of the chin–lip crease and the nasolabial grooves or creases becoming more well defined. An increase in the bulk of tissue around and under the chin will further modify the overall appearance; in those who remain thin around the face, the lines may become more marked and the cheeks appear hollow. The skin around the chin and neck will become loose, with a tendency to sag and fold, a prelude to the marked folds of skin so often seen in extreme old age. Hardly noticed, indeed hardly noticeable, is the slow increase of the cartilaginous content of the nose and the ears, yet such change must make its own contribution to the overall look of any face. It does seem, however, that increases in the size of the ears are more noticeable in the male than the female.

OLD AGE

All these alterations will continue at an accelerated rate from 60 to 70 years of age. At the end of this period, in addition to the well-established major creases and lines, there is likely to be an increase in the number of very fine lines covering most of the skin surface. Further modifications to the bone of the maxilla and the mandible will alter the appearance of the chin. The contour of the jaw slims down and becomes more rounded. The mouth will undergo numerous subtle alterations as the muscular lips lose

some of the elasticity, permanent creases forming. The upper lip frequently becomes quite thin, and the lower lip has a tendency to protrude forwards. At some stage during this decade, the slow progressive changes that occur to the cartilaginous portions of the nose during life become visible. The nose becomes slightly wider and more flattened. It may also be noticed that the ears have enlarged slightly. The surface of the skin may develop blemishes in the form of clusters of small vessels or blotches of pigmentation. For those with upper eyelids that tend to droop in earlier life, this phenomenon will become quite marked in some cases. It may become so extreme that their drooping eyelids start to impinge on their field of view.

The eighth and later decades reveal further degeneration of the tissues of the face that are an extension of those discussed above. However, just as very small children have a face that can only be said to look like that of a baby, the very elderly eventually develop a face that can only be described as typical of the very old. In some instances, the proportions of the face in the elderly are similar to those found in the very young. This reflects the loss of muscle and bone in the elderly at the very sites at which it was built up in the young as they progressed to adulthood.

Conclusion

The process of ageing of the face can therefore be described as a predictable series of changes that will take place at an unpredictable rate but in a roughly predictable order.

There is no mistaking the appearance of a very young child; the proportions alone are enough to ensure this. There is no mistaking the appearance of extreme old age as the proportions are again unmistakable. It is in the path between these two extremes of age that the uncertainties of facial form are to be found.

The pattern of ageing of the face that this chapter has endeavoured to outline cannot be considered in any way definitive. It represents merely a series of signposts that may help to bring some understanding and order to what at first seems to be a series of arbitrary changes that are hard to quantify yet somehow easily recognized. We are all different, and we will all age differently. However, we will all experience the same sort of general changes to our face as we do so.

PART 4

Medico-legal issues

CHAPTER 18

Forensic 'art' in human identification

W HAGLUND

Introduction	235	Information to the public	242
Reliability and success of facial approximations	236	Handling the response	242
Reliability and success	240	Conclusion	242
Information provided to the artist	240		

Introduction

Forensic art has become a 'catch-all' term for many different techniques used to generate leads to the identities of unknown individuals. Such techniques include the ageing of missing person photos, composite drawings of suspects and displays for courtroom purposes (Eliopulos, 1993). This chapter focuses on the use of forensic art for publicizing the existence of unidentified individuals in order to generate leads to their identity. Definitions and the reported utility of various techniques to create visages from skulls are discussed and recommendations made for maximizing their use.

There has been debate in the literature over terminology for the various processes to create or compare visages (George, 1987; Rhine, 1990; Haglund and Reay, 1991). Terms in usage for the creation of a facial image from a skull, skull radiograph or skull photograph have been labelled 'facial reconstruction', 'facial reproduction', 'facial restoration' and 'facial approximation'. Some of these terms duplicate descriptions used in other forensic areas while others are misleading (Caldwell, 1981; Rhine, 1984; George, 1987; Haglund et al., 1987). The following conventions are used throughout this chapter (Goyne and Haglund, in press).

Facial reconstruction is the technique of reassembling or conjoining fragmented skeletal remains. (Reconstruction of skulls is not covered in this chapter, but the text may be of help when the reassembling of bone fragments is necessary to interpret trauma or is required before other techniques to recreate a visage can be applied. For a review, see Goyne (1988).

Facial restoration refers to the repair of damaged soft tissue.

Facial approximation indicates the creation of a sketch or model of the average soft tissue expected from a defined skull type. The term 'facial reproduction' is not used here because it implies a perfect replication or copy, which is never the case (George, 1987).

Skull photo superimposition is a method that involves comparison between an image of the skull and an image of photographs taken during life by superimposing the images. It differs from restoration and approximation methods in that it is a collaborative technique used to confirm the identity of an individual whose identity is already suspected.

When, then, to use facial approximation? Except for skull photo superimposition, facial approximation techniques are not generally considered techniques to confirm identity; rather, they are used to advertise a case of unidentified human remains to the public in order to generate leads to their identification. However, facial approximations have been used, in concert with collaborative information, to increase the 'comfort' level of identifications (Rhine, 1984). As lead-generating techniques, facial approximations should be undertaken only after traditional identification methods have been exhausted. If checks of missing persons, fingerprints and dental databases have not been made, or descriptions of clothing and other items descriptive of the remains have not previously been presented in the media, it would be a premature and unnecessary expenditure of time and resources to have an approximation rendered.

Reliability and success of facial approximations

Attempts to evaluate the potential success of facial approximations in identification can be divided into discussions of: (1) the recognition value of various facial features; (2) agreement between different artists' versions of the same skull; (3) agreement between artists' approximated versions with photographs of the deceased taken during life or with death masks; and (4) reported rates of success of facial approximations in making identifications of unidentified dead (Snow *et al.*, 1986).

A recent study by Helmer *et al.* (1993) made systematic comparisons between two different investigators' sculptured renditions of casts of the same individual's skull and compared these renditions in turn to photographs of the deceased taken during life. This serves as an ideal format for the illustration of points 1–3 listed above. Three-dimensional sculptures were rendered for 12 individuals on identical casts of their skulls. These individuals had previously been identified. Each investigator was provided with eyeball prostheses and information regarding sex, age and constitutional type of the individual. Helmer predetermined 'individualized' tissue depth measurements, in accordance with sex, age and constitutional type, for 34 measuring points. In addition, investigators operated from compulsory guidelines compiled from the literature. Neither investigator had artistic training but each had comparable technical and sculptural skill. Problems that arose during preparation of the clay-sculpted rendition of the face were discussed individually between the investigator and the team director (Helmer).

Independent evaluators were asked to compare each pair of facial sculptures of the same skull and then make comparisons between the sculptures and life photographs of the deceased. Evaluators rated

their general impressions with regard to age, sex and body constitution, and the overall impression of the approximation efforts. Evaluations of specific components of the profile, eyes, nose, mouth and chin were made (Table 18.1). Results of these evaluations are tabulated in Table 18.2. Age and sex were the areas showing the most agreement between different sculptures and resemblance to the deceased during life. Areas of least agreement were the mouth and eyes. The latter are locations where the skull provides less reliable predictive value for features. Helmer states that, 'A replica without hair has limited resemblance to most individuals. Intuitive interpretation of hair style can result in similarity to an individual only by chance, and is not dependable.'

Interestingly, Helmer concluded that, over the course of the study, the technical ability of the investigators, although it improved, did not influence results. He further stated that it was not necessary to have trained artists or sculptors. In fact, the results, according to Helmer, can be negatively influenced by creative influence. Helmer emphasized the need for compulsory, standardized guidelines in order to predict soft tissue features from the skull (Fig. 18.1). When these standardized principles were followed, the two renditions were in close resemblance; when investigators deviated from standardized principles, greater deviation occurred. Such deviations resulted either from deficiency or vagueness of standards or from individualized interpretations of the investigator. The compulsory guidelines, compiled from the literature, used by the investigators and considered 'essential' by Helmer, were not specifically stated. Exactly what formed the criteria for the guidelines is not clear as they were drawn from a variety of sources (Merkel, 1885–90; Kollman, 1910; Wilder, 1912; Stadtmüller, 1921–22; Gerasimov, 1955, 1968; Lebedinskaya, 1957; Ullrich, 1959, 1966; Krogman, 1973).

Each of Helmer's control measures removed considerable freedom of choice from the investigators. In all likelihood, this increased the potential for similar likenesses to be produced by the investigators. Several issues come to mind that are not clarified in the report of this study. It would be interesting to know the nature of questions and problems that arose during the course of producing the reconstructions. It is unclear whether or not the make-up and hair were applied to the sculptures by a make-up artist before or after evaluations were rated. If applied before the evaluations, considerable bias would have resulted. It is also important to know the original condition of the remains at the time of discovery. Were they completely skeletonized or was their condition such that residual soft tissue remained to be documented to give further guidance to the forensic investigators?

In most investigations in which artists are used to

Table 18.1 Specific areas rated by evaluators in Helmer's comparisons

Profile	Eye region	Nose	Mouth region	Chin region
Region above the nose	Run of the margin of the eyelid	Length of the nose	Position of the mouth	Fullness
Middle part of the face	Length of the margin of the eyelid	Width of the nose	Width of the mouth	Form (width, length, point)
Lower part of the face	Upper eyelid	Shape of the root of the nose	Fullness of the lips	
	Lower eyelid	Run of the bridge of the nose	Curve of the lips	
	Width of the palpebral fissure, including the position of the canthus	Shape of the sides of the nose	Run of the oral fissure	
	Position and run of the eyebrow			

Data compiled from Helmer *et al.* (1993).

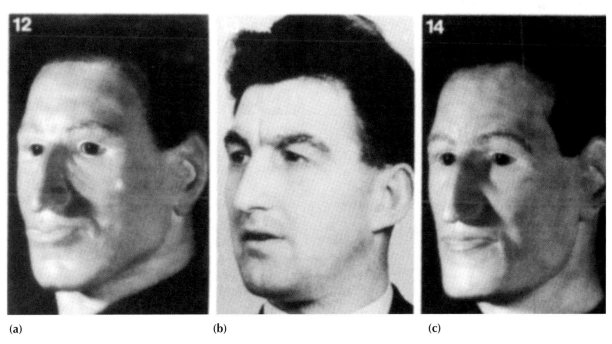

(a)   (b)   (c)

Fig. 18.1 Reliability of approximations showing two different artists' sculptured version (a and c) of the same individual portrayed in ante mortem photograph (b). Reproduced from Helmer *et al.* (1993) with the permission of John Wiley & Sons, Inc., New York

perform facial approximations, the guidelines are open ended and left to the discretion of the individual artist rather than tightly controlled, as in Helmer's study. Areas of most difficulty include lack of skin depth standards for various races, age and body builds, and the inability to predict soft tissue features of noses, ears, lips and eyes (Rathbun, 1984). Helmer *et al.* (1993) suggested that a better appreciation of the accuracy of 'reconstruction' would be a series of tests with portraits by experienced investigators. For insight to the utility of facial approximations in a 'real' field situation, in which various artists were

Table 18.2 Assessment of resemblance between two different investigators' renditions of the same skull and between the renditions and an ante mortem photograph of the deceased during life (numbers represent the percentage of responses)

Resemblance	Comparison of reconstructed pairs with each other					Comparison of 12 reconstructed pairs with living photographs									
						First examiner					Second examiner				
	Great	Close	Approx.	Slight	None	Great	Close	Approx.	Slight	None	Great	Close	Approx.	Slight	None
General impression with regard to age	50	33	17			42	42	8	8		42	33	17	8	8
General impression with regard to sex	75	17		8		84	8		8		92				
General impression with regard to constitution	25	42	17	17		33	67				25	33	25	17	
Profile	17	42	33	8		8	67	25				67	25	8	
Eye region	8	25	8	59			25	50	17	8		42	42	17	
Nose	8	50	25	17		25	50	25			8	67	8	17	
Mouth region		25	8	50	17	8	17	42	33			50	42	8	
Chin region	17	8	50	25			75	17	8			33	50	8	
Overall impression		33	50	17			42	8	50			33	25	33	8

Adapted from Helmer *et al.* (1993).

used to make approximations for skulls of the same individuals, we can turn to the Green River serial murder investigation in the Pacific Northwest of the USA (Haglund *et al.*, 1987, 1991; Rothwell *et al.*, 1989).

The Green River murder investigation has to date encompassed recovery of the bodies of 41 young women, killed between July 1982 and March 1984 and recovered between July 1982 and February 1990. The majority of the remains were recovered as skeletons from rural areas. Many of them had been scavenged and scattered by animals. The victims were young women with a connection to prostitution. The efforts to generate identifications included 26 renditions of nine of the remains by nine different artists. Approximations were attempted only after traditional investigative techniques, extensive publicity in the media, missing person searches and comparisons

with known missing person dental and medical records had been exhausted.

The use of nine different artists in the Green River case demonstrates the variability of results that can be expected when there is a lack of standardization, as insisted upon in Helmer's study. Although the artists were provided with the same estimates of sex, race and age for each individual skull, interpretation of these parameters, the choice and use of tissue depth, the alignment of features and the choice of parameters for the construction of noses and mouths were left to the artists. Results often yielded dissimilar interpretations for the same skull. Comparison between visages (Fig. 18.2) illustrates notable variation between interpretations of the eye region, nose and profile, with some consistency of the prominent cheek and chin region. Note also the significant difference of age representations for the individual.

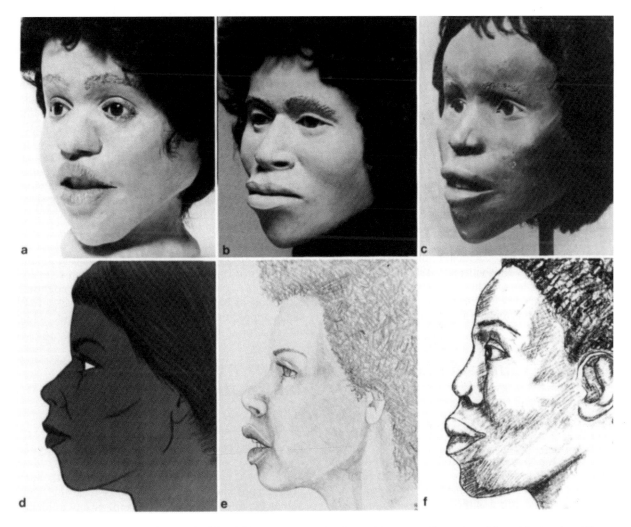

Fig. 18.2 Interpretations of same skull by different artists in the Green River case. Reproduced from Haglund and Reay (1991) with the permission of Raven Press, Ltd, New York

Of the five individuals for whom approximations were rendered and who were eventually identified, leads for the identification were stimulated through news reports of missing persons in two cases, release of a previously unmentioned well-healed hip fracture in one case, follow-up of a previously identified person's aliases in another and media coverage of the discovery of an unconnected, unidentified body in yet another. No leads to identification were attributed to facial approximations. Four individuals for whom facial approximations were carried out remain unidentified. In all fairness, the Green River victims presented extremely elusive individuals to identify. Identification of the victims had been pursued exhaustively by investigators for months and sometimes years before approximations were attempted. Aspects of the victims that contributed to difficulties in identification in the Green River cases were: (1) the delay in discovery of the bodies; (2) the condition of the remains; (3) the age of the victims; (4) their mobile lifestyle; (5) their status as missing persons; and (6) problems encountered in location of ante mortem dental and medical records (Haglund *et al.*, 1987).

The dichotomy of 'philosophical' approaches taken by different artists towards their final products should also be pointed out. There was, on the one hand, an emphasis on individuality, such as specific hairstyle and jewellery, and on the other, a generalist approach. The rationalization given by artists for the first approach was to gain as specific an image as possible. That for the second is that, since the skull cannot dictate such specifics, their inclusion is misleading. It was also apparent that students of certain teachers of forensic art shared stylistic predilections in approach. Artists employed in producing the Green River faces demonstrated different artistic abilities, which was particularly evident in the artists' abilities to produce more finished and lifelike images, and less distracting heads. This was apparent in skin texture and in the production of necks and shoulders, which eliminated 'unnatural' distractions.

Reliability and success

Helmer's study and experiences with the Green River investigation demonstrate that different levels of 'success' are being evaluated. First is the reliability with which different artists can produce a similar face from the same skull. Second is how predictably visage renditions based on a particular skull compare with the deceased during life. A third level measure of success is the utility of the facial approximation in generating the lead to the deceased's identity.

To further confuse the meaning of 'success,' there have no doubt been facial approximations that have

elicited leads to identification without closely resembling the deceased in question. In other words, resemblance has in some cases turned out not to be critical. It may have been the fact that a face purported to be that of some unidentified individual, accompanied by additional information, was presented to the public and yielded a clue to the actual identity. Therefore, success for the investigative agency can result from a poor resemblance. Conversely, an approximation bearing close resemblance to the deceased may fail to stimulate leads to identification: an artistic success can be an investigative failure. This might result, for example, from insufficient exposure to the target population in the news media.

Practitioners of forensic art have reported successful identifications for individual cases (Rhine, 1977, 1990; Charney *et al.*, 1978). Other reports indicate rates of 'success' of between 50% (Caldwell, 1981) and 75% (Haglund *et al.*, 1991). For many of these reported 'successes', it is unclear whether success indicates that the facial approximation stimulated the lead to identification or that the identification would have been made whether or not the approximation played a part in the identification. According to Neave (1980), 'It appears that success of facial approximation depends as much upon the circumstances pertaining to the subject under investigation as it does upon the accuracy of the technique.' Examples of such circumstances might be inadequate preapproximation investigation, newly reported missing persons or simply the fact that a previous attempted lead has finally resulted in identification. Demographics of the victim, such as mobility or transience, few social contacts or drawing from a large target population make for less likelihood of recognition. Conversely, being long established in a community, investigators thereby drawing from a smaller population, increases the odds of recognition (Haglund *et al.*, 1991). To maximize results from facial approximations, it is essential to provide sound information to both the artist and the public.

Information provided to the artist

Photographs should be provided to show the original condition of any persistent (existing) facial tissue present at the time the body was recovered. Such photographs should be mandatory both at the scene and at the time of the initial receipt of any unidentified remains at the mortuary. Facial approximations are usually not attempted until traditional identification techniques have been played out weeks, months or even years after the original discovery. By this time, decomposition or cleaning processes may have eradicated tissue that could have provided clues to the artist about details of features. Photographs should include overall true frontal views of any residual tissue of the face, and profile and close-ups of the hairline, nose, eye and mouth areas. Any skull photographs or radiographs should be taken in the Frankfort horizontal position. Photographs should be taken with obtuse lighting in order to best demonstrate surface features. Figure 18.3 demonstrates an initial photograph of a decomposed homicide victim in which the hairline was crucial in recognition by family members.

Meticulous scene processing is often necessary to recover hair and teeth from the scene of skeletal remains. This may require extensive screening and searching of the immediate area surrounding the skeletal remains. This should include examination of bird nests, into which hair may have been incorporated (Howard *et al.*, 1988). The colour, length, texture and style of hair are important to this type of identification.

The remains should be analysed by a forensic anthropologist and forensic odontologist to ensure that the artist is provided with a sound assessment of race, sex, age of the decedent at time of death,

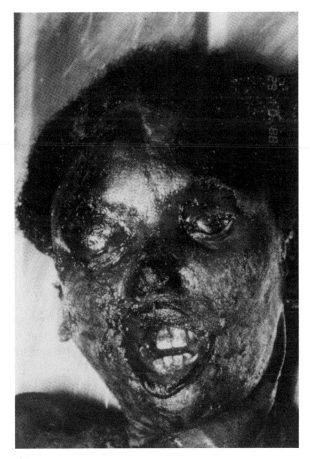

(b)

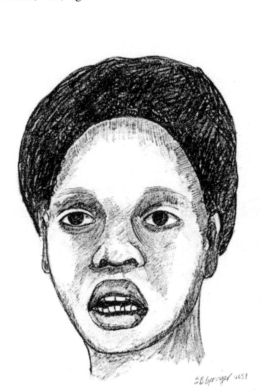

(a)

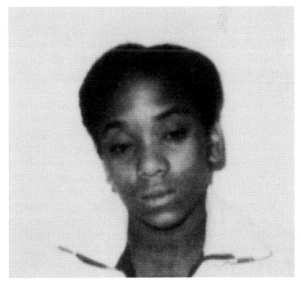

(c)

Fig. 18.3 Drawing (a) was rendered from a photograph of the decomposed remains (b) and compared with an ante mortem snapshot of the deceased (c). The high hairline was important in the recognition of the deceased

body habitus and a best estimate of the range of time since death. Reporting of any asymmetries of the face, facial idiosyncracies or trauma is most helpful. The artist should produce profile views of drawings and 'open-mouthed' renditions, with teeth visible if possible.

Information to the public

A basic power of facial approximations is their ability to intrigue the general public and act as a 'hook' to media interest. When an unidentified body is initially found, the news media has high interest. Once the initial attention dies down, rekindling that interest is often difficult unless there is a new twist to the case. Approximations handily provide such a twist.

Investigators should provide their own photographs of approximations to the media; this way, they can control lighting and perspective. A fact sheet should accompany any release of photographs. A disclaimer stating that the approximation may not be an exact likeness of the deceased and that it represents an artistic opinion is crucial. The lay public has high expectations of techniques presented in the guise of science. They must know that the approximation might range anywhere from a close resemblance to the deceased to little or no resemblance at all. If possible, multiple renditions of same skull are desirable to make this point. Other considerations are the target of dispersal and the duration of exposure. The longer the facial approximation is before the public, the greater will be the number of people viewing it, but one has a very narrow window of exposure with the media. If the identities of multiple unidentified individuals are being sought, renditions of multiple victims should not be released simultaneously: each additional release of a new victim expands the exposure.

When information on a missing person is reported, it should be captured by investigators, even if it does not have direct bearing on the particular identification being sought. Identification of unidentified persons is not necessarily a local problem but often necessitates a regional, transjurisdictional campaign to advertise the unknown remains. Responses to such appeals often additionally pertain to other remains, and unidentified persons, perhaps in different jurisdictions, who can then be identified by capturing such information. Facial approximations also offer the opportunity to capture previously unreported missing persons. Therefore, appeals accompanying an advertisement of facial approximations should encourage the viewer who knows of anyone missing to report them.

Handling the response

Eliopulos (1993) makes some excellent suggestions for handling responses to facial approximations. One person should act as liaison to handle or supervise calls. This should preferably be the person who knows the most about the case. A call-in sheet to formalize collection of information should be used. Other persons who might inadvertently get a call should be aware of the appeal effort so it does not succumb to the 'fall through the crack' syndrome. It is also important to maintain archived records collected on 'located persons'. Many individuals reported missing and subsequently located fall into high-risk groups and may become missing again: during the Green River investigation, three individuals were identified through records on 'located' persons.

Conclusion

What is the best that can be hoped for from facial approximations? George (1987) states that visualization of a face from a skull is a lofty goal. However, as Gatliff underscores, facial approximations are a last-ditch effort. The outcome is uncertain in every case, but if the sculpture is done correctly and is as accurate as possible within the limitations of the technique, it is usually worth a try (Gatliff, 1984). The challenge for artists is to refine and agree upon standards; the challenge for investigators is to analyse and recognize those circumstances which have served to make specific identifications more likely.

References

Caldwell MC. 1981: The relationship of the details of the human face to the skull and its application in forensic anthropology. Unpublished MA thesis, Arizona State University.

Charney M, Snow CC, Rhine JS. 1978: The three faces of Cindy M. Paper presented in the Physical Anthropology Section of the 30th Annual Meeting of the American Academy of Forensic Sciences, February 20–25, St Louis, Missouri, USA.

Eliopulos LN. 1993: Death investigator's handbook: a field guide to crime scene processing, forensic evaluations, and investigative techniques. Boulder, CO: Paladin Press.

Gatliff BP. 1984: Facial sculpture on the skull for identification. *American Journal of Forensic Medicine and Pathology* **5**(4), 327–32.

George RM. 1987: The lateral craniographic method of facial reconstruction. *Journal of Forensic Sciences* **32**(5),1305–30.

Gerasimov MM. 1955: *Vosstalovlenie lical po cerepu (Wiederherstellung des Gesichts aufgrund des Schädels)*, Moscow: Akademie Nauk [in Russian].

Gerasimov MM. 1968: *The face finder*. New York: Lippincott.

Goyne TEW. 1988: Reconstructing skulls: techniques, materials, and interpretation. *Medico-Legal Bulletin* **37**, 1–10.

Goyne TEW, Haglund WD. Variants of visual identification. In Fierro MF. (ed.) *CAP handbook for postmortem examination of unidentified remains: developing identification of well-preserved, decomposed, burned, and skeletonised remains* (2nd edn). Schachowa, IL: College of American Pathologists (in press).

Haglund WD, Reay DT, Snow C. 1987: Identification of serial homicide victims in the 'Green River Murder' investigation. *Journal of Forensic Sciences* **32**(6), 1666–75.

Haglund WD, Reay DT. 1991: Use of facial approximation techniques in identification of Green River serial murder victims. *American Journal of Forensic Medicine and Pathology* **12**(2), 132–42.

Helmer RP, Röhricht S, Pebrson D *et al.* 1983: Assessment of the reliability of facial reconstruction. In Iscan MY, Helmer RP. (eds) *Forensic analysis of the skull: cranial analysis, reconstruction, and identification.* New York: Wiley-Liss, 229–46.

Howard JD, Reay DT, Haglund WD, Fligner CL. 1988: Processing of skeletal remains: a medical examiner's perspective. *American Journal of Forensic Medicine and Pathology* **9**(3), 258–64.

Kollman J. 1910: Plastische Anatomie des menschlichen Körpers. 3. Abschnitt: *Schädel* (3rd edn). Leipzig: Veith.

Krogman WM. 1973: *The human skeleton in forensic medicine.* Springfield, IL: Charles C. Thomas.

Lebedinskaya GV. 1957: On the problem of reproduction of the actual shape of the eyes in reconstructions of the face on the skull. *Short communications of the Ethnographic Institute of USSR Academy of Sciences* **27**, Moscow [in Russian].

Merkel F. 1885–90: *Handbuch der topographischen Anatomie.* Bd 1, Braunsweig.

Neave R. 1980: Facial reconstruction of skeletal remains: three Egyptian examples. *MASCA Journal* **1**(6), 175–7.

Rathbun TA. 1984: Personal identification: facial reproduction. In Rathbun TA, Buikstra JE. (eds), *Human identification: case studies in forensic anthropology.* Springfield, IL: Charles C. Thomas, 347–56.

Rhine JS. 1977: A comparison of methods of restoring living facial features to the skull. Presented at the Pan American Conference of the International Reference Organization in Forensic Medicine and Sciences, Mexico City.

Rhine JS. 1984: Facial reproduction in court. In Rathbun TA, Buikstra JE. (eds) *Human identification: case studies in forensic anthropology.* Springfield, IL: Charles C. Thomas, 357–62.

Rhine JS. 1990: Coming to terms with facial reproduction. *Journal of Forensic Sciences* **35**, 960–3.

Rothwell BR, Haglund WD, Morton TH. 1989: Dental identification in serial homicides: the Green River murders. *Journal of the American Dental Association* **119**, 373–9.

Snow CC, Gatliff BP, McWilliams KR. 1986: Reconstruction of facial features from the skull: an evaluation of its usefulness in forensic anthropology. *American Journal of Physical Anthropology* **33**, 221–7.

Stadtmüller F. 1921–22: Zur Beurteilung der plastischen Rekonstruktions methode der Physiognomie auf dem Schädel. *Zeitschrift fur Morphologie Anthropologie* **22**, 337–72.

Ullrich H. 1959: Die methodischen Grundlagen des plastischen Rekonstruktionsverlfahren nach Gerasimov. *Zeitschrift für Morphologie und Anthropologie* **49**, 245–8.

Ullrich H. 1966: Kritische Bemerkungen zur plastischen Rekonstruktionsmethode nach Gerasimov aufgrund persönlicher Erfahrungen. *Ethnogr-Archöl-Z* (Berlin) **7**, 111–23.

Wilder H. 1912: The physiognomy of Indians of southern New England. *American Anthropologist* **14**, 415–36.

CHAPTER 19

Reporting and presentation of evidence

DL RANSON

Introduction	245	Medico-legal analysis	251
Communication	245	During the trial	252
Environment of the court	248	After the trial	255
In the witness box	248	Court equipment	255
Preparation	250		

Introduction

Many witnesses view appearing in court with apprehension, and this is true for both ordinary witnesses of fact and expert witnesses. While the role of the expert witness in court should be clear cut and straightforward, giving expert evidence can in practice, be a taxing and demanding process. Much of the difficulty experienced by expert witnesses in court relates to the fact that they are operating in an alien environment without ready access to the tools and materials that would be available to them in their laboratories. In addition, for the first time in an investigation, they are required to present and explain their findings to a group of people who have little or no knowledge of the scientific, medical or dental principles involved.

Communication

For most scientists, the output of their work is their analytical results, and the quality of analysis depends on both scientific accuracy and reliability. This is also true for the forensic scientist and the forensic medical and dental practitioner. However, in forensic matters, communication of the meaning of the results becomes a critical aspect of the scientific and medical work. A forensic scientist may have carried out the most scientifically rigorous examination to a high standard of quality, but if the implications of the results are not effectively communicated to the court, such that a judge and lay jury can comprehend them, the scientific and medical work performed is rendered valueless. It is often hard for the non-forensic scientist, dentist or doctor to appreciate the importance of communication in forensic practice as it goes far beyond the issues included in traditional scientific and medical training.

In considering aspects of communication for the medical witness, we need to consider communication to four audiences: oneself, one's colleagues, lawyers and the public.

COMMUNICATION TO ONESELF

The most significant issue of communication for the forensic medical practitioner is communication to oneself by means of notes and specialist reports. At first glance, this seems somewhat trite, but when one considers how the practice of forensic medicine interacts with the justice system, communication to oneself takes on a greatly increased significance. In practice, the original forensic medical work is carried out as part of an investigation for some aspect of the justice system. Despite the attempts by judicial administration systems to speed up the processes by which matters are investigated and brought to trial, the delays are, in practical terms, considerable. The investigation of criminal and civil cases can be prolonged; setting down matters for trial and obtaining the attendance of the necessary witnesses at a convenient time adds further delays to the process. As a result, it is not unusual for forensic scientists or medical practitioners to step into the witness box to give evidence many months, and sometimes years, after they carried out the associated medical examination. In such a situation, the quality of the original scientific notes and medico-legal report takes on an enormous significance. It is important to be able to refresh one's memory from high-quality notes made at the time of the original examination. Since the court permits such contemporaneous notes to be used, forensic practitioners should take advantage of this by ensuring that their notes are of high quality and provide the best possible information.

The availability of comprehensive contemporaneous medical notes makes it easy for the investigator to prepare detailed medico-legal reports. A wide range of individuals working within the civil and criminal justice systems require such reports. It is important to recognize that the quality of such reports often determines the nature of subsequent legal procedures and may influence whether a scientist, dentist or medical practitioner is eventually called to give evidence as a witness.

Before any criminal or civil trial, it is not uncommon for expert witnesses to be engaged in pretrial discussions with the legal parties involved, and such discussions may again take place many months or years after the original examination. Detailed, comprehensive medical notes and reports place the medical practitioner in an excellent position to deal with any technical or scientific issues that are raised by the parties in pretrial discussions.

It is in the witness box itself that well-structured, comprehensive, detailed notes and reports come into their own. The witness box is a lonely place for scientists, dentists and doctors. They have no direct access to library resources and no administrative or secretarial support on hand. Their ability to perform effectively as witnesses and to deliver their evidence in an organized and intelligible fashion is enhanced by their possession of a set of comprehensive records within which information can be quickly found.

Efficiency in organizing materials also reinforces credibility and professional standing in the eyes of the court.

COMMUNICATION TO COLLEAGUES

Forensic medical examinations are most often carried out by one medical practitioner working alone. However, some cases involve several specialists. Even where only one doctor makes the original examination, several medical practitioners involved in the justice process may scrutinize the results. In both civil and criminal jurisdictions, parties acting for the Crown/plaintiff and the defendants may all seek further medical information, often in the form of expert opinion evidence. In these situations, the medical expert to whom the matter is referred usually only has access to the report made at the time of the original medical examination or scientific tests. For the best possible results to be obtained from referrals for such medical opinions, it is essential that the original doctor's notes and reports are comprehensive and detailed. The aim of medical records in forensic case work is to place another doctor in the same position, with regard to the quantity and quality of the information, as the original doctor when the examination was performed. In practice, this is, of course, impossible. Despite this, the existence of high-quality notes and medico-legal reports eases the task of the other medical specialists to whom the matter is referred.

Language and terminology play an important part in communication to one's colleagues. The medical profession, like the legal profession, is often accused of using complex technical language riddled with jargon. Such language can cause considerable problems in court. However, the use of such specialist terminology increases the accuracy and quality of communication with medical and scientific colleagues. Technical terms are thus justified when they increase communication and accuracy on specific medical issues. The use of inexact lay expressions in a medico-legal report leads to imprecision and confusion, although they can improve communication of complex issues to lay members of the community, including juries. The correct balance between the use of technical terms and lay expressions can be hard to achieve, but due consideration should be given to this issue when compiling medical notes and medico-legal reports.

COMMUNICATION TO LAWYERS

Lawyers vary greatly in their medical knowledge. There are a few practising lawyers who are also medical or dental practitioners, and such individuals have a wide understanding of related medical issues. However, even lawyers who hold medical qualifications do not necessarily have specialist medical knowledge in a particular subdiscipline. The identity of the lawyers dealing with a particular case is often hard to ascertain at an early stage of the proceedings. Indeed, in many cases, the legal personnel may change as a result of, for example, conflicting professional commitments. It follows that medical notes and reports should provide accurate and comprehensive communication to lawyers who may have no knowledge of the medical matters involved. The importance of accurate communication to lawyers cannot be overemphasized. The rationale of the entire forensic medical report is the use to which the information can be put in the legal process. The key players in the legal process are lawyers, so for the report to have maximum impact on the legal process, it must be intelligible to lawyers.

Informed communication between lawyers and medical, dental and scientific specialists is vital to the justice system. Decisions on whether to prosecute or to bring actions in law are made by lawyers on the basis of their understanding of the evidence that is presented to them. Medical matters can be demanding and complex. One may understand the technical terms used in a medical or scientific report by referring to an appropriate glossary, but to comprehend their meaning in the correct scientific and medical context is far more difficult.

The terminology used in communicating to lawyers is a combination of the language used in communicating with medical colleagues and with the public. However, when explaining a medical report to a lawyer, the significance of medical observations needs to be emphasized in order that the correct medico-legal inferences can be drawn.

COMMUNICATION TO THE PUBLIC

In the case of criminal trials in the higher courts, communication of complex issues to the public (as the jury) is a major concern for the expert. For a jury to comprehend and draw the appropriate inferences from a medical witness's evidence, the language must be accessible. Lawyers are particularly concerned to ensure that the judge and jury understand the language used by medical witnesses. It must be remembered, however, that a lawyer, without formal medical knowledge, who has been working on a particular case for some time is likely to understand many of the specialist issues of the medical evidence and to be familiar with the medical language employed. It is difficult for such a person to put herself in the position of a lay jury member and to be aware of the range of knowledge that such an individual might have.

Jury members vary in the extent of their specialist knowledge, their educational attainment spanning a wide range. A jury might be composed of individuals with no secondary or tertiary education or of individuals with tertiary qualifications in medically related disciplines such as anatomy or biochemistry. During the course of a trial, it is important for both medical witness and lawyers to gain an impression of the success or failure of the communication of issues to a jury. For the medical witness, this is not as difficult as it may appear. Witnesses can use various techniques to increase their communication to a lay jury. These techniques are those used in an ordinary medical consultation with patients, during which the practitioner explains to the patient the nature of the disease or illness and the issues associated with it. If medical witnesses keep in mind that a jury is no different from many of their patients, and can indeed span the intellectual knowledge range of their patients, they should have little difficulty in getting their message across. If, however, the medical witness engages in a technical discussion or argument with particular lawyers, there is a risk that the jury will be left out and will understand little of the matters being discussed.

It is important not to underestimate a lay jury. The range and depth of coverage of scientific and medical forensic matters by the media has educated members of the community in a variety of technical issues. Knowledge by lawyers and medical practitioners of the existence of such information in the general media can be of great value in assisting in the process of communication to lay people in court and particularly to juries.

Communication in the courtroom usually takes the form of words delivered as evidence by the witnesses, but this is not the only way to achieve good communication. The use of charts, videos, diagrams, photographs and physical models should always be considered. Where evidence relating to the human body is concerned, the medical witness often has the best physical model available: their own body.

A well-informed jury who have had the medical issues clearly explained to them in an accessible and intelligible way by an expert witness are in the best possible position to evaluate the medical evidence and come to a valid conclusion. Medical practitioners should always remember that it is the lay jury, judge or magistrate who assesses their evidence, and it is this assessment rather than the private opinions of their colleagues or the lawyers that determines the forensic outcome of the medical evidence.

To communicate successfully to a court takes careful planning and preparation. In many ways, preparing to give evidence in court is similar to preparing a lecture. The information must be presented to the audience in such a way as to retain their interest in what is said and to permit them to comprehend and analyse what they see and hear. The development of analogies that can be used to explain complex medical and scientific notions in lay terms is useful. Such explanatory analogies are a feature of the oratory of good communicators and part of the armoury of experienced forensic medical practitioners.

Environment of the court

For those who frequently appear in court as witnesses, the concept of the courtroom as a stage immediately suggests itself. The barristers and judges, with their wigs and gowns, resemble actors in costume. Just as actors convey the emotion and atmosphere of the events they are portraying to the audience with their acting skills and the way in which they interact with the set, so the barristers convey to witnesses and the jury the seriousness of the task in which they are engaged. Part of this skill involves recreating the emotions that surrounded the events of the case even when they originally occurred some months or years before. The structure of the courtroom and the costumes of the lawyers are indeed both alien and intimidating. In the past, such intimidation was in part intended to ensure that witnesses spoke only the truth. The physical location of witnesses in an isolated witness box (Fig. 19.1), exposed so that the whole court can see them, is also unnerving as it allows witnesses to be scrutinized not only with regard to what they say but also with regard to their appearance, dress, stance and gestures. The demeanour of witnesses is critical with regard to the evidence that they give. The impression of the evidence that a witness communicates to a jury is significantly influenced by the witness's behaviour and demeanour in giving evidence.

In the witness box

The process of presenting evidence in court, includes examination-in-chief, cross-examination and re-examination.

EXAMINATION-IN-CHIEF

The party who has required the doctor or dentist to attend at court to give evidence initially requests that the doctor be called to the witness box, identifies them to the court and then proceeds to ask a series of questions that are designed to elucidate the facts and opinions set out in the medico-legal report. The information that is sought from the witness at this time is the information which the party calling the witness wishes to have placed before the court. The questions may cover all of the material contained in the original statement or only some of it. In cases in which a doctor is called to give evidence on behalf of the prosecution in a criminal matter, the questions will relate to the specific elements of the crime that the prosecutor wishes to prove. There may be features of the medical examination that the prosecution does not require the doctor to give in evidence. This may be because other witnesses will give such evidence or because the matter has already been agreed by the parties. The witness should therefore answer only the specific questions asked.

If a doctor or dentist is to give expert opinion evidence during examination-in-chief, it is the task of the party calling them to set out the nature of their expertise and to prove to the court that they have sufficient expertise to give opinion evidence in the matter. Because the barrister who carries out the examination-in-chief knows the details of the witness's evidence, he or she is not usually permitted to ask leading questions of the witness. That is, the barrister can ask only open questions that seek to elicit the evidence at issue but may not ask a question that tends to suggest the answer. Thus the question will be 'What did you see when you arrived at the house?' rather than 'Did you see a dead body lying at the foot of the stairs when you arrived at the house?' In certain circumstances, however, with the consent of both parties and the judge, a court may permit leading questions during examination-in-chief in order to speed up the court process with regard to evidence that is non-controversial or not a significant issue in the case.

During examination-in-chief, the judge will occasionally ask the medical witness questions to elucidate or clarify some point of the evidence. The witness should note these questions by the judge most carefully. In most circumstances, the judge is attempting to ensure that the evidence that the witness has given can be understood by the jury. If a witness finds that the judge is asking a number of questions on matters relating to evidence that they have already given, the judge probably considers the witness's previous answers confusing or too technical in nature. The witness should use the opportunity offered by the judge's questions to clarify the evidence and to deliver parts of it again in a manner that lay people will find easier to understand. Very occasionally, a judge will ask about new matters that have not been covered, but these questions are usually left to the end of a witness's evidence. When the party calling the witness considers that they have obtained all the evidence needed for their case, the examination-in-chief comes to an end. As the court process is adversarial, the opposing party now has a turn.

CROSS-EXAMINATION

After the completion of examination-in-chief, the process of cross-examination commences. In criminal matters in which the medical witness has been called to give evidence by the prosecution, it is the defence counsel who cross-examines the witness. The defence counsel has access to the witness's statements made prior to the court case and, in addition, has usually taken detailed notes of the evidence given during the examination-in-chief. These notes may well include a record of specific words and phrases used by the witness in the previous answers.

The extent and nature of cross-examination are extremely variable, and much depends on the nature of the defence that is being raised by the accused person. Several approaches and techniques are used in cross-examination, and a medical witness may experience one or more of these in any particular case. It is important to remember, however, that in many

cases the evidence-in-chief given by the medical witness in response to questions put by the prosecutor is not an issue for the defence at all. For example, in the case of an alleged murder in which the body of the victim was found in a skeletonized state, the forensic odontologist who examined the dental remains may not be cross-examined on the process of the dental examination or on the opinion they have formed as to the identity of the victim. The defence may accept that the victim is the person alleged. In such a situation, the main defence argument might be that the injuries to the skull suggest an accidental rather than a deliberate application of force. In other such situations, the cross-examination of the medical witness on their findings may be minimal, and in some cases, there is no cross-examination at all.

The process of cross-examination is potentially detailed, exacting and challenging for the medical witness. The questions may be open or leading. It is not uncommon for counsel to put forward a hypothetical situation in which a particular set of events has occurred and to ask the witness whether such a scenario might explain the facts observed. Considerable latitude is available to the cross-examiner concerning the manner in which questions are put and

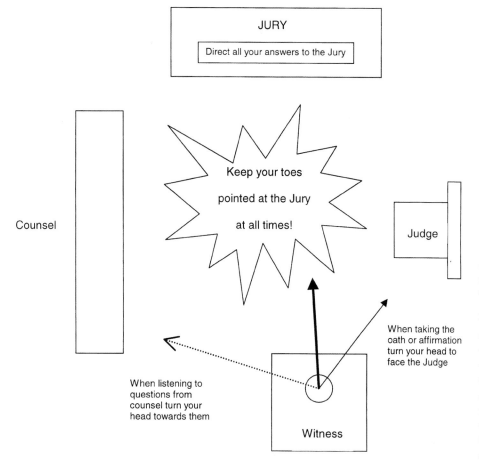

Fig. 19.1 This plan view of a stylized courtroom shows the position of the witness in relation to the judge, jury and counsel. The witness should stand with the toes pointing at the jury and simply turn their head when taking the oath or listening to questions or comments from the judge or counsel. (In courts without a jury, they should face the judge or tribunal chairman)

the range of material that can be covered. The cross-examination may seek to clarify points that have been covered in the examination-in-chief, particularly those points which have been damaging to the cross-examiner's case. A witness's opinion, veracity and competence may be challenged, and prior statements made by the witness may be compared and contrasted with their current evidence. A cross-examiner who is unable to shake or successfully challenge the witness's evidence, or to demonstrate that the witness lacks skill or credibility, will quickly end the cross-examination in order to prevent the witness presenting further evidence damaging to their case.

RE-EXAMINATION

At the conclusion of cross-examination, the party who originally called the witness may re-examine the witness in relation to the issues that arose in cross-examination. New evidence may not normally be introduced during re-examination, but this may occasionally occur with the permission of the court and usually with the acquiescence of the other party. Re-examination is used to shore up the original information gained through examination-in-chief and to minimize any damage done to the witness's evidence during cross-examination. Re-examination can demonstrate real artistry on the part of a barrister, but the best re-examination is often no re-examination at all. If damage has been done to a party's case during cross-examination by the other side, it is often better not to show up the weakened case by asking further questions. It is better to sit back and ask nothing, thereby implying that no damage has been done.

In some situations, further cross-examination and further re-examination may occur with the permission of the judge. When both parties have finished with a witness, the judge may ask questions; in some cases, the jury may be permitted to ask the witness questions through the judge. If any important issues arise out of the answers given by the witness to questions from the judge or jury, the barristers for both parties may be permitted to ask follow-up questions. The witness, after completing the evidence, is permitted to step down from the witness box; in most cases, the party calling the doctor will ask that the doctor be excused. The judge usually agrees to this, and the witness may then go, having been excused from further attendance in the matter.

While this description of procedures in the giving of evidence may seem complex and potentially threatening, the experience is made easier and more enjoyable if the witness is well prepared. It is also helpful if the witness is aware of the roles of the various parties in court and their own place in the court proceedings. It is sometimes said that the training of

witnesses is unnecessary as all they have to do is answer the questions put to them from their own knowledge, professional background and training. However, this is not the case. The processes involved in a legal proceeding and the legal techniques employed during a trial are alien to most dentists and doctors. Without some experience and training in the delivery of such expert evidence, the witness's ability to assist the court is compromised. There is no doubt that training and skill in the art of being a witness help to ensure that complex medical evidence is delivered to the court in a clear, concise and competent fashion.

Preparation

The presentation of evidence in court is generally the end point of forensic odontology and forensic pathology. It follows that preparing to appear in court is an essential activity for all expert witnesses.

LONG-TERM PREPARATION

Long-term preparation merges with the original forensic work performed in a particular case. It includes ensuring that the work has been appropriately carried out and that the original documentation and notes are complete in all relevant particulars. Mistakes and omissions made at this time cannot usually be rectified without considerable embarrassment to the witness, and the need for such amendments may seriously damage the witness's credibility in the eyes of the court. It is important, even at this early stage, to canvass the possible need for court attendance as a witness and the likely civil issues or criminal charges involved. Notes, potential exhibits and relevant materials should be stored in a secure place for retrieval during the later stages of pretrial preparation.

MEDIUM-TERM PREPARATION

At the completion of the substantive casework, together with the medical notes and records, the main preparatory work commences. This should initially include presentation of the case material to one's peers in order to gather feedback on the quality of the casework performed, obtain advice on relevant recent advances in the area, and gain experience of previous cross-examination on the opinions one has expressed and the conclusions one has reached. The medical literature should be reviewed at this time and articles dealing with the subject matter of the case obtained and analysed. If special illustrations or models are considered to be useful in communicating the evidence in court, they should be prepared and their use discussed with the lawyers during any pre-trial conferences.

At the completion of these processes, the medical witness puts the notes and materials together. Well-prepared witnesses can give evidence confident that:

- they have all the documents and materials they need to communicate their findings;
- they understand what the legal system requires of them in the particular case;
- the legal representatives understand the nature of the evidence the witness can give.

SHORT-TERM PREPARATION

If the early preparation has been adequate, short-term preparation should be limited to reviewing the materials, organizing the illustrations, assembling any equipment and ensuring that the court attendance has been included in the witnesses' work schedule. A few days before appearing at court to give evidence, the witness should read their original statement carefully and cross-reference the material in it with their notes, the relevant photographs, charts, radiographs and information obtained from literature searches. At the completion of this review process, the witness should be able to find any relevant item of information quickly in the notes. The models, charts and other illustrations should be packaged appropriately for transport to court and for subsequent storage by the court as exhibits. If the witness has given evidence in the matter before, perhaps at a preliminary hearing, it is advisable to obtain a transcript of the evidence given on that occasion. This transcript should be studied carefully prior to giving any further evidence. The work involved in preparing for a trial can vary from a few hours of reading to days of planning, research and conferences. Similarly, depending on the time a case takes to come to trial, these phases of preparation can occur over a few days or several years.

One of the main organizational matters to which a medical witness must attend relates to notes and records. While a barrister has the bar table upon which to arrange documents and materials, the witness has often just a small lectern on which to arrange any notes. For most witnesses, this small space is all that is required as they are asked to give nearly all their evidence from personal recollection without reference to written materials. In contrast, the forensic medical witness may have to juggle a medical report, a set of personal notes, hospital records, photographs and radiographs on a tiny area.

To cope well in this situation requires a high degree of organization of the witness's materials. Filing of papers in an orderly fashion in a binder or folder is a very useful way of preparing documents. The witness should be so familiar with the materials that finding information in them while being questioned is a swift and efficient process that causes minimum disruption to the flow of evidence. Modern courtrooms provide far more space for the witness to lay out notes and materials, which is a far more satisfactory situation.

While the giving of evidence in court does not ordinarily require the witness to perform analyses or examinations, a medical witness is occasionally asked to look at an exhibit and to demonstrate a feature of it to the court. The court will normally have the required equipment, such as examination gloves, available for the witness, but this is not always the case; the forensic medical practitioner should take to court such items of equipment. Not only is it useful to the court if the medical witness is prepared in this way, but it also demonstrates the witness's professionalism with regard to the court work. Useful items include examination gloves, a pocket calculator, a magnifying glass, a ruler, a pointer, and pens and pencils, including whiteboard and overhead projector markers.

With the completion of the case file, the doctor or dentist should ensure that the court attendance is correctly entered into the diary at their practice or usual place of employment and that their staff know where they are and how to contact them. Mobile telephones or pagers must be switched off when giving evidence as there is nothing that irritates a court more than to hear pagers beeping and mobile telephones ringing. Such an event is likely to earn a rebuke from the judge.

Medico-legal analysis

It is not sufficient for a medical or dental practitioner who has been called to give evidence to consider only the scientific issues that the evidence involves. Since forensic medicine is that area of medicine performed and practised for the benefit of the court, the forensic medical witness must be aware of the courts' requirements and the particular legal and associated issues that arise in the case before the court. The dentist or doctor does not have to become a lawyer in order to do this but should be aware of the legal principles at issue. In a criminal matter in which the medical witness is appearing on behalf of the prosecution, the witness should be aware of the charge that the defendant faces and the legal and evidential elements that go to make up the alleged offence. In addition, the medical witness needs to be aware of the potential general or specific defences that might be appropriate to such a charge and how such defences might be introduced during the court proceedings. With these matters in mind, the witness, in preparing to give evidence, should identify in this evidence points of possible or probable contention with regard to fact or opinion and consider these areas in advance.

During the trial

For the forensic medical practitioner, the trial represents the end stage of all the effort that has gone into the investigation. It is in the delivery of oral testimony that the success of the forensic medical casework will be seen. As a result, the forensic practitioner should treat the appearance in court as a witness with the same attention to detail given to their clinical or pathological examination.

From the perspective of the medical witness, the issues surrounding the giving of oral evidence in court can be divided into several areas.

ATTENDANCE

If a witness has been subpoenaed to attend at court and has been informed that their evidence will be required at a particular time on a particular day, they must attend on that date at that time. There are very few situations in which a court will excuse lateness or non-attendance. Personal sickness is one of these, but a medical certificate will almost certainly be required. Formal legal requirements aside, punctuality is a courtesy of all aspects of professional life, and the courts are no less deserving of such courtesy than are a dentist's or doctor's patients.

Unfortunately, while medical witnesses are usually punctual at court, the courts themselves are not always able to guarantee that the witness will in fact be called to give evidence at the appointed time. If delays appear to be developing, medical witnesses are usually contacted by the party calling them and arrangements made to contact them again closer to the new time they will be required.

These issues of attendance at court apply not only to the initial calling of a medical witness to give evidence but also to the recommencement of evidence after a break. A doctor or dentist who is giving evidence when a court adjourns for lunch must be present when the court resumes after lunch so that their evidence can proceed without delay. The same applies where a court adjourns at the end of a day: the witness must re-attend at the commencement of the hearing on the next day on which the court sits. A judge occasionally permits another witness to be interposed during a doctor's evidence so that the court can continue to hear evidence while the doctor attends to other matters. However, such a procedure is extremely unusual and should never be anticipated.

While the procedures and principles involved appear strict, medical expert witnesses are in practice afforded a high level of courtesy by courts, one which goes beyond that given to other witnesses in legal proceedings. Doctors and dentists should be careful, therefore, not to abuse the privileges they are afforded at court by displaying a lack of courtesy.

CONVERSATIONS OUTSIDE THE COURT

The court wishes to hear from each witness their own information unmodified by conversations with other witnesses. A medical witness waiting outside the court should, therefore, refrain from talking to other witnesses about the case. General conversations regarding the weather or the nearest restaurant are acceptable. However, such an innocent conversation may be observed by the party who has not called the witness and may be raised in court to discredit the witness's evidence. Even if one convinces the court that all that was being discussed was the weather, it is an unnecessary interruption to court proceedings and does nothing to put one in a good light.

This matter is even more important where a medical witness is in the midst of giving evidence when the court adjourns. During the break, the medical witness should not communicate with other witnesses, the media or other persons regarding the evidence given, the questions asked or the evidence to be given at a later stage. If the lunch break or end-of-day adjournment occurs during cross-examination of a witness, the witness has at that stage been made aware of a number of the defence issues in the case. These issues should not be made known to the other witnesses, including other medical witnesses who have not yet been called.

With regard to the issue of communication, it should be remembered that there is no formal property in a witness. If the party calling you, or the opposing party, wishes to talk to you in advance about matters in relation to the evidence that you will be giving, you are not prevented from doing so. However, there is no obligation upon a witness to discuss their evidence with any party: the only obligation is to answer the questions put to them in the witness box. In practical terms, however, most expert witnesses are there to assist the general process of the court and there is little point in obstructing either party. As a matter of legal courtesy, if an opposing party wishes to discuss the evidence a witness will give in advance, they should inform the party calling that witness of their intention to do so.

APPEARANCE AND BEHAVIOUR

How the witness looks, behaves and interacts with the people in the court all affects the attitude of a jury toward them. The ideal attributes of medical witnesses are a series of contradictions. They must not be boring but neither must they be flamboyant entertainers; they must not display 'left-wing' politics, nor 'right-wing' politics; they must not dress too informally, or too formally. Finding the middle ground can be difficult. However, there are some general principles that are of use in this area.

DRESS

Juries expect the medical witness to fulfil their own views of how a doctor or dentist should dress. Juries, like patients, may be suspicious of a practitioner who wears a T-shirt or jeans, or intimidated by one who wears a very formal dark pin-striped suit and a bow tie. Most members of the community believe that dentists and doctors should be smartly dressed. Sometimes the doctor's clothes need to be in tune with the type of evidence they are giving. Thus a specialist giving rarefied information on complex surgical techniques may dress somewhat formally, whereas a doctor giving evidence relating to everyday family medicine practice may dress in a more casual or middle-of-the-road fashion. For men, an ordinary suit or sports jacket and trousers, and for women a smart skirt and blouse, with or without a jacket, is the most appropriate. Clothing that is controversial for any reason is best avoided. Stories abound regarding what jurors have said about people and their clothing: 'I don't trust a doctor who wears a bow tie', and so on. While the witness should not simply blend into the background, their clothing should not be distracting to a jury such that it draws attention away from what they are saying. Jangling flashing jewellery should not be worn. While it may go against a witness's personality, a slightly casual version of formal dress is usually the most appropriate clothing.

Entering and leaving the court

The first time a jury sees a witness is when the witness is called into court and walks from the entrance to the court to the witness box. Those first few seconds are all-important. When walking to the witness box, witnesses should carry themselves in a business-like manner, concentrating their gaze on the witness box itself and avoiding the temptation to look all around the court to see who is there. It is often useful to visit the courtroom prior to giving evidence to become familiar with the layout and the position of the witness box. It is important not to dawdle or become distracted while walking to the witness box but at the same time not to give the impression of haste. Perhaps this latter point is more important in relation to the act of walking out of the courtroom!

When a medical witness has completed giving their evidence, they will in most instances be formally excused by the judge from further attendance or otherwise asked to stand down. It is only after this that the witness should close the file, put away the notes and leave the witness box. The witness should then leave the court in the same manner in which they entered it, walking in a calm and dignified fashion regardless of the experience they have had in the witness box.

As we have seen, medical witnesses may have to bring a number of items into court. In some cases, these include bulky charts and presentation aids that are hard to handle in the confined space of the witness box. If the medical witness mentions the problem to the court staff, the court clerk or usher may be able to assist.

THE WITNESS BOX

When the witness has arrived in the witness box, all eyes in the court are focused on them. The witness is asked to state their name and then to take the oath or affirmation. This is the first time that the medical witness's voice has been heard in the courtroom, and first impressions can be important for the jury. It may also be the first time that the witness has heard their own voice speaking in that particular courtroom.

The taking of the oath is a moment of great formality and importance in the eyes of the court. It is hard to know how a jury views the taking of an oath, but the medical witness should, in any event, treat it with the utmost seriousness. Even if the medical witness is aware of the wording of the oath, they should always allow themselves to be led through it by the court. Each phrase should be declared loudly and clearly, and in a manner implying that the witness understands the terms of the oath. It does not require a theatrical performance, but the jury should be left with the impression that the witness's only concern is to tell the truth. As well as the manner of speaking, the witness's stance and attitude need to be appropriate. The oath is spoken to the judge, magistrate or tribunal chairman, who should be faced at all times. The witness should not slouch, fidget or look around in a distracted fashion, and the Bible or other religious work should be held up in a formal but not rigid pose. While a witness is being sworn in, all people present in the court should remain completely silent and neither move nor create any form of disturbance. Indeed, a court usually waits for silence and the attention of all people present before the oath is administered. No person should enter or leave the court while the oath is being administered. As a result of these requirements, the eyes of most people in the court, in particular those of the jury, are focused on the witness who is taking the oath.

The aim of the barristers for both parties is to seek from the witness evidence that supports their own client's view and to ensure that that evidence is addressed appropriately to the jury. If the witness gives evidence that does not support their client's case, the significance of that evidence needs to be minimized in the eyes of the jury. An effective technique is for a barrister to request that the witness gives answers that are favourable to their client directly to the jury while answers that are unfavourable are directed to the barrister so that the jury loses eye contact with the witness. The witness should, of course, stand or sit in such a way that ensures that they address all answers to the jury and the judge, as it is they who have to evaluate and decide upon the evidence.

There are other important physical factors in relation to stance while giving evidence. While the witness should maintain a relaxed demeanour, it is important not to slouch in the witness box while giving the answers or during any interruptions or minor breaks in the delivery of evidence. Similarly, the witness should not fidget or fiddle with objects while giving evidence. It is all too easy to use a pen as a pointer to illustrate a feature on a chart or photograph and then to continue holding and fiddling with the pen, which may be a source of great distraction for the jury. If a pointer or other aid is used, it should be replaced on the witness box shelf as soon as it is no longer required. The maintenance of a professional physical attitude while giving evidence should not be underestimated. The development of a few simple habits and effective techniques can vastly improve the quality and effectiveness of evidence given by a medical witness.

CONTENT

What a medical witness says in the witness box is often crucial to the outcome of the legal process. It goes without saying that the medical witness, like all witnesses, should always tell the truth. Any lies or innocent errors are likely to be discovered at some stage, and the worst possible connotation will be immediately applied to the inaccurate statement.

Several techniques can be used by the expert witnesses to deliver information to varied audiences. For the sake of the transcript, it is important to use correct technical terms and the appropriate medical jargon. However, the communication value of such evidence to the people in the courtroom may be limited. In order to address this, the witness needs to translate the technical terms smoothly and transparently into appropriate lay expressions or to explain them with examples or analogies. In the case of anatomical terms, it is convenient to use the correct medical term and then to point to the anatomical area on one's own body and use the lay expression at the same time. This can be done as part of a natural explanatory gesture that does not appear to be demeaning to a jury. A medical witness who believes that their evidence may be difficult for a jury to understand should prepare explanatory charts or anatomical models to use as illustrations.

In addition to the issues of communication centered on the technical nature of medical terminology, there are other important aspects to the use of language in the witness box. Light-hearted analogies, jokes and puns can be efficient means of communication, but they may be inappropriate in a court of law. Jokes, in particular, have a great ability to offend as well as lighten and reveal important information. It is easy to ridicule a tragic and serious situation by the use of an inappropriate joke.

One of the greatest difficulties that the expert medical witness faces in adversarial trials is the situation in which the questions by the barristers for both parties do not address the key scientific issue or, if they do, do not adequately deal with the issue with respect to its important ramifications or associated relevant issues. In some cases, the failure of barristers to ask questions relating to specific issues has the potential to lead to a miscarriage of justice. If the medical witness is aware of this potential for the court to be misled, what is their responsibility?

On the one hand, the expert witness is continually reminded that it is not their task to formulate the questions but merely to answer the questions put to them. They are also reminded to answer just the question rather than add any riders to their answer or engage in discussion in co-related areas. On the other hand, the modern view of the forensic scientific and medical witness is that they have a broad duty to the court that is equal to or above the duty they owe to the party that called them to give evidence. Where a witness feels that the manner in which they have given their evidence has the capacity to mislead the court, they should raise this matter with the judge, who then can explore the issue with both counsel. In the book *Forensic science and the expert witness* (Phillips and Bowen, 1985), the authors state:

> In the court room the witness is very largely a captive of the questioner. It is not an exaggeration to assert that a satisfactory result depends just as much on the skill of the questioner as on the skill of the witness. The manner of the questioning conditions the form

and often the content of the answers and when, as sometimes happens, the questioner does not really understand the subject matter, questions may be put in ways which either confound or restrict the witness. Questions are sometimes asked which are unanswerable because, to a scientific witness, they have no rational basis, and not infrequently, the wood is lost in the trees.

After the trial

AUDIT

For the forensic medical practitioner, performance in the witness box is such a critical component of their professional work that it requires regular audit and review to ensure that the work in giving evidence to the courts meets the needs of the justice system. This process is no different from the health care audits relating to medical treatment, in which clinical medical practitioners are regularly involved as part of their ordinary medical practice. It is not always easy to get effective feedback in relation to one's performance as a witness. Judges are probably the best people to provide such an assessment because they do not view the witness from the partisan perspective of the barristers who have been examining the witness during the court proceedings.

Court equipment

- Ring file binder or other file organizer.
- Notes, charts, photographs and other materials related to the forensic medical examination, collated and assembled into a file that can be easily referred to in court. (Copies of the contents of this file should be made as the original may have to be submitted as an exhibit in court.)
- Latex examination gloves.
- Gloves, if the witness is expected to pick up exhibits (for example, bloodstained clothing) and indicate their findings on them.
- Pen-knife.
- Multipurpose pen-knife with attachments, which may be useful for opening packets or wrapped exhibits.
- Magnifying glass. This can be useful if the witness is asked to examine photographs.
- Calculator, as the witness will occasionally be asked to calculate a value or convert units of measurement.
- Pens.
- Pencils.
- White board and overhead projector markers.
- Rulers.
- Pointers.
- Notepaper.

Reference and recommended reading

Forbes TR. 1985: *Surgeons at The Bailey: English forensic medicine to 1878*. Yale: Yale University Press.

Freckelton I, Selby H. 1993: *Expert evidence*. North Ryde, NSW: Law Book Company.

Gee DJ, Mason JK. 1990: *The courts and the doctor*. Oxford: Oxford University Press.

Medical Protection Society. 1992: *Medico-legal reports and appearing in courts*. London: Medical Protection Society.

Phillips JH, Bowen JK. 1985: *Forensic science and the expert witness*. Sydney: Law Book Company.

Smith R, Wynne B (eds). 1989: *Expert evidence: interpreting science in the law*. London: Routledge.

Winfield R (ed.). 1989: *The expert medical witness*. Sydney: Federation Press.

CHAPTER 20

Identification and the law

I FRECKELTON

Introduction	257	Coroners' inquests	260
Definition of death	258	Criminal law	260
Actions in tort	258	Crimes compensation	262
Contractual arrangements	259	Proof of death	263
Property in a dead body	259	Identification of the living	263
Probate	259	Conclusion	264

Introduction

The ascertainment of the identity of persons, alive and dead, is of significance to the law in many ways. In 1765 Blackstone proclaimed that, 'The law not only regards life and member, and protects every man in the enjoyment of them, but also furnishes him with everything necessary for their support.'[1] He followed this observation by noting that 'These rights of life and member, can only be determined by the death of the person; which is either a civil or natural death.' He said little of natural death but noted that civil death is to be regarded as occurring when a person is banished from the realm, or enters into religion, that is to say, goes into a monastery, at which point 'he is absolutely dead in law; and his next heir shall have his estate'.[2]

In contemporary civil law, the determination of the deceased's death and the time of his or her passing is vital for the viability of actions on behalf of plaintiffs and the enforcement of rights by the survivors of the deceased. Many contractual obligations simply lapse upon the death of a party. As Oliver Wendell Holmes in the USA noted, 'The only thing which can be transferred is the benefit or burden of the promise, and how can they be separated from the facts that gave rise to them? How, in short, can

a man sue or be sued on a promise in which he had no part?',[3] Thus, in this context too, the proof of both death and time of death can have major financial repercussions.

In terms of probate law, proof of death is a prerequisite for the granting of probate, and there are presumptions that assist in the task. However, the law is understandably demanding in relation to proof of death having occurred in order to avoid the embarrassing scenario of distribution having taken place over a living person's estate.

In the criminal law context, proof of identity, through either visual or aural identification, is an integral part of many prosecutions, particularly in relation to robberies and assaults. Moreover, it is a fundamental element of a murder or manslaughter prosecution that the person who is alleged to be the victim is human and is actually dead. This much is elementary, but the time of the death of the deceased may also be vital to the resolution of the criminal proceedings in terms of proving the potential for a suspect to be implicated. Furthermore, in some jurisdictions, if the deceased died more than a year after the infliction of injury, this may result in the acquittal of the accused. Issues of proof of causation of death can be complex and heavily contested in criminal, civil and coronial jurisdictions.

This chapter analyses a range of legal contexts in which proof of identity, death and time of death are relevant.

Definition of death

The legal criteria for death have only troubled the legal system in comparatively recent times with the growing sophistication of medical technology.[4] Even today in England, there is no statute that defines death and only a little caselaw that concerns the definition of death. Traditionally, death was regarded as the stoppage of the circulation of blood.[5] It was only in the 1981 English case of *R. v. Malcherek, R. v. Steel*[6] that Lord Lane CJ acknowledged that 'Modern techniques have undoubtedly resulted in the blurring of many of the conventional and traditional concepts of death' and noted that 'There is, it seems, a body of opinion in the medical profession that there is only one true test of death and that is the irreversible death of the brain stem which controls the basic functions of the body such as breathing. When that occurs it is said that the body has died, even though by mechanical means the lungs are being caused to operate and some circulation of blood is taking place.'

By 1993 the English Court of Appeal was prepared to go further, and it was held by the majority in the tragic case of *Airedale NHS Trust* v. *Bland,*[7] involving a survivor of the Hillsborough Stadium collapse who was in a permanent vegetative state, that death occurs when the brain stem has been destroyed.[8] This is generally regarded now as also being the law in Australia, New Zealand, Canada and the USA. In Australia, the Law Reform Commission recommended that death be defined in human tissue legislation in terms of either the irreversible cessation of blood circulation or the irreversible cessation of brain function.[9] All jurisdictions in due course enacted this legislation in their human tissue legislation.

Actions in tort

Death can both create and extinguish liability in tort. At common law, an action died along with the deceased. So far as the defendant was concerned, this was partly associated with the retributive character of an action in tort. However, by 1934 in England and a little later in Australia and New Zealand, reforming legislation came to provide that, despite the death of a litigant, all causes of action subsisting against or vested in him or her survive against or, as the case may be, for the benefit of the deceased's estate. Actions involving dignitary interests generally form an exception to this principle; these may be, for example, actions for damages for adultery, seduction, defamation and enticement of spouses. However, the amount of damages may be reduced as the courts do not generally award exemplary damages when the tortfeasor (or the victim) is deceased. Some legislation also limits claims for non-pecuniary losses, on the basis that such awards should be limited to actions actually brought by a living person[10] rather than by their relatives.

Where it is the tortfeasor who has died, early legislation in many jurisdictions provided that actions in tort against an estate that survived pursuant to legislation had to be pending at the time of death or that the cause of action had arisen not earlier than 6 months before the death of the deceased and proceedings had been instituted quickly. These requirements have now been liberalized in most places, with the periods being extended. However, the time frames are still short enough to be problematic if there is substantial delay in determining whether a tortfeasor has actually died.

At common law, actions did not exist for wrongfully inflicted death. It was cheaper for a tortfeasor to kill than it was to maim. In 1846 Lord Campbell's Act in England sought to remedy this defect by making it an actionable wrong, at the suit of defined relatives, to cause another's death 'by a wrongful act, neglect or default which is such as would (if death had not ensued) have entitled the party injured to maintain an action and recover damages in respect thereof, notwithstanding that the death was caused under circumstances amounting in law to felony'.[11] The relatives protected by the Act are broadly defined in most jurisdictions that have enacted comparable provisions to include spouses, parents, grandparents, step-parents, children, posthumous children, grandchildren and step-children. Divorced spouses, blood relationships, illegitimate children, adoptive and foster children are also included in some jurisdictions. Actions must usually be commenced within a shorter time of death than applies under ordinary periods of limitation.[12] Recovery is limited in such actions to economic or material advantages for survivors;[13] thus the criterion is loss rather than need. The issue is dependency. Dependants are generally only entitled to an amount that will give them an annuity for the period of what was likely to have been their dependency. Even funeral expenses are often not allowed.

Error in identification is another way in which death can come into issue in the realm of tortious actions. In the notorious case involving the death of Lieutenant Colonel Thomas Hart, for example, his widow successfully sued for infliction of severe emotional distress arising out of a botched identification of remains.[14] The deceased was believed to have been one of 14 men shot down over Pakse, Laos, during the Vietnam conflict. In the summer of 1985, the

United States Army released what it said were Hart's remains, but his widow was not confident that she could trust the identification. She took the remains for re-analysis to a forensic anthropologist at Colorado State University who expressed the view that it was impossible for the remains to be sufficient for anyone to be identified from them. In October 1988 Lieutenant Colonel Hart's widow was awarded US$632 000 damages.[15]

Contractual arrangements

By and large, the death of one of the parties to negotiations has the effect of terminating any offer that might otherwise have been operative at the time of death. In 1876 it was regarded as 'admitted law' that 'if a man who makes an offer dies, the offer cannot be accepted after he is dead'.[16] However, there may be situations in which a court could conclude that the offeror intended that an offer should remain open after his or her death. In such circumstances, the death may not have any impact upon the currency of the offer.

As a general rule, rights under a contract pass to personal representatives upon death,[17] but, of course, where the obligations of the deceased are personal to him or her, resulting in an inability for ongoing compliance with the contract, the contract terminates.[18]

Property in a dead body

In Anglo-Australian law, a corpse has been held to be somewhat analogous to wild animals in that a human being, alive or dead, cannot be the subject of property[19] so cannot be stolen.[20] Even the heir has no property in the bodies of his or her ancestors and can bring no action in respect of them.[21] Although executors do not have property in a body, they may obtain an action to compel another to hand it over for burial. After burial, a corpse forms part of the land in which it is lawfully buried, and the right of possession goes with the land. It has also been suggested that the law of England has traditionally been that a person is guilty of a misdemeanour if they prevent the burial of a dead body or, without lawful excuse, dissect a dead body, even if their motives are laudable, or if they have the means and obligation to bury a dead body and neglect to do so.[22]

In the USA, the law varies from jurisdiction to jurisdiction on the 'no property principle'. In the old case of *Larson* v. *Chase*[23] the Supreme Court of Minnesota held that a widow was entitled to damages for the dissection of her dead husband on the basis that she had a right to possession of the deceased's body without medical procedures being unlawfully executed upon it. A number of courts have found excuses for ignoring the absolute no property principle and have spoken in terms of 'quasi-property' to describe relatives' rights in a dead body.[24] A determination of who holds possessory rights to a dead body can prove vital as that person may have to consent to an evidentiary autopsy, and the general tendency has been for autopsy statutes and cases to vest possessory rights in relatives of the deceased for the purpose of authorization of autopsies to be conducted on the deceased.

Probate

Where there is no available evidence of a person's having been alive at some time during a continuous period of 7 years or more, an important presumption of death can come into play. However, this only occurs if it can be shown that there are people who would be likely to have heard of the person over that period, that they have in fact not heard of him or her and, finally, that all due inquiries have been made.[25] The presumption is simply that the deceased is no longer alive, rather than that he or she died at or before any other given date. However, it is always open for a court to receive evidence that it is likely that a person died at a particular time, such as in an aeroplane or maritime accident.

For the purposes of determining entitlement under a will, it may be important to determine the order of persons' deaths. This is not always easy because of the circumstances of death, for example, in time of war or even in a car or train accident. Craniofacial identification may have a role to play in this context. There is no presumption of law based upon age or sex. The question is one of fact, depending entirely upon evidence that can be adduced of the circumstances of the deceased persons' deaths. Many different statutory provisions in different jurisdictions apply to assist with the evidentiary predicament.

On occasions, it is known that two persons have died, and the cause of their death may also be known, for example, as a result of an aeroplane accident. Yet it may be unclear but important to determine who was the survivor – who died before whom. The common law provides little assistance: there is no presumption arising from age or sex as to survivorship. The question is one of fact, and if evidence cannot prove who died first, the law will treat the matter as incapable of determination. The onus is on the person seeking to prove that one person died before the other.[26] To resolve the problem, a statutory presumption has been created in many jurisdictions. The provision in Victoria, Australia, is typical:

In all cases where ... two or more persons have died in circumstances rendering it uncertain which of them survived the other or others, such deaths shall (subject to any order of the court), for all purposes affecting the title to property, be presumed to have occurred in order of seniority, and accordingly the younger shall be deemed to have survived the elder.[27]

In South Australia, it is provided that 'Where an intestate and his spouse die within twenty-eight days of each other, this Part applies as if the spouse had not survived the deceased'.[28] In contrast, in New Zealand, the law is that where any two persons have died at the same time or where there is reasonable doubt about who survived whom, the property generally of each person 'shall devolve, and if he left a will, it shall take effect unless a contrary intention is shown thereby, as if he had survived the other person or persons so dying and had died immediately afterwards'.[29]

Coroners' inquests

Coroners have jurisdiction to conduct inquests into deaths, fires and, in some places, into other phenomena. New Zealand aside, a coroner cannot hold an inquest simply because he or she is of the view that such a step would be in the public interest.[30] The death of a person is a precondition to death inquests. This is a matter of evidence. If the coroner is not satisfied as to whether a person has died, he or she will either not hold an inquest at all (as in the case of a person who is simply missing in unsuspicious circumstances) or, if an inquest is held, will not make the preliminary finding of death.[31]

It is generally regarded that neither a non-viable fetus nor a stillborn child can properly be the subject of an inquest.[32] In addition, a number of practical problems can be posed to the exercise of the coroner's jurisdiction. As is pointed out in the 10th edition of *Jervis on Coroners*:

In the case of the discovery of partially destroyed bodies or parts of bodies, or pieces of tissue, there are a number of difficult problems which may be encountered, since it cannot automatically be assumed that the body to which the piece of tissue or part belongs is dead. Certainly a severed arm or leg is not conclusive evidence that the body from which they come is dead. Similarly with a piece of tissue not sufficiently vital as to demonstrate the inevitability of death.[33]

Ultimately, it is a question of evidence. This was illustrated in the gruesome New South Wales case of *Re Oram; ex parte Brady,*[34] in which it was held that the finding of a tattooed arm, severed from a human trunk by a sharp knife, was not sufficient to constitute a body for the purpose of endowing the coroner with jurisdiction since an arm may be removed from a body without loss of life.

Criminal law

It is necessary in a murder case for the prosecution to prove beyond reasonable doubt that the victim at the time of death was a living human being. This raises the troubled question of when life begins and ends. Partial resolution of the issue is to be found in the 1953 Victorian case of *R.* v. *Hutty,*[35] in which it was held that a 'baby is fully and completely born when it is completely delivered from the body of its mother and it has a separate and independent existence in the sense that it does not derive its power of living from its mother.' It was held by Beach J that this could occur before the umbilical cord was cut and that the crucial question was whether the child was fully extruded from the mother's body 'and is living by virtue of the functioning of its own organs'.[36] In Australia, the jurisdictions of Victoria, New South Wales and South Australia are governed by the common law, while in Queensland, Western Australia and Tasmania there is a supplementary rule that an accused is deemed to have killed a child who dies in consequence of anything done or omitted to be done by the accused either before or during its birth.

The Infant Life (Preservation) Act 1929 (UK) was passed to create the offence of 'child destruction'. In doing so, it too, in effect, provided a definition of human identity. The aim of the legislation was to protect unextruded babies during the birth process. Its provisions find a mirror in many jurisdictions and serve, to an extent, to define the commencement of human life for the purposes of the criminal law. In similar terms, s.10(1) of the Crimes Act 1958 (Vic) provides that 'Any person who with intent to destroy the life of a child capable of being born alive, by any wilful act unlawfully causes such child to die before it has an existence independent of its mother' is guilty of the offence of destruction of a child. Section 10(2) provides that if a pregnancy has subsisted for 28 weeks or longer, that is prima facie proof that the fetus was 'capable of being born alive' for the purposes of determining whether an offence has been committed. In England, however, it has been held that a 27-week-old fetus was capable of being born alive if it was capable of 'breathing and living by reason of its breathing through its own lungs alone'.[37]

It is not necessary for the remains of the deceased to be found in order for a prosecution for murder, manslaughter or infanticide to be successful. Nor has it been necessary under most legal systems.

Antiphon, in approximately 419 BC, wrote a defence of Helos, who was accused in Athens of the shipboard murder of Herodes on the journey from Athens to Mytilene, the chief town of the island of Lesbos. On behalf of the accused, Antiphon did not take the point that no body had been found so no murder could be proved. Instead, he stressed that no bloodstains could be found in spite of assiduous investigation – save those discovered to be of sheep blood – so it was unlikely that the deceased was the victim of foul play at the hands of the accused.[38]

As Fisse points out, 'There is no rule that the defendant cannot be convicted of criminal homicide merely because the victim has disappeared. If there were, the absurd consequence would follow that there could be no conviction for a murder committed on a ship before a hundred witnesses if the defendant happened to kill the victim by dropping her overboard with a weight attached to her feet'.[39] The issue came before the New South Wales Court of Criminal Appeal in the case of *R. v. Margaret Burton*[40] where it was noted that, in Hale's *History of the pleas of the Crown*,[41] the author had stated, 'I would never convict any person of murder or manslaughter, unless the fact were proved to be done, or at least the body found dead.' The Court, however, held that convictions of murder or manslaughter where no body has been found are not necessarily to be denied validity because no body has been found: 'But the absence of a body, and a case in which the Crown is compelled to rely for proof of death upon circumstantial material, necessarily merit a significant degree of caution before verdicts of guilty of murder or manslaughter can be recognised as soundly based'.[42] It comes down to the probative value of the evidence available as to whether the victim is actually dead.

A further problem exists in determining the culpability of an accused where a victim dies a long time after an assault. In terms of causation, it becomes logistically problematic to evaluate the nexus between assault and death, particularly where there are intervening medical factors. The courts developed a rule that if death followed more than a year and a day after an assault, the defendant was not accounted criminally responsible.[43] In Australia, this rule was incorporated in legislation in the code states of Queensland, Western Australia and Tasmania.[44] In the USA, the rigidity of the rule was relieved by determinations that it functioned as no more than a presumption that could be displaced by appropriate evidence.[45] With growing sophistication in terms of medical diagnosis and treatment, the rule is becoming more and more anachronistic. It has been abolished in a number of jurisdictions[46] and will probably no longer exist in most places by the turn of the millennium.

However, it remains incumbent upon the prosecution to prove that an assailant substantially contributed to the death of the victim.[47] It has been held in this regard that foresight by the accused of the possibility or probability of death or grievous bodily harm to the victim by the accused's act is irrelevant: 'The question to be asked is whether an act or series of acts (in exceptional cases an omission or series of omissions) consciously performed by the accused is or are so connected with the event that it or they must be regarded as having a sufficiently substantial causal effect which subsisted up to the happening of the event, without being spent or without being in the eyes of the law sufficiently interrupted by some other act or event'.[48] The issue currently arises in relation to charges of conduct endangering life when persons suffering from HIV or AIDS engage in unprotected sex with a partner without fully informing them of their medical status. The courts continue to grapple with the extent to which a person's acts must have been the *causa causans* or the *causa sine qua non* of death. In the end, much comes down to the probabilities that are reasonably foreseeable by the offender of the infliction of death or serious injury.

Four approaches to the test for causation may historically be discerned in the criminal law:

1 the 'operating and substantial cause' test;
2 the 'natural consequence' test;
3 the 'reasonable foresight of the consequences' test;
4 the '*novus actus interveniens*' test.

The latter is used sometimes in conjunction with and sometimes independently of the other three tests.[49]

The most prominent Australian case applying the 'operating and substantial cause' test was *R. v. Hallett*,[50] in which the South Australian Court of Criminal Appeal noted that there had been a tendency toward confusion:

> between the factors relevant when considering causation and those relevant when considering the necessary mental element to constitute the crime of murder... Foresight by the accused of the possibility or probability of death or grievous bodily harm from his act, though very relevant to the question of malice afterthought, has nothing to do with the question of causation. The death of the deceased is the material event. The question to be asked is whether an act or series of acts (in exceptional cases an omission or series of omissions) consciously performed by the accused is or are so connected with the event that it or they might be regarded as having a substantially causal effect which subsisted up to the happening of the event, without being spent or in the eyes of the law sufficiently interrupted by some other act or event.[51]

The key question is whether something happens which is sufficient to break the chain of causation, be it an extraordinary act of nature or something more pedestrian as a result of unforeseeable external involvement. Put another way, Lord Parker CJ in *R.* v. *Smith*,[52] held that, 'if at the time of death the original wound is still an operating cause and a substantial cause, then the death can properly be said to be the result of the wound, albeit that some other cause of death is also operating'.[53] He held that only if it can be said that the original wounding is no more than the setting in which another cause operates, the death does not result from the wound. Lord Parker CJ held that only if 'the second cause is so overwhelming as to make the original wound merely part of the history can it be said that death does not flow from the wound.'[54]

In contrast, a number of cases have determined that if a person's behaviour, ultimately causing them injury or death, was not the 'natural consequence' of what was done by the accused, the accused cannot be said to have caused it.[55] A variant of the test prescribes that the accused must have been able reasonably to have foreseen the consequence of what he or she did for the accused to have caused what later transpired: 'Where the injuries are fatal, the attempt [to escape] must be the natural consequence of an unlawful act and that unlawful act 'must be such as all sober and reasonable people would inevitably recognise must subject the other person to, at least, the risk of some harm resulting therefrom, albeit not serious harm.'[56]

The law on causation in Australia's criminal law remains none too clear after the most significant consideration of the issue – that occurring in the High Court decision in *Royall*.[57] In that case, McHugh J conceded that 'Judicial and academic efforts to achieve a coherent theory of common law causation have not met with significant success.' However, of relevance in the context of coronial law, he noted that the object of the civil law is not the same as the object of the criminal law:

> But both areas of law use principles of causal responsibility to limit liability for the consequences of wrongful acts. Tort and contract law do so, inter alia, by rules of remoteness of damage which are based on notions of justice and morality: cf Overseas Tankship (UK) Ltd v Morts Dock & Engineering Co Ltd (The Wagon Mound (No 1)) [1961] AC 388 at 422–433. Criminal law does so by reference to rules which are based on notions of moral culpability. Speaking generally, the broad principles of causation applicable in civil cases should be equally applicable in criminal cases.

His Honour accepted that the law of negligence has used the doctrines of reasonable foreseeability and *novus actus interveniens* to limit responsibility for negligent acts and omissions that are causally connected with the injury suffered. He found that, similarly in criminal law, a person should not be held liable for a wrongful act or omission 'which has caused harm in a but for' sense if the harm was the product of a *novus actus interveniens* or was not a reasonably foreseeable consequence of the act or omission. He rejected the 'natural consequence' test and the 'operating and substantial cause' test, accepting that 'for the purposes of the criminal law, causation cannot be separated from questions of moral culpability.' In this, he was joined by Brennan J, who also identified the foreseeability of the consequences of an accused's conduct as the key criterion of causality.[58] In contrast, Toohey and Gaudron JJ expressed concerns about the potential for juror confusion if the concept of foreseeability were introduced into the assessment of causation,[59] while Deane and Dawson JJ accepted that 'On occasions foreseeability may play some part in a jury's inquiry into cause of death' but preferred to 'keep causation and intent separate as far as possible and to avoid the introduction of questions of foreseeability in relation to causation.'[60]

Thus, in Australia in the criminal context, there is no clear criterion for determining whether an act caused a death. It appears that in the criminal law, as in the civil, issues of public policy, such as culpability in the form of capacity to foresee consequences of behaviour, play a significant role in determining causation.

In sentencing hearings, too, the issue of causation plays a prominent role. Difficulties occur in the context of injuries that come into being, or death that ensues, as a secondary complication of an initial assault. For example, in *R.* v. *Thomas McKnoulty*,[61] the victim was savagely assaulted by the accused, but after admission to hospital the victim suffered complications – her condition deteriorated and an episode of vasospasm (contraction of small blood vessels, in this case inside the brain) occurred. The blood supply to the brain was cut off, and a considerable part of her brain died. In the circumstances of the case, the vasospasm was determined to be a delayed complication owing to the victim's injuries and thus a complication for which the accused was properly to be held responsible. It was taken into account as an aggravating feature of the sentencing process, the accused being regarded as responsible for all the medical sequelae of his conduct. If, however, the major cause of the victim's deterioration was the negligence of a doctor at the treating hospital, it is likely that the sentencing court would not have taken into account as an aggravating factor the aspects of the victim's condition for which the doctor was responsible.

Crimes compensation

In some jurisdictions, criminal injuries compensation awards of substantial proportions may be made 'for expenses actually and reasonably incurred and pecuniary loss suffered by dependants as a result of a victim's death.'[62] Once again, proof of death is a prerequisite of entitlement, as is proof of a connection between the criminal act and the pain and suffering later suffered by secondary and other victims.[63] Such matters can be far from straightforward because of difficulties in proof and can have a fundamental impact upon a dependant's entitlement to compensation from a state fund.

Proof of death

Proof that a person has died or that a person's remains are those of the deceased can frequently only be resolved by expert evidence. In this regard, the standard rules of expert evidence apply: the person giving evidence must properly be able to be classified as possessed of specialized knowledge in relation to the evidence to be given, whether by virtue of skill, experience or training; the evidence must emanate from an area of expertise, namely not be so out of step with the views within the intellectual marketplace as to be unreliable or not generally accepted amongst relevant experts, and the data upon which the expert opinions are based must be proved by relevant evidence.[64]

These issues are not always straightforward, and expert evidence in controversial areas of novel scientific endeavour is from time to time ruled inadmissible. For example, expert evidence in relation to bite-mark identification was ruled inadmissible in both Queensland and the Northern Territory of Australia on the ground that evidence in relation to bite-mark analysis was not yet to be accounted as more probative than prejudicial in the particular circumstances of the evidence offered.[65] This form of discretionary exclusion of evidence that is not sufficiently proved to be susceptible of effective evaluation and worthy of being relied upon is likely to become more common in many jurisdictions.[66]

It is vital that a straightforward picture of the parameters of expertise and of certainty in relation to the identification of remains or the construction of identity and mode and time of death be presented to courts. Opinion evidence should not function as an excuse for speculation unfettered by data.[67] Expert evidence is frequently only part of the attempt to reconstruct the identity of remains and the time of death. The expert evidence forms just one part of the mosaic of the information presented to the court. Some of it will consist of evidence of fact, some, of evidence in the form of inferences to be drawn from fact. The task of the cross-examiner is to make both forms of evidence properly accountable by exploring the logical connections between data and opinion, the potential for alternative hypotheses, the expertise of the witness and the soundness of the bases of the testimony.[68]

Identification of the living

The law has traditionally regarded identification of persons by witnesses, be they eyewitnesses or earwitnesses, as fraught with the potential for error. In one of England's most notorious miscarriages of justice, Alfred Beck, who was picked out in identification parades by 12 women, served 7 years and was then released. He was later again picked up and identified by 4 women in a line-up, and was convicted and awaiting sentence when the real offender was finally apprehended.[69] The case led to the establishment of the English Court of Criminal Appeal in 1908. Similarly, the case of Oscar Slater, who served 18 years following a wrong eyewitness identification, led to the establishment of the Scottish counterpart of the Court of Criminal Appeal in 1926.[70] In 1987 the Australian Law Reform Commission recommended that, so serious were the dangers of unreliable eyewitness identification and the risk of mis-estimating its weight, such evidence should not be admissible in criminal proceedings unless an identification parade had been held or it was not reasonable to have held such a parade before the identification was made.[71]

It has been held necessary to warn juries of the special need for caution before convicting on identification evidence, to instruct juries on the reason for this need and to refer juries to the fact that a mistaken witness can be most convincing, and that even a number of witnesses can inadvertently fall into error in the realm of identification.[72]

Many cases have stressed the importance of the holding of identification parades in due form, rather than dependence upon other forms of less reliable identification.[73] Justice Stephen of the Australian High Court has described photo-identification as inherently unreliable as well as beset by serious evidentiary disadvantages. In the most important case on the subject in Australia, it has been held, however, that there is no rule that requires the quashing of a conviction when evidence has been admitted from identification from photographs and an identity parade could have been, but was not, held. The question is whether the conviction is safe in all the circumstances.[74]

In spite of the dangers posed by mistaken eyewitness and aural identification, courts have been loathe to allow expert evidence on the dangers to go before juries. In Australia's leading case on the subject, *R. v. Smith*,[75] Vincent J disallowed such evidence:

In circumstances in which proof of events, the substance of conversations, and the identity of perpetrators may be dependent upon the evidence of ordinary people, there is obvious concern detectable in the judgments relating to the use of expert evidence, that by refined analysis of the processes involved in the reception, retention and repetition of information, substantial complexity will be introduced into the conduct of a criminal trial without significantly increasing the reliability of fact finding by juries. Indeed the authorities clearly indicate that there has been some apprehension by appellate courts that juries will be confused by jargon and less capable of employing the common sense with which the law accepts they are endowed: see *R.* v. *Turner* [1975] QB 834.

In doing so, he was upheld by the Australian High Court.[76] The practical consequence of the decision is that expert evidence in relation to the general principles of unreliability of identification, both visual and aural, and also the operation of memory, remains inadmissible. However, it may be that, in a specific factual scenario, evidence about particular risks attendant upon a particular form of identification may be admissible.

Conclusion

Proof of death, the identity of the deceased and that of the offender, the connection between tortious or criminal acts and death, the manner of death and the time of death are fundamental in determining both civil and criminal liability. This places a premium upon the quality and accuracy of a number of forms of expert testing and, ultimately, evidence. Where evidence from forensic pathologists, odontologists, psychologists and experts in craniofacial reconstruction is able to supply clear answers, courts will make rulings in accordance with the probative value of the evidence. Where the state of development of the techniques employed, or the condition of the samples available, do not permit clarity of answer, or the deterioration in remains or the results of the testing lead only to equivocal results, it is essential, as a matter of professional ethics, if not the operation of law, that these uncertainties be disclosed by expert witnesses. This may sometimes lead to such evidence being withheld from the trier of fact on a determination of inadmissibility but will more often result in reduced weight being given to the evidence. The reliability of the fact-finding that takes place in the civil, criminal and coronial justice processes ultimately rests upon the two factors: first, integrity of the evidence and the witnesses, and second, the extent to which trial lawyers can make witnesses, both lay and expert, accountable.

References

1. Blackstone W. 1765: *Commentaries on the laws of England*, vol. 1. Oxford: Clarendon Press, 127.
2. Blackstone W. 1765: *Commentaries on the laws of England*, vol. 1. Oxford: Clarendon Press, 128.
3. Holmes OW. 1882: *The common law and other writings*. Birmingham: Legal Classics Library, 342.
4. Galbally F. 1981: Death by statute. *Australian Law Journal* **55**, 339; see also Australian Law Reform Commission. 1977: Report No. 7, *Human tissue transplants*, Canberra: AGPS.
5. See, for example, *Black's law dictionary*, 4th edn, p. 488.
6. [1981] 2 All ER 422.
7. [1993] 1 All ER 821; see Freckelton I. 1993: The persistent vegetative state conundrum. *Journal of Law and Medicine* **1**(1), 35.
8. See also *Re A* [1992] 3 Med LR 303. For useful discussions of this issue, see Skegg P. 1988: *Law, ethics and medicine*. Oxford: Clarendon Press, 188ff; Kennedy I, Grubb A. 1994: *Medical law*. London: Butterworths, 1383ff; Singer P. 1994: *Rethinking life and death*. Melbourne: Text Publishing, 20ff.
9. Australian Law Reform Commission. 1977: Report No. 7, *Human tissue transplants*. Canberra: AGPS, para 133–6.
10. See, for example, *Jaksic* v. *Cossar* (1966) 85 NSWR (Pt 1) (NSW) 102.
11. In due course, this provision was applied in many jurisdictions in the common law world: see, for example, Compensation to Relatives Act 1897(NSW); Wrongs Act 1958, Pt III (Vic).
12. It can be as short a period as 12 months, as for example, in Western Australia.
13. See *Sheils* v. *Cruikshank* [1953] 1 All ER 874.
14. Baden M. 1991: *Unnatural death*. London: Sphere Books, 78ff.
15. Baden M. 1991: *Unnatural death*. London: Sphere Books, 82; see also the case of Major Fanning detailed by the same author on pp. 79ff.
16. *Dickinson* v. *Dodds* (1876) 2 Ch D 463 at 475 per Mellish LJ; see also *Reynolds* v. *Atherton* (1921) 125 LT 690 at 695.
17. See *Stubbs* v. *Holywell Railway Co* (1867) LR 2 Ex 311.
18. See *Farrow* v. *Wilson* (1869) LR4CP 744.
19. 3 Coke Inst 215; *Haynes' Case*, 12 Rep 113; *Peirce* v. *Swan Point Cemetery*, 14 Am Rep 667 at 677; *Doodeward* v. *Spence* (1908) 6 CLR 406 at 408; see Jones JTR. 1990: Evidentiary autopsies. *University of Colorado Law Review* **61**, 569.
20. See *Stephen's Digest of Criminal Law*, 5th edn, p. 252, cited in *Doodeward* v. *Spence* at p. 419.
21. 2 Blac Comm, c.28; save sometimes to apply for an autopsy, exhumation or inquest.
22. *Doodeward* v. *Spence* (1908) 6 CLR 406 at 414, a case involving an action for conversion and detinue of a corpse of a stillborn two-headed child.
23. 28 Am SR 370.
24. See *Peirce* v. *Swan Point Cemetery*, 10 RI 227 (1872);

Bogert v. *City of Indianapolis*, 13 Ind 134 at 138 (1859); *Pettigrew* v. *Pettigrew*, 56 A 878 at 879 (1904); *Koerber* v. *Patek*, 102 NW 40 at 42 (1905).

25. Stone X. 1981: The presumption of death. *Modern Law Review* **44**, 516; *Chard* v. *Chard* [1956] P 259; *Axon* v. *Axon* (1937) 59 CLR 395; *Rinley Martin* v. *The Queen*, unreported, Western Australian Court of Criminal Appeal, 4 April 1996 interpreting s.269 of the Western Australian Criminal Code.

26. See *Wing* v. *Angrave* (1860) 8 HLC 183; 11 ER 397; see also *Hickman* v. *Peacey* [1945] AC 304 at 341.

27. Property Law Act 1958 (Vic), s.184.

28. Administration and Probate Act 1919 (SA), s.72e.

29. Simultaneous Deaths Act 1958 (NZ), s.3(1)(a); see also Property Law Act 1969 (WA), s.120(a); Administration and Probate Ordinance 1929 (ACT), s.49P.

30. See *R.* v. *Poplar Coroner; ex parte Thomas* [1993] 2 WLR 547; Freckelton I. Inquest law. in Selby H. (ed.), The inquest handbook. Sydney: LBC (in press).

31. See generally Freckelton I. 1995: Coronial law. In Linden S. *Health and guardianship*, The Laws of Australia (TLA), vol. 20. Sydney: LBC.

32. Matthews P, Foreman JC. 1986: *Jervis on the office and duties of coroners*, 10th edn, London: Sweet and Maxwell, 47–8.

33. Ibid at pp. 48–9.

34. (1935) 52 NSWWN 109.

35. [1953] VLR 338 at 339.

36. See also *Paton* v. *British Pregnancy Advisory Service Trustees* [1979] QB 276; *C* v. *S* [1988] QB 135; *Attorney-General for the State of Queensland (Ex rel Ker)* v. *T* (1983) 57 ALJR 285; *K* v. *Minister for Youth and Community Services; Re Infant K* (1982) 8 Fam LR 250.

37. *Rance* v. *Mid-Downs Health Authority* [1990] NLJ 325 at 326.

38. Freeman K. 1946: *The murder of Herodes and other trials from the Athenian law courts*. London: Macdonald and Co., 70.

39. Fisse B. 1990: *Howard's criminal law*, Sydney: LBC, 30.

40. (1987) 24 A Crim R 169.

41. Vol 2, p. 290.

42. At 174.

43. Yale. 1989: A year and a day rule in homicide. *Cambridge Law Journal*, **48**, 202; *Dyson* [1908] 2 KB 454; *Evans (no 2)* [1972] VR 523.

44. It also found expression in coronial legislation in a number of Australian jurisdictions: see Freckelton I. 1995: Coronial law. In Linden S. *Health and guardianship*, TLA vol. 20. Sydney: LBC.

45. See, for example, *Commonwealth* v. *Lewis*, 409 NE 2d 771 (1980).

46. See, for example, the Crimes (Year and a Day Rule) Act 1991 (Vic).

47. See *Hallett* v. *The Queen* [1969] SASR 141; *Butcher* [1986] VR 43 at 55–6.

48. *Hallett* v. *The Queen* [1969] SASR 141 at 148–9.

49. Freckelton I. 1997: Causation in coronial law. *Journal of Law and Medicine* **4**(3), 289; Freckelton I. 1996: Coronial law. In Linden S. *Health and Guardianship*, vol. 20, *The Laws of Australia*, Sydney: LBC.

50. [1969] SASR 141. See along similar lines, *Lawford and Van de Wiel* (1993) 69 A Crim R 115 at 122. However, see *Royall* (1991) 54 A Crim R 53 at 78 per Deane and Dawson JJ.

51. A 'substantial cause' has been held to be 'a convenient word to use to indicate to the jury that it must be something more than de minimis': *Hennigan* (1971) 55 Cr App R 262 at 264–5 per Lord Parker CJ.

52. [1959] 2 QB 35 at 42–3.

53. See also *Dalby* [1982] 1 WLR 425.

54. Ibid. See also *R* v. *Blaue* [1975] 3 All ER 446.

55. See, for example, *Beech* (1912) 7 Cr App R 197 at 200; *Roberts* (1971) 56 Cr App R 95 at 102.

56. *Mackie* (1973) 57 Cr App R 453 at 459–60.

57. (1990) 54 A Crim R 53.

58. At 68.

59. At 87.

60. Ibid at 78.

61. Unreported, NSW Supreme Court, 6 July 1995 per Abadee J.

62. See, for example, the former Criminal Injuries Compensation Act 1983 (Vic), s.17.

63. See *Martin* v. *Crimes Compensation Tribunal* (1994) 8 VAR 39.

64. See generally Freckelton I, Selby H. (eds) 1993: *Expert evidence*, Sydney: LBC.

65. See *Lewis* v. *The Queen* (1987) 29 A Crim R 267; *Carroll* v. *The Queen* (1985) 19 A Crim R 410.

66. This is particularly so in Australia where ss.135 and 137 of the Evidence Act 1995 (Cth) and the Evidence Act 1995 (NSW), amend the rules of expert evidence have been rationalized to give the judicial discretion to exclude greater sway in admissibility determinations.

67. *Straker* v. *R* (1977) 15 ALR 103 at 114.

68. See generally Freckelton I. 1996: Wizards in the crucible: making the boffins accountable. In Nijboer H. *New trends in criminal investigation and evidence*, Leiden; Freckelton I, Selby H. 1993: Cross-examination of the expert witness. In Freckelton I, Selby H. (eds), *Expert evidence*, Sydney: LBC.

69. See Australian Law Reform Commission. 1975: Report No. 2, *Criminal investigation*, Canberra: AGPS, para 118.

70. See Australian Law Reform Commission. 1985: Report No. 26, Evidence, Canberra: AGPS, para 416.

71. Australian Law Reform Commission. 1995: Report No. 38, *Evidence*. Canberra: AGPS, para 192. See also Evidence Act 1995 (Cth), s.114.

72. See *Turnbull* (1976) 63 Cr App R 132; see also *Dixon* v. *R* [1983] 1 VR 227; *Pattinson and Exley* [1996] 1 Cr App R 51 at 54ff.

73. See, for example, *R* v. *Siega* (1961) 45 Cr App R 220.

74. *Alexander* v. *R* (1981) 145 CLR 395; see also *R* v. *Pavic*, unreported, NSW Court of Criminal Appeal, 21 August 1995; *R* v. *Codey*, unreported, NSW Court of Criminal Appeal, 1 November 1995.

75. [1987] VR 907 at 911.

76. *Smith* v. *The Queen* (1990) 64 ALJR 588. See further Freckelton I. 1993: The common knowledge rule. In Freckelton I, Selby H. (eds), *Expert evidence*, Sydney: LBC.

Recovery of remains

CA BRIGGS, WB WOOD

Introduction

The increasing demands of the law courts for improved processing, recording and preservation of evidential material, including human remains, requires improved field management techniques. The results of laboratory investigations of recovered remains are completely dependent on the quality of the recovery process. The traditional role of the rake, pick, shovel and backhoe in many police recoveries of bodies or skeletonized remains, and the almost complete dependence on photography alone for the recording of evidential context and relationships, is being overtaken by the need to apply accepted and proven archaeological methodology to the field recovery and recording process.

The purpose of any recovery process is to:

- identify the victim or victims;
- determine the time since death;
- determine the circumstances of death;
- gather and preserve evidence.

The identity of victims can only be definitively established from the remains themselves. Circumstantial evidence may be provided in the form of associated cultural artefacts, for example wallets, clothing and jewellery, known to belong to the victim. Information on the time since death and the circumstances of the death may be deduced from the remains but is more frequently provided by the context of the remains. It is important to appreciate that the actual recovery process destroys contextual evidence, and hence every effort must be made to observe, sample and record the context, prior to starting any recovery.

All evidential material must first be recorded *in situ* before recovery. This includes a written description of the evidence and its orientation, together with mapping and photography. To be able to reconstruct the scene in the laboratory, it is essential to be meticulous in both the recording and the recovery process.

The context of remains

The location and condition of the remains, and the nature of the surrounding physical environment, greatly influence the recovery process. Within buildings, and with fresh or relatively recent remains, the investigative authorities have standard procedures for the recording and collection of evidential material. This tends to be meticulous and exhaustive. In external exposed situations, or with burials in confined spaces, for example within basements below buildings, and especially when dealing with badly decomposed or skeletonized remains or with charred remains from fire scenes, the recovery and recording procedures tend to be dealt with less methodically, with a consequent loss of evidence.

Suspected burial sites

The exact locations of remains is not always known to crime investigators. Acting on suspicious circumstances or the reports of informants, a search of a potential crime scene and even exploratory excavations and test holes may have to be made. Soil probes, trained cadaver dogs, sophisticated geophysical techniques or aerial photography are other options that might need to be considered. Body disposal locations are usually within reasonable access by roads, walking tracks, water, etc.

Burial indicators

These are clues to the possible disposal site and presence of human remains. Any or all of the following indicators may be obvious and should be noted during a search.

SURFACE DEPOSITION

- Exposed bones, which may be bleached, weathered, stained, charred, compact or scattered.
- Camouflage materials, including collections of bush debris, logs, rocks, etc.
- Cultural artefacts, including clothing, jewellery, blankets or other wrapping materials, wallets, discarded food remains, containers, cigarette stubs, etc.
- Vegetation damage, suppression, regrowth or enhanced growth.
- Insect activity, such as flies, odour, maggots or pupal cases.
- Animal activity, consisting of scattered bones, gnawed ends of bones and animal scats or tracks.

With isolated bones recovered within or close to water courses, the possibility of considerable movement from the original deposition site must be considered, and a thorough search of the upstream areas carried out for other bones and cultural artefacts. In other situations, isolated or scattered and fragmented bones suggest the possibility of animal interference.

SUBSURFACE DEPOSITION

- Soil disturbance, soil scatter, subsoil exposure, organization of a surface mound, subsidence and soil separation at grave margins are all evidence of burial just beneath the surface.
- Vegetation: in relatively recent disposal situations, associated vegetation within and surrounding a grave site will usually show signs of damage from trampling and the associated soil disturbance. In older locations, and especially if the times of deposition and recovery are separated by intervening periods of rainfall, vegetation damage may still be apparent in the surrounding areas, but the grave location itself is more likely to demonstrate vigorous new growth owing to moisture collection within the grave fill. This is even more likely with soil subsidence due to compaction of the grave fill and decomposition of the corpse. The breakdown products of decomposition also may act as an additional nutrient source, enhancing the new growth even further. In wooded locations, the division of tree roots during grave preparation may result in new growth shooting directly from the roots and hence outlining the grave margins.
- Insect activity: particularly during the warmer months, decomposition odours are likely to attract blow-flies. In the later stages, beetles and pupal cases may be found.
- Animal intrusion – evidence of digging.
- Odour, particularly in superficial burials.

Search methods

The most commonly used technique is a visual, random or systematic line or grid search of the suspect area, looking for burial indicators. This may be combined with soil probing of any suspicious areas. The use of cadaver dogs requires special training to identify the odours of decomposition. Dogs should only be used when the search area is not too extensive. Ground-penetrating radar and magnetometry are geophysical techniques for the location of subsurface soil disturbance and require expensive equipment and skilled operators. Not all locations are suitable for this technology, and a pre-search assessment of the location by a geophysicist is highly desirable. The use of gas detectors for the detection of methane and other gas emissions from decomposing organic materials may occasionally be useful. Aerial photography, especially using infra-red or thermal techniques, is appropriate if the search area is extensive and relatively open countryside. As a last resort, heavy equipment for surface soil removal or trenching to expose soil intrusion and/or grave outlines may be required.

History of the site

Background information about the events leading to the discovery and/or reporting of the remains, and any known interference with the remains or their context, must be noted. Knowledge of past utilization of the site can also be important. Any history of Aboriginal usage or Aboriginal artefactual material being located or recovered nearby, historical use of the site for farming, commercial, domestic or other applications and any history of excavation or landfill activity should be noted.

Site appraisal

The site should be appraised for any real or potential problems that might adversely influence the recovery. These may be of varied types:

- Geophysical: terrain type, isolation or access, power and water availability, lack of shade, density of vegetation, threat of fire, flood, tidal activity, wild animals, snakes, crocodiles, spiders, midges, mosquitoes, etc.
- Legal: permits for access to private property from owners or managers. If there is any prospect of property damage or destruction, for example of fences, paving or building foundations, compensation or restoration must be anticipated.
- If there is any suspicion that human remains may be of Aboriginal origin, the assistance of a Heritage officer should be sought.
- Economic: all police investigations are subject to budgetary constraints. Some assessment of the cost of the recovery procedures must be made.
- Personnel and equipment.
- Time.

Pre-recovery conference

Discussions between the crime scene officer and forensic pathologist or anthropologist will assist with site appraisal and the recovery by providing the best selection and use of available resources and appropriate recording and recovery processes.

ESTABLISH THE LIMITS OF THE CRIME SCENE

- A grid search: 'emu' parade.
- Mark all surface evidence, including the remains, and record them photographically.

  For site survey and mapping:

- determine and record the map reference co-ordinates (1/25 000);
- survey, map and record the general site features: roads, fences, buildings and geological features;
- carry out specific or detailed surveying and mapping of the burial location and other evidential material.

ESTABLISH SPATIAL CONTROLS

- Set a reference datum point.
- Map a grid layout: vegetation may have to be cleared.
- If possible, plot the north/south orientation of the grid margins.
- Use triangulation to establish the grid margins and corners.

- Use more than one grid if there are several separated concentrations of remains or evidence.

Surface remains: exposure, recovery and recording

- Clear excess vegetation (except trees) to 1–2 cm above the soil surface and remove any loose surface vegetation debris.
- Visually scan the site and flag all material evidence and physical remains.
- Use a metal detector to scan the site, and flag the location of positive recordings.
- Photograph the cleared area, including the site board with identification, date, scale and North arrow.
- Map all the evidential material *in situ*, with a description and location.
- Take general and close-up photographs of all bones and evidence *in situ*.
- Lift and package and record all evidential material (producing an inventory). For skeletonized remains:
  - collect, bag or package in units if at all possible and label fully;
  - record them on a skeletal record table or chart.
- Evidence material outside the grids should be photographed and mapped (by triangulation to one grid corner) before lifting.
- Excavate the positive metal detector readings with non-metal tools.
- Screen the surface dirt within the grid using water pressure and plastic screens with a 2–3 mm mesh.
- Entomological evidence may be located some distance (meters) from the remains as insect larvae tend to migrate before pupating.
- Collect soil samples from beneath any major skeletal collection.
- Screen the dirt for 10–15 cm under the skeletal remains.

Classification of burial

1. *Individual or co-mingled.* A grave may contain the remains of one person buried alone or the co-mingled remains of two or more persons buried either at the same time or over a period of time.
2. *Isolated or adjacent.* An isolated grave is separate from other graves and may be excavated without concern about encroaching on adjacent graves. Adjacent graves, as in a crowded cemetery, need to be approached with caution as the wall of one grave is also the wall of another.

3. *Primary or secondary.* If primary, the grave contains the remains of the deceased as they were first buried. If the remains are secondary, they have been removed from the original site and reburied.

Buried remains: excavation, exposure, recovery and recording

Excavation methodology is dependent on the site context and the type and condition of the grave fill. In deeper graves, one wall may have to be sacrificed for ease of recovery:

- Excavate the grave fill in 5–10 cm soil levels.
- Expose, map and record each piece of new evidence *in situ* before lifting, packaging and labelling.
- Screen all dirt from the grave fill (not from the walls), noting soil changes such as those of pH, colour and grain size.
- Scan each new level with a metal detector, marking all findings as above.
- Use wooden tools to excavate metal (so they will not mark the metal).
- Record all evidence, locate it on the grid, map it and photograph it before lifting.
- If possible, expose the whole skeleton before lifting. This may entail the exposure of the skeleton on a soil pedestal.
- Remove any soft tissue intact by undercutting and placing it on a board or blanket.
- Make an inventory of the bones as they are removed and package them in units.
- Take soil samples from the grave fill and the abdominal regions of the remains for pH and toxicology.
- Scan the dirt for 10–15 cm below the burial with a metal detector, then remove the dirt and screen for loose bones and teeth, cultural artefacts and entomological or other evidence.
- The empty grave should then be cross-sectioned, photographed and drawn to scale to record its vertical shape.

Recording in situ

This is important for determining the position and orientation of remains, the interrelationship of remains to artefacts, the possibility of animal or other interference, etc.

Sampling

- Soil for decomposition byproducts, drugs, hair, pH and pollen.
- Vegetation.
- Insect larvae/pupae.
- Establish care in collection, handling and preservation in order to avoid contamination or injury.
- Employ correct sampling and packaging procedures for the preservation of sample materials.
- Produce a sample inventory.

Cataloguing, packaging and transport

The aim is to allow ease of identification in the laboratory and to prevent loss, damage and deterioration, contamination or confusion or mixing with other evidential material.

Chain of custody

It is absolutely essential to maintain continuity for the prevention of contamination, loss or interference. Fastidious attention must be given at all times to the maintenance of the chain of custody.

Field diary and written records

These are an essential accompaniment to mapping and photographic records, providing a later reference (memory) of field personnel involved and of recovery procedures and events.

Special recovery situations

These may include:

- water locations: sea, river, lake, dam, canal, water course, storage tanks;
- cremated remains at fire scenes: buildings, vehicles, bushfires;
- bodies enclosed in paving materials;
- bodies buried in dumps.

Further reading

Bass WM, Birkby WH. 1978: Exhumation: the method could make the difference. *FBI Law Enforcement Bulletin* **47**, 6–11.

Burke M. 1987: Eaten alive. *Australian Police Journal* Jul–Sep, 83–9.

Mcdonald J, Ross A. 1990: Helping the police with their inquiries: archaeology and politics at Angophora reserve rock shelter, N.S.W. *Archeol Oceania* **25**(3), 114–21.

Morse D, Dailey RC, Stoutamire J, Duncan J. 1984: Forensic archaeology. In Rathbun TA, Buikstra JE. (eds) *Human identification*. Springfield, IL: Charles C. Thomas, 53–64.

Rathbun TA, Rathbun BC. 1984: Human remains recovered from a shark's stomach in South Carolina. *Journal of Forensic Sciences* **29**(1), 269–76.

Wolf DJ. 1986: Forensic anthropology scene investigations. In Reichs KJ. (ed.) *Forensic osteology*. Springfield, IL: Charles C. Thomas, 3–23.

Wood, WB. 1987: Recent fatal crocodile attacks in Northern Australia. Paper delivered at the Australasian and South West Pacific Islander Police Medical Officer's Conference, Gold Coast.

APPENDIX II

Packaging of evidence

MA RAYMOND, WJ ASHLEY

Exhibit	Packaging medium
Adhesive tape	Roll in a plastic bag
	Loose tape in a box or paper bag
Acids	Sealed glass container
Blood (liquid)	Sequestrene tube
Blood (wet)	On cotton fabric or thread and in a petri dish
Blood (dry)	Paper container in a plastic bag
Blood (clothing)	Paper bags
Bones	Paper bags
Bullets	Plastic bags
Fired bullets/cartridges	Plastic bags (a separate bag for each)
Charred documents	Packed securely in a rigid container (box)
Clothing	Paper bags
Drugs	Sealed plastic bags
Dentures	Semirigid sealed plastic container
Fibres/hairs	Sealed plastic or folded paper bag
Firearms	Wrapped in paper or in a large plastic/paper bag

Exhibit	Packaging medium
Glass	Rigid cardboard or plastic container
Gunshot residue	Collected on double-sided sticky tape and sealed in a suitable plastic container
Paint	Plastic bag or solid container
Shoes	Paper bags
Shoeprint lifts	Rigid paper or plastic container
Shoe/tyre casts	Paper or plastic bag
Teeth (dry)	Semirigid sealed plastic container (packed in gauze)
Teeth (burnt)	Stabilize with low-viscosity, self-polymerizing resin and place in a semi-rigid sealed plastic container (packed in gauze)
Teeth (wet)	Semirigid sealed plastic container (containing saline)
Toolmarks	Plastic bags or containers
Soils and minerals	Plastic bag or container

Commonly used dental charts

DH CLARK, E DYKES

The majority of dental charts used throughout the world contain a pictorial layout of the dentition known as an odontogram. An odontogram is divided into 32 sections, one section for each tooth, and may be depicted pictorially in 17 different ways, in either arch or exploded geometric form. The most common types are indicated in Fig. III.1.

All geometric dental charts should be read as though the viewer is looking at the mouth from the front. Thus the left-hand side of the chart is the patient's right side. In the exploded design, the vertical line indicates the midline, above the horizontal line the upper teeth, and below it the lower.

Upper right	Upper left
Lower right	Lower left

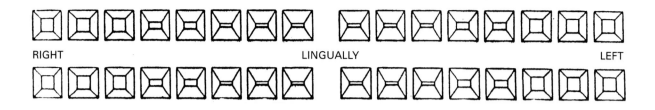

RIGHT LINGUALLY LEFT

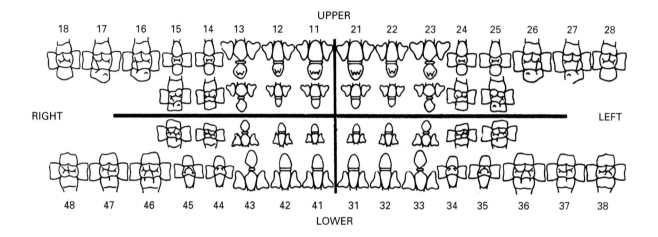

UPPER

18 17 16 15 14 13 12 11 21 22 23 24 25 26 27 28

RIGHT LEFT

48 47 46 45 44 43 42 41 31 32 33 34 35 36 37 38

LOWER

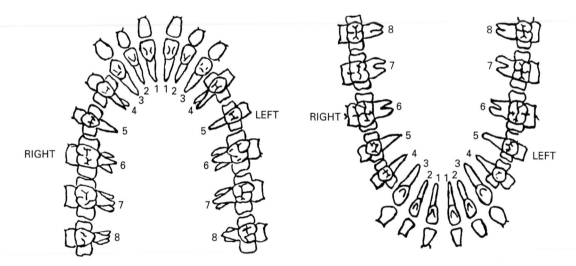

Fig. III.1 The three most common types of odontogram

Added to the odontogram is an alphanumeric notation that enables the dentist to indicate individual teeth in his/her records. Unfortunately, there are several different notations in use throughout the world, with a number of modifications to each notation.

FDI notation

In 1971 the Federation Dentaire Internationale adopted Theilman's notation, which is now known as the FDI notation (Fig. III.2) and used fairly widely throughout the world. Each quadrant of the jaws is numbered from 1 to 4, starting on the upper right in a clockwise direction. The last (third) molar is designated 8, the central incisor 1, in each quadrant; thus a single tooth is designated by two numbers, the first being the quadrant number, the second being the position of that tooth in the quadrant. The deciduous quadrants are numbered 5 through to 8. Thus a record indicating 16 and 55 present indicates the upper right first permanent molar and the upper right second deciduous molar.

Forensic odontologists communicate internationally using this notation even when it is not used in their own country. For example, British and American forensic odontologists should pass information for identification purposes using this notation even though both use different notation systems in their respective countries.

When speaking this notation, both numbers are spoken, i.e. 'one eight', not 'eighteen'.

Permanent dentition

18 17 16 15 14 13 12 11	21 22 23 24 25 26 27 28
48 47 46 45 44 43 42 41	31 32 33 34 35 36 37 38

Deciduous dentition

55 54 53 52 51	61 62 63 64 65
85 84 83 82 81	71 72 73 74 75

Fig. III.2

Palmer/Zsigmondy notation

In parts of Europe, Africa and China, the Palmer/Zsigmondy notation is used (Fig. III.3). This is the only notation used in the British Health Service.

Permanent dentition

87654321	12345678
87654321	12345678

Deciduous dentition

EDCBA	ABCDE
EDCBA	ABCDE

Fig. III.3

Thus 8 is the last tooth in the each quadrant – the third molar or wisdom tooth. E is the last deciduous molar in the each quadrant.

During the eruption of the permanent dentition, there will be a period when both deciduous and permanent teeth will be present in the mouth, and this will be indicated by a mixture of numbers and letters. Individual teeth are indicated by a line above or below and to the right or left of the letter or number. For example, ⌊8 indicates the upper left third molar.

Modifications to the standard chart may be the use of lower case letters or Roman numerals I to V, equivalent to A to E.

Universal notation

Starting at the upper right thrid molar, the teeth are counted in a clockwise (Fig. III.4) direction. As each tooth has a separate number (or letter for the deciduous), there is no requirement to indicate side or upper and lower, as is the case in Palmer/Zsigmondy notation described above.

Permanent dentition

1 2 3 4 5 6 7 8	9 10 11 12 13 14 15 16
32 31 30 29 28 27 26 25	24 23 22 21 20 19 18 17

Deciduous dentition

A B C D E	F G H I J
T S R Q P	O N M L K

Fig. III.4

When speaking, teeth are referred to as a whole number, ie. 'thirty-two' rather than 'three two', as in the FDI notation. The reader should note this point as the numbers 11 to 32 are common to both notations but refer to completely different teeth.

The main variation to this notation is the reversal of the lower numbering, 17 to 32 going from left to right. The Universal notation is used almost exclusively in the USA.

These are the the three major notations in current use. There are 40 notations said to be in use throughout the world, a number of which are variations of the main three above.

Anthropological notation

The anthropological notation (Fig. III.5) is never used by dentists in forensic or clinical practice, but dentists involved in assisting anthropologists should be conversant with this notation. Upper case lettering

Permanent dentition

M3 M2 M1 Pm2 Pm1 C I2 I1	I1 I2 C Pm1 Pm2 M1 M2 M3
M3 M2 M1 Pm2 Pm1 C I2 I1	I1 I2 C Pm1 Pm2 M1 M2 M3

Deciduous dentition

m2 m1 c i2 i1	i1 i2 c m1 m2
m2 m1 c i2 i1	i1 i2 c m1 m2

Fig. III.5

denotes permanent teeth, lower case lettering deciduous teeth, the first letter of the tooth type being used as the abbreviation. Each single entry using this notation must be accompanied by a line to the left or right and above or below (as in the Zsigmondy/Palmer notation).

Chronology of dental development

E DYKES, DH CLARK

Deciduous dentition

MAXILLARY AND MANDIBULAR CENTRAL INCISOR

Calcification begins	3–5	months *in utero*
Crown complete	4	months
Eruption	6–8	months
Root complete	1–2	years
Root resorption begins	4–5	years
Tooth exfoliated	6–7	years

MAXILLARY AND MANDIBULAR LATERAL INCISOR

Calcification begins	4–5	months *in utero*
Crown complete	4–5	months
Eruption	7–8	months
Root complete	1–2	years
Root resorption begins	4–5	years
Tooth exfoliated	7–8	years

MAXILLARY AND MANDIBULAR CANINE

Calcification begins	5–6	months *in utero*
Crown complete	9	months
Eruption	16–20	months
Root complete	2–3	years
Root resorption begins	6–7	years
Tooth exfoliated	9–12	years

MAXILLARY AND MANDIBULAR FIRST MOLAR

Calcification begins	5	months *in utero*
Crown complete	6	months
Eruption	12–16	months
Root complete	2–2.5	years
Root resorption begins	4–5	years
Tooth exfoliated	9–11	years

MAXILLARY AND MANDIBULAR SECOND MOLAR

Calcification begins	6	months *in utero*
Crown complete	10–12	months
Eruption	20–30	months
Root complete	3	years
Root resorption begins	4–5	years
Tooth exfoliated	10–12	years

Permanent dentition

CENTRAL INCISORS

Maxillary				**Mandibular**		
Calcification begins	3–4	months		Calcification begins	3–4	months
Crown complete	4–5	years		Crown complete	4–5	years
Eruption	7–8	years		Eruption	6–7	years
Root complete	10	years		Root complete	9	years

LATERAL INCISORS

Maxillary				**Mandibular**		
Calcification begins	10–12	months		Calcification begins	3–4	months
Crown complete	4–5	years		Crown complete	4–5	years
Eruption	8–9	years		Eruption	7–8	years
Root complete	11	years		Root complete	10	years

CANINES

Maxillary				**Mandibular**		
Calcification begins	4–5	months		Calcification begins	4–5	months
Crown complete	6–7	years		Crown complete	6–7	years
Eruption	11–12	years		Eruption	9–10	years
Root complete	13–15	years		Root complete	12–14	years

FIRST PREMOLARS

Maxillary				**Mandibular**		
Calcification begins	1–1.75	years		Calcification begins	1–2	years
Crown complete	5–6	years		Crown complete	5–6	years
Eruption	10–11	years		Eruption	10–12	years
Root complete	12–13	years		Root complete	12–13	years

SECOND PREMOLARS

Maxillary				**Mandibular**		
Calcification begins	2–2.25	years		Calcification begins	2–2.25	years
Crown complete	6–7	years		Crown complete	6–7	years
Eruption	10–12	years		Eruption	11–12	years
Root complete	12–14	years		Root complete	13–14	years

FIRST MOLARS

Maxillary				**Mandibular**		
Calcification begins	At birth			Calcification begins	At birth	
Crown complete	2–3	years		Crown complete	2–3	years
Eruption	6–7	years		Eruption	6–7	years
Root complete	9–10	years		Root complete	9–10	years

SECOND MOLARS

Maxillary				**Mandibular**		
Calcification begins	2–5.3	years		Calcification begins	2–5.3	years
Crown complete	7–8	years		Crown complete	7–8	years
Eruption	12–13	years		Eruption	11–13	years
Root complete	14–16	years		Root complete	14–15	years

THIRD MOLARS

Maxillary				**Mandibular**		
Calcification begins	7–9	years		Calcification begins	8–10	years
Crown complete	12–16	years		Crown complete	12–16	years
Eruption	17–21	years		Eruption	17–21	years
Root complete	18–25	years		Root complete	18–25	years

Laboratory materials

JL LEDITSCHKE, RG TAYLOR, CJ SCANE

The following information has been collected to provide a database of key suppliers for the techniques used in this book. These suppliers are all based in Australia but have equivalent companies in your area and in some cases a direct branch or outlet. Available Internet and E-mail addresses have also been included.

Dental materials

Tooth-coloured acrylic powders

Purchased in Australia from:
Dentex Australasia Pty Ltd
55 Cleeland Road
Oakleigh South VIC 3167

Telephone: +613 9548 9366
Facsimile: +613 9548 9377

Or any major dental supply company in your area.

Modelling or potter's clay – range of colours

Purchased in Australia from:
Northcote Pottery
85A Clyde Street
Thornbury VIC 3071

Telephone: +613 9480 4799
Facsimile: +613 9480 3075

Or any major pottery supply company in your area.

Q3 silastic 3481; Q3 thixotropic 3482; modelling clay; micropolystyrene filler (Dow Corning)

Dow Corning Australia Pty Ltd
16 Hall Street
Hawthorn East 3123 VIC

Telephone: +613 9822 0010
Facsimile: +613 9824 7760
Internet: http://www.dow.com/main.html
See branches in your location

Purchased in Australia from:
Polymer/Daystar
51 Stephen Road
Dandenong 3175 VIC

Telephone: +613 9793 5444
Facsimile: +613 9792 2684

Vertex s.c. powder, vertex s.c. liquid, dental impression material – dental plaster, dental modelling wax

Purchased in Australia from:
Halas Dental Limited
423 Smith Street
Fitzroy 3065 VIC

Telephone: +613 9419 7944
Facsimile: +613 9416 3853

Or any major dental supply company in your area

Casting epoxy resin (c.d.) kit, including hardener 1.5 kg, also known as Araldite m

Purchased in Australia from:
R.F. Services Pty Ltd

60 Lothian Street
North Melbourne 3051 VIC

Telephone: +613 9329 0111
Facsimile: +613 9329 0646

Or any major fibreglass outlet in your area.

Mortuary supplies

Gloves (post mortem, examination, sertex and conform)

Purchased in Australia from:
Ansell International
530 Springvale Road
Glen Waverley 3150 VIC

Telephone: +613 9264 0888
Facsimile: +613 9264 0886
E-mail: info@ansell.com
Internet: http://www.ansell.com/

Or any major surgical glove supplier in your area.

Eye protection

Hogies Eye Wear
Purchased in Australia from:
Advanced Surgical Technologies
142 Stawell Street
Burnley 3121 VIC

Telephone: +613 9428 0101
Facsimile: +613 9428 1404

Or any major safety, mortuary or pathology supplier in your area.

Safety shields, nitrile aprons

Purchased in Australia from:
Alltech Associates (Australia) Pty Ltd
852 Canterbury Road
Box Hill 3128 VIC

Telephone: +613 9897 4355
Facsimile: +613 1300 362411

Or any major safety, mortuary or pathology supplier in your area

Postmortem sewing needles, lipshaw – part 411–3

Shandon Lipshaw
171 Industry Drive
Pittsburgh, PA 15275, USA

Telephone: +1 412 788-2460
Facsimile: +1 412 788-2480
Internet:
http://database.sweets.com:8080/sweets/p1/pg14/99/
11700XXZ/8213.HTM

Purchased in Australia from:
Edward Keller Pty Ltd
3 Walker Street
Braeside 3195 VIC

Telephone: +613 9580 1666
Facsimile: +613 9580 6872

Or any major mortuary or pathology supplier in your area.

Suturing twine (body closure and reconstruction)

Purchased in Australia from:
RH Minter Pty Ltd
17 Park Street
Oakleigh 3166 VIC

Telephone: +613 9568 6999
Facsimile: +613 9568 1813

Or any major mortuary or pathology supplier in your area.

Feature builder and solvent ('mortician's wax')

Dodge Chemical Company
165 Cambridge Park Drive,
Cambridge, MA 02140, USA

Telephone: +1 617 661-0500

Purchased in Australia from:
RH Minter Pty Ltd
17 Park Street
Oakleigh 3166 VIC

Telephone: +613 9568 6999
Facsimile: +613 9568 1813

Or any major mortuary supplier in your area.

Radiographic supplies

Radiographic developer g153 a and b and fixer g354; product code fn4si

Purchased in Australia from:
Agfa-Gevaert Ltd

376 Whitehorse Road
Nunawading 3131 VIC

Telephone: +613 9264 7711
Facsimile: +613 9264 7890

Or your local outlet for Agfa-Gevaert products or radiographic chemical supplier.

Dental radiographic films

- Extaspeed size 1, ep-11p, cat 888 712; extaspeed size 2, ep-21p, cat 896 0007.
- Extaspeed size 4, eo-42p, cat 883 1828.
- Ultraspeed size 1, df-55, cat 127 372; ultraspeed size 2, df-57, cat 165 8210.

Purchased in Australia from:
Kodak (Australia) Pty Ltd
173 Elizabeth Street
Coburg 3058 VIC

Telephone: +613 9353 2520
Facsimile: +613 9353 2011
Internet:
http://www.kodak.com/hiHome/dental/index.shtml

Or your local outlet for Kodak products or radiographic film supplier.

Miscellaneous

Plastic bags (used to hold the property of the deceased and for other laboratory uses)

Polypac Converting
21 William Street
Balaclava 3183 VIC

Telephone: +613 9527 5081
Facsimile: +613 9525 9162

Or from any major plastic goods distributor in your area.

Body bags (used as an outer covering)

Anchor Packaging
11 Salsbury Street
Botany 2018 NSW

Telephone: +613 1800 814 458
Facsimile: +612 9666 3326

Or from any specialist packaging distributor in your area.

Tube body bags (used as a final wrap)

Beaver Plastics
Cremorne Street
Richmond 3121 VIC

Telephone: +613 9429 2377
Facsimile: +613 9429 0381

Or from any specialist plastics packaging distributor in your area.

Guides for post mortem cranial radiography

JG CLEMENT

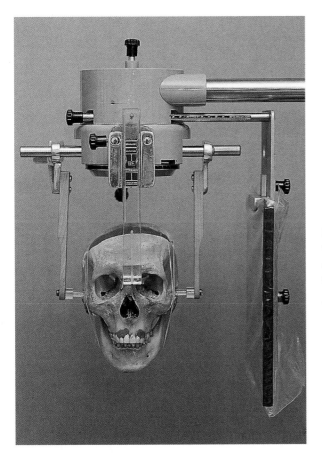

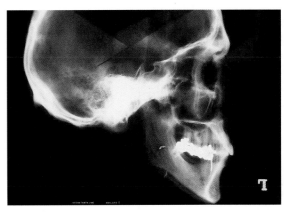

Fig. VI.2 Typical post mortem lateral cephalometric view of a skull disarticulated from the axial skeleton. The absence of soft tissue negates the need for an aluminium step wedge over the face, and considerable adjustments need to be made to typical exposure settings (see Table VI.1). Two radiographic exposures may still be required to image all parts of the specimen adequately

Fig. VI.1 Skull in a cephalostat. The mandible has small pads of silicone rubber replacing the lost cartilaginous discs of the temporomandibular joints. The anterior teeth are temporarily held in their sockets using Plasticine. The film cassette is on the right of the field

Table VI.1 Suggested initial settings for X-ray equipment when used for post mortem radiography

Anatomical area		Radiological exposure factors			
		Living patient/Intact body area		Dissected/Dry bony specimen	
		mAS	kVp	mAS	kVp
Calvarium	Anteroposterior/posteroanterior	20	70	8	70
	P–A ↓ 25°	16	70	6	70
	Townes (A–P ↓ 3.5°)	16	70	6	70
	Lateral	16	70	6	70
	Inferosuperior	16	70	6	70
Facial bones	Posteroanterior	20	70	8	70
	P–A ↓ 25° (orbits etc)	16	70	6	70
	Waters (P–A; 35° ↑ head tilt)	20	70	8	70
	Reverse Townes	16	70	6	70
	Inferosuperior	12	70	4	70
	Lateral	8	70	3	70
Maxillae (with teeth)	Posteroanterior	20	70	8 (4)[b]	70
	Lateral	8	70	3 (1.5)	70
	Waters	20	70	N/A	N/A
	Inferosuperior	12	70	3 (1.5)	70
Mandible (with teeth)	Posteroanterior	16	70	3 (1.5)	70
	Lateral	8	70	1.5 (0.75)	70
	Lateral oblique[a]	8	65	1.5 (0.75)	65
Teeth (individually)	Dental X-ray unit, 40 cm focus–film distance, D-speed dental film	N/A	N/A	1–2	70

[a] All exposure factors, except lateral oblique mandible, disected maxillae/mandible and teeth, assume modern radiographic equipment, 100 cm focus–film distance, bucky/stationary grid and regular green-emitting intensifying screens. Factors are for *guidance only* and will vary according to variations of equipment, film types and intensifying screen speed/sensitivity (if used).

[b] Bracketed values are for use with a dental radiographic unit and dental/occlusal film, D speed.

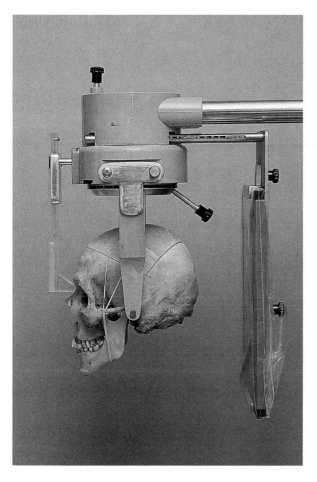

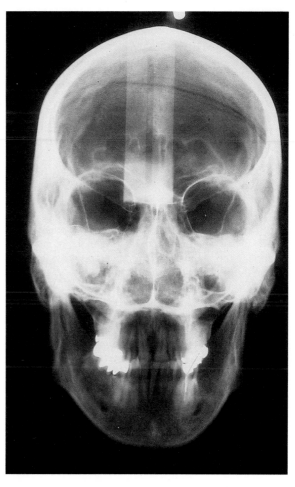

Fig. VI.3 Skull in a cephalostat aligned for an antero-posterior view. The skull can be rotated 180 degrees to facilitate posteroanterior views, which are more likely to correspond with available ante mortem records

Fig. VI.4 Radiograph of the skull. The radio-opacity of dental restorations obscures some detail in this projection. Similarly, the aligning rod placed at the root of the nose masks the frontal sinus outline. If this is removed, care needs to be taken to stabilize the skull and prevent rotation about the ear rods

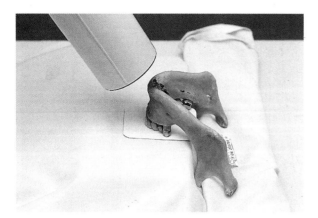

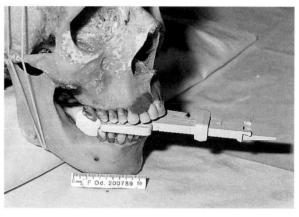

Fig. VI.5 Mandible disarticulated from the skull making it easier to take anterior occlusal views of the mandibular dentition. Note the use of boxes covered with a towel to achieve the necessary orientation of the jaw

Fig. VI.7 A human skull showing the position of an intra-oral film holder. This demonstrates the use of Plasticine to hold the teeth within their sockets and rubber bands to mimic the muscles of mastication

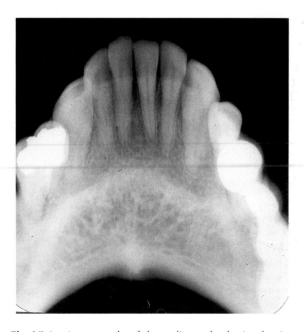

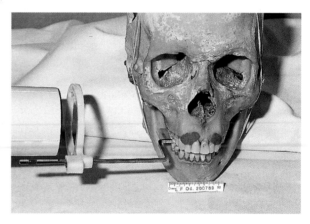

Fig. VI.8 Same skull as that shown in Fig. VI.7, demonstrating the position and use of a cone-centring device. This ensures the production of consistent, reproducible radiographic projections during test exposure

Fig. VI.6 An example of the radiograph obtained using the configuration and positioning of the specimen in Fig. VI.5. Radiographs of the skeleton divested of all soft tissue show excellent contrast and fine bone and dental details

Guides and checklists for medico-legal reports

DL RANSON

Principles

All forensic medical examinations, whether performed in a dental, anthropological or pathological setting, are focused on the eventual compilation of a forensic scientific/medical report. It is a feature of forensic scientific examinations that they should satisfy the requirements of the justice system as well as the ordinary requirements of medical and scientific practice. The scientific investigator's notes in this respect are of particular significance. While the requirement to compile and maintain a set of examination notes is common to all areas of scientific practice, the contents of notes taken during a forensic scientific/medical examination often have a different focus from those made in a non-forensic scientific setting. The following points should be borne in mind when recording the results of medico-legal investigations.

- It is essential that an investigator's notes should take into account the requirements of the relevant legal system with respect to the laws of evidence and procedure as well as the need to record the conduct and results of the medical and/or scientific examination.

- The notes should include all of the information that forms the basis of the eventual medico-legal report. In addition, it should indicate the source of any additional information that became available during the examination and was subsequently relied upon.

- The notes should be set out in an orderly fashion and be legible and tidy. The use of abbreviations for medical terms and phrases should be avoided.

- Notes, charts, photographs and other materials related to a forensic medical examination should be collated and assembled into a file that can be easily referred to in court. (Copies of this file sometimes need to be made, as the original may have to be submitted as an exhibit in court.)

The following are suggested headings for the composition of medical notes.

PRELIMINARY MATTERS

Personal details (of investigator)

Name:

Qualifications:

Position:

Professional address:

Contact telephone/fax numbers:

TEMPORAL MATTERS

Date and time called (original call out):

Date and time of arrival:

Date and time of commencement of each examination:

Date and time of completion of each examination:

Date and time of completion of medical notes:

Date and time of departure:

If more than one examination is performed or other locations are attended, record the above times for each attendance and examination. Where the examination of a specimen takes place over a protracted period of time, the length of time should be noted.

PHYSICAL MATTERS

Place of principal examination:

Nature of scene:

Location within scene:

Address of scene:

Quality and suitability of the environment:

Security of specimen:

Examination facilities available:

If more than one place is attended or utilized, describe each individually. Use photographs, sketches and diagrams, including scales and orientation features.

OBSERVERS PRESENT

Name:

Role:

Position (rank, profession or status):

Time of presence:

Include these details for all the observers who were present, regardless of how long they were in attendance.

CIRCUMSTANCES

From person requesting call-out:

From medical/paramedical personnel:

From co-investigators (police, etc.):

From coroner:

Record separately the information provided by different individuals relating to the same examination. If further information becomes available after the scene or laboratory examination has been completed, this factor should be specifically noted.

MEDICAL HISTORY (OF POTENTIALLY DECEASED, MISSING PERSONS)

Past history of medical illness:

Past history of surgical treatment:

Past history of mental illness:

Past history of dental and oral disease:

Past history of trauma:

History of recent episodes of trauma:

Past history of medication:

Family history (including relevant history of the above):

FORENSIC MEDICAL/ ANTHROPOLOGICAL/DENTAL EXAMINATION

Record injuries by means of a written description and a sketch on an appropriate body or skeletal chart. The numbering of injuries in the notes and chart can aid in cross-referencing and commenting upon the findings in a subsequent medico-legal report.

In describing a wound, consideration should be given to the following features:

- site
- size
- shape
- surrounds
- colour
- contours
- course
- contents
- age
- borders
- classification.

SPECIALIST INVESTIGATIONS

Pathology examination:

Dental examination:

Anthropological examination:

Radiological examination:

Visible light photography:

Invisible light photography:

Others as relevant:

SPECIMENS

- Foreign extracorporeal material
- Biological human material.

Receipt of specimens

Details of specimen provider:

Time and date of hand-over of specimens:

Place of hand-over of specimens:

Place of storage of specimens:

Provision/disposal of specimens

Details of specimen recipient:

Time and date of hand-over of specimens:

Place of hand-over of specimens:

METHODS USED TO RECORD FINDINGS

- Charts
- Photography
- Video
- Radiology.

FORENSIC MANAGEMENT

Initial information provided to investigators:

Name of informant:

Signing and dating of notes:

Written material:

Sketches:

Charts:

Photographs:

Others:

The means used to record the examination as it progresses must be scrupulous. This material will be used in compiling the subsequent forensic scientific/medical report.

Sample forensic scientific/ medical report

The following report sets out one of the many ways in which a forensic report can be constructed. In it, a fictitious investigator, Dr Jane Bloggs, reports on the examination of the remains of a fictitious John Smythe and describes essentially normal anatomical findings without evidence of significant natural disease. The report structure used is similar to that of an

autopsy report. Dental and anthropological reports will clearly differ in content, but the overall framework and structure of all such medico-legal reports are similar.

Forensic pathologists differ in the method by which they describe the normal appearances and abnormalities seen during an autopsy. This proforma does not purport to represent an ideal method of describing individual pathological features but instead represents one style of autopsy reporting.

The structure of this report is based on a body systems approach, grouping the autopsy observations and findings under body system headings such as 'Central nervous system' and 'Respiratory system'. The tissues and organs that comprise the system are described together, regardless of their anatomical location. For example, under 'Respiratory system', head structures such as the nose, sinuses and nasopharynx are described along with chest structures such as the bronchi and the lungs.

Another approach is the anatomical one, in which sections of the report each cover an anatomical region. Descriptions under these anatomical headings necessarily involve organs and tissues from several body systems. For example, in the section headed 'The chest', tissues from the cardiovascular system (heart) and the respiratory system (lungs) would be described.

It cannot be overemphasized that the task of the medico-legal report is to communicate effectively all the relevant information that may possibly be required by the justice system. In this regard, the medico-legal autopsy report varies in style and content from the routine hospital-style clinical medical report.

This Document Details the Nature and Results of the Medico-legal Investigation of the Death of 'John Smythe' Case No. 0000/96

My name is Jane BLOGGS, and my professional address is the Coronial Investigation Centre, 101 Mortuary Drive, Boneville.

I am a Medical Practitioner practising as a specialist in forensic anthropology and pathology.

My qualifications are: Bachelor of Medicine (MB), Bachelor of Surgery (BS). I hold the Diploma of Forensic Anthropology of the Society of Anthropologists. I am a Fellow of the College of Forensic Pathologists by examination in forensic pathology.

I am employed as a Forensic Pathologist and Anthropologist at the Coronial Investigation Centre, Boneville.

Prior to taking up my current appointments, I was a Lecturer in Anatomy and an associate in the Department of Pathology at the University of Boneville.

My practical experience in forensic pathology and human anatomy commenced in 1970. I have been engaged in professional practice in forensic pathology and anthropology since 1975.

CIRCUMSTANCES

At 0900 hours on 1 January 1998 at the Coronial Investigation Centre, Boneville, I performed an examination of the human remains of a body whom I believed to be that of John SMYTHE aged 25 years.

Information available to me at the time of the autopsy examination comprised the Police Report of Death to the Coroner provided by Senior Detective Jones (form COR/83), my own observations of the scene of death and the medical records from New Hospital, Boneville.

OBSERVERS PRESENT

Mr Peter Helpful, Forensic Technician, Coronial Investigation Centre
Detective Sergeant Boss, Homicide Squad, Boneville Police
Detective Constable Dogsbody, 'A' Division, Boneville Police
Constable Pic, Photographer, Boneville Police
Constable Trace, Crime Scene Department, Boneville Police

PRELIMINARY INVESTIGATIONS

Scene of death

At 2000 hours on 31 December 1997, I was contacted by the Coroner's Office and requested to attend at 1 Novel Street, Boneville. I arrived at 1 Novel Street, Boneville, at 2030 hours on 31 December 1997 where I met:

Inspector Smith, Divisional Inspector, Boneville Police
Detective Sergeant Boss, Homicide Squad, Boneville Police
Detective Constable Dogsbody, 'A' Division, Boneville Police
Constable Pic, Photographer, Boneville Police
Constable Trace, Crime Scene Department, Boneville Police

Next give a detailed account of the observations and procedures performed at the scene.

After completion of my examination of the scene, I made arrangements for the body to be transferred to the mortuary of the Australian Forensic Medicine Institute, 101 Mortuary Drive, Boneville and for an autopsy to be performed the next day.

At 2100 hours on 31 December 1997, I departed from the scene at 1 Novel Street, Boneville.

The following list of headings and subheadings represents a suggested layout for a medico-legal report. In practice, the need for particular sections of the report will vary from case to case depending on the circumstances.

Clothing:

Jewellery:

Extracorporeal material:

Radiology:

List the details of the radiographic views of the body used for identification or injury documentation purposes.

EXTERNAL EXAMINATION

Body:

Body morphometry:

Skin:

Body hair:

Hands and feet:

Eyes and eyelids:

External ears (pinnae):

Nose:

Lips:

Mouth:

Dentition:

Rigor mortis:

Livor mortis:

Features of decomposition:

IDENTIFYING FEATURES, INCLUDING MARKS AND SCARS

Labels:

Hair:

Marks:

Numerically list tattoos, old injuries and skin marks, other than scars and recent injuries, arranged by surface region.

Scars:

Numerically list scars, surgical or otherwise, arranged by surface region.

SIGNS OF RECENT MEDICAL INTERVENTION

Each category has a numbered list of therapeutic attachments or interventions arranged by surface region.

Cannulae, tubes and catheters:

Needle puncture sites:

Dressings and patches:

Surgical intervention:

SIGNS OF RECENT INJURY

Each category has a numbered list describing each injury.

Head and neck:

Chest:

Abdomen:

External genitalia:

Right upper limb:

Left upper limb:

Right lower limb:

Left lower limb:

Back:

INTERNAL EXAMINATION

Organ weights

Brain: grams

Right lung: grams

Left lung: grams

Heart: grams

Liver: grams

Right kidney: grams

Left kidney: grams

Spleen: grams

Central Nervous System

Scalp:

Skull and cranial vault:

Cerebral vessels:

Dura:

Leptomeninges:

Brain:

Spinal cord:

Spinal column:

Cardiovascular System

Pericardium:

Heart:

Epicardium:

Endocardium:

Myocardium:

Ventricles:

Atria:

Cardiac valves:

Coronary arteries:

Aorta:

Great veins:

Pulmonary arteries:

Pulmonary veins:

Mediastinum:

Respiratory system

Nasopharynx and sinuses:

Larynx:

Trachea and bronchi:

Lungs:

Pleural cavities:

Diaphragm:

Thoracic cage:

Gastrointestinal system

Tongue and oropharynx:

Oesophagus:

Stomach:

Intestines:

Liver:

Bilary system:

Pancreas:

Peritoneal cavity:

Genitourinary system

Kidneys:

Bladder:

Prostate:

Testes:

(Uterus:)

(Fallopian tubes:)

(Ovaries:)

External genitalia:

Reticuloendothelial system

Spleen:

Lymph nodes:

Endocrine system

Thyroid gland:

Pituitary and adrenal glands:

Musculoskeletal system

The detailed skeletal examination could be included here or, if performed by an external consultant, their report could be referenced here.

SPECIMENS

Chain of evidence

At 1200 hours on 1 January 1998 at the Coronial Investigation Centre, Boneville, I handed the following specimens to Constable Trace (Crime Scene Department, Univille Police):

Results

Histology (see attached report):

Toxicology (see attached report):

Neuropathology (see attached report):

Odontology (see attached report):

Anthropology (see attached report):

SUMMARY OF MEDICAL, ODONTOLOGICAL, ANTHROPOLOGICAL AND PATHOLOGICAL FINDINGS

List the major autopsy findings by category.

COMMENTS

Numerically list the major medico-legal issues arising from the medical investigation and your interpretation of them.

Cause of death

List the diseases, injuries or conditions directly leading to death under the headings I(a), I(b) and I(c) or by means of a textual conclusion.

Contributing factors

List additional factors contributing to death but not related to the causes stated in I(a), I(b) or I(c) above.

GLOSSARY OF TERMS

Insert the relevant legal jurat appropriate to the local jurisdiction.

ACKNOWLEDGEMENT

I hereby acknowledge that this statement is true and correct, and I make it in the belief that a person making a false statement in the circumstances is liable to the penalties of perjury.

Jane Bloggs MB BS FRCPA
Senior Staff Specialist
Coronial Investigation Centre, Boneville

E-mail: bloggsj@cic.boneville.edu.au
Tel: 9999 4444
Fax: 9999 7777

Acknowledgement made and signature witnessed by me at..a.m. / p.m.

on .... /............ /............

at the Coronial Investigation Centre, 101 Mortuary Drive, Boneville.

Signature: ....

Name: ....

Officer or rank and number: ....

Glossary

ala (pl. **alae**) **nasi**   literally 'a wing'; curved lateral walls of the nostrils (nares).

alveolar prognathism   forward projecting bony margins of the jaws, which carry the dentition.

anterior nasal spine   a sharp, pointed, bony protruberance located in the midline at the base of the nose.

anthropometric   pertaining to the measurement of human shape and form.

auditory meatus (pl. **meatii**)   ear canal; from the outside to the eardrum.

bony exostosis   an extra, often abnormal, local overgrowth of bone.

brachycranic   a short head (cephalic index above 80).

brachyfacial   short-faced.

bregma   midline point of intersection of the sagittal and coronal sutures.

buccinator   literally 'trumpeter'; the muscle of the cheeks that blends with those of the throat posteriorly and the lips anteriorly.

calvarium   the upper part of the skull.

canthus   the angle of the eye.

cephalostat   a device for restraining the head to ensure a reproducible head position for serial radiographs.

cervix   neck.

chondrocranium   cartilaginous parts of the developing skull.

datum point   a point from which measurements are made, a fiducil marker.

deciduous dentition   the primary dentition that is shed and replaced by the permanent teeth.

degloving   the removal of the outer layers of the skin or the investing soft tissues from underlying skeletal structures.

diaphysis (adj. **diaphyseal**)   the shaft of a long bone.

dolichocephalic   having a long head (a cephalic index below 75).

dolichocranic   dolichocephalic.

dolichofacial   having a long face.

ectocranial   relating to the external surface of the cranium.

endochondral   within cartilage.

endocranial   within the cranium.

entomological   pertaining to the study of insects.

epiphysis (adj. **epiphyseal**)   a secondary centre of ossification at the end of a long bone.

f stop   aperture setting on a camera; the higher the number, the smaller the aperture and the less the amount of light admitted to the film.

fontanelle   literally 'a small spring, fountain or source of water'; the temporary discontinuities in the bony plates of the vault of the skull, which, being growth centres, are obliterated by growth.

foramen magnum   the largest opening of the skull, through which the spinal cord passes.

Frankfort plane   a line between the lower border of the orbit and the porion of the external auditory meatus.

gingivae   gums.

glabella   most forward projecting point of the forehead in the midline above the nasion and between the supraorbital ridges.

gnathion   lowest point in the midline of the lower border of the mandible.

goniometer   a device that allows objects to be tilted into any orientation.

gonion   lowest posterior and most outward point of the angle of the mandible.

head somitomeres   the segments of the primitive mesoderm that contribute to cranial musculoskeletal structures.

incompetent lips   lips which, at rest, do not seal the mouth.

intercanthal distance   horizontal distance between the contralateral corners of the eyes.

lambda   midline point of intersection of the sagittal and lambdoidal sutures.

lordosis   curvature (secondary) of the lumbar spine.

mastoid process   large protruberance of the skull behind and below the external ear, to which the sternomastoid muscle is attached.

menton   lowest point of the lower jaw under the chin.

mesenchyme   non-epithelial cells between the embryonic ectoderm and endoderm (Greek: *meso* middle).

metopic suture   midline fibrous joint between the two bones of the forehead, usually obliterated by the growth and fusion of bones by the age of 8.

modus operandi the common pattern of action for a particular person; the way of doing something.

morph, morphing progressively to change the shape of an object so that it comes to be something else; each step may be so small as to be difficult to detect.

morphology the study of shape and form.

nasion bony landmark in the midline at the root of the nose where it joins the forehead.

neurocranium skull structures enclosing the brain and the organs of smell, sight and hearing.

obicularis oculi ring of muscle that surrounds the eye.

obicularis oris ring of muscle that surrounds the mouth.

occipitofrontalis thin layer of muscle found in the scalp and only loosely attached to the skull; embryologically formed from the same origins as the muscles of expression and the anterior sheet of muscle in the neck (platysma).

occiput back of the skull (literally 'against the head').

opisthocranion midline point on the posterior aspect of the skull most distant from the glabella (excluding the external occipital protuberance).

orthodontics a study of cranial growth and dental development for the correction of abnormal tooth position.

orthoganism projecting jaw.

orthogonal mutually at right angles.

petrous literally 'stony'; part of the temporal bone found in the base of the skull.

pharyngeal (branchial or **visceral) arch** arch of embryonic mesenchyme giving rise to the muscles, cartilage and bone of the oropharyngeal structures.

philtrum midline furrow of the upper lip.

photogrammetry an optical technique for mapping a scene to establish the relative positions of its components.

plagiocephaly asymmetrical deformity of the skull owing to premature closure of the lambdoidal and coronal sutures.

pneumatization process by which some bones of the skull come to have air-filled spaces formed within them as they grow.

porion uppermost, outermost point of the bony external auditory meatus.

prognathism forward projection of one or both jaws from their normal relationship.

sclerotomes the ventromedial part of a somite; aggregates of mesenchymal cells in the embryo from which the musculoskeletal system develops.

sella turcica literally 'Turk's saddle'; a midline depression in the upper surface of the sphenoid bone, clearly visible on radiographs, the fossa for the pituitary gland.

somite embryonic body segment (Greek: *soma* = body).

sprue a channel in the investment through which molten materials are poured to make a casting.

sternocleidomastoid a large strap muscle of the neck that joins the sternum to the mastoid process on the skull.

sternum the breastbone, to which the collar bone and ribs are attached.

synchondrosis cartilaginous (hyaline- or fibrocartilage) union of two bones.

temporalis a fan-shaped muscle on the side of the head, which is attached to the coronoid process of mandible and which has an important role in closing the jaws.

thixotropic referring to a material that can be made to become more fluid if subjected to physical disturbance, for example, stirring.

tibia one of the two major bones of the leg below the knee.

tooth cusps major elevations on the biting surfaces of the molar and premolar teeth.

torus rounded, bony prominence.

tragus literally 'goat'; a small tag of soft tissue that is part of the external ear located in front of the external auditory meatus.

tuber knob, protuberance or swelling.

vignetting (intentional) a technique in photographic printing in which the picture is faded away towards its margins to give a soft-edged border and emphasize the central subject.

vignetting (unintentional) can arise by using a lens of too short a focal length for the film format, the margins of which are then not exposed. A similar defect can arise if too long a lens hood infringes on the angle of view for any given lens.

viscerocranium (splanchnocranium) facial skeleton surrounding the respiratory and digestive tracts.

voir dire a court hearing of sworn evidence held in the absence of the jury; often used to enable the judge to decide upon the credentials and knowlede of a potential expert witness.

vomer literally 'plowshare'; a thin pentagonal plate of bone that forms the posterior part of the midline structures of the nose.

Index

aboriginal, cranial traits 40, 51
acrylic resin in replica modelling 88, 90–3
adipocere (grave wax) 86
adolescents, craniofacial identification 6–7
aerial photography 119–20
age estimation
  anthropological assessment 55–9
  atlas and axis 57
  auricular surface 59
  craniofacial anatomy 55–9
  dental identification 75–9
  epiphyses 56
  Haversian units (osteons) 59
  immature skeletons 56
  non-dental, cranium 56–8
  occiput 57
  ossification pattern and timescale 42, 56
  osteoarthritic changes 59
  postcranial skeleton 58
  pubic symphysis 58
  sternal rib 58–9
anatomical landmarks 170–1
  computerized version 198
  determination 192
  facial shape registration 191–2
  soft tissue thickness data 180
  stomium, gonion, gnathion, nasion, bizygion 208
anatomy *see* craniofacial anatomy
anthropological assessment 49–59
  age determination 55–9
  cranial traits, Caucasoid, Mongoloid, Negroid 51
  craniometry 52
    distinguishing (American) Caucasians from Negroes 52
  cultural indicators of race in skeletons 53
  racial affiliation determination 49–50
  racial characteristics, postcranial skeleton 53
  racial identification

    adults 50–2
    juvenile bones 50
  sex determination 53–5
appendices 267–98
arcus senilis 231
arsenic 87
art, facial approximation *see* forensic art
arterial injection 86–7
aspartic acid, *levo-dextro* conversion, dentine 79
assault, and subsequent death, criminal law 261
atlas and axis, age estimation 57
audit, post trial 255
automatic face recognition systems 168–9
autopsy 25–36
  aims 29–30
  craniofacial region 32–3
  external examination 32–4
  health and safety 32
  human identification 25–36
  identification of the body 30–1
  internal examination 34–5
  post autopsy procedures 35–6
  post mortem radiology 31–2
  post-cranial region 33–4

basilar suture *see* spheno-occipital synchondrosis
Bertillonage 168
birth, and criminal law 260–1
bizygomatic diameter 208, 210
bloodstains, pattern interpretation 19–20
body *see* remains
bone
  age assessment 59, 214–16
  endochondral and membrane bones 42, 45
  FELS method of scoring bone age 216
  Haversian units (osteons) in age estimation 59, 214–16
  incineration, changes 64
  long bones, age-related changes 59

bone (*cont.*)
  ossification pattern and timescale 42
    closure of sutures 44–5, 57
botanical material, examination 20, 21
brachycephaly 44, 219
brachyfacial growth pattern 220–1
buildings, controlled entry
  identification by 3D surface recordings 190–1
    limitations 193
    registration method 191–2
    shape analysis method 192–3
burial sites 267–71
  chain of custody 270
  classification of burial 269
  excavation and recording 270
  indicators 268
  pre-recovery conference 269
  search methods 268
  see also corpse
burning and incineration
  damage to face 96
  dental changes 64

camera
  accessories 108–9
    case 108–9
    extension tubes and bellows 108
    ladder 109
    tripod 109
  aperture and depth of field 141–2
  choice 105–6, 123–4, 138, 145
  close-up photography 126
  depth of field 130–1, 141–2
  dual-camera system 144–9, 147–9
    cameras 145
    face aligning system 146–7
    infra-red shutter release 146
    lighting 139–41, 146
    subject photography 147–9
    support stand 144–5
  equipment, preparation 112
  exposure 109–10, 128–30, 141
  film 107, 126–7, 142–3
    reciprocity failure 127
  filters 108
  lenses 106–7, 124, 126, 138, 145
  light
    artificial light sources 107–8
    synchro-sun 110
  light behaviour 109
  light meters 125
  maintenance 109
  motor drives 108
  perspective 131–2, 139
  scale 133
    identification number 131
  see also photography
Camper's plane 166
canthi
  intercanthal distance 46, 207, 297
  photographic superimposition techniques 159–60
Carabelli's trait, crown form 75

case management 19
Caucasoid cranial traits 40, 51
causation, and foreseeability 261–2
cephalic index 205
cephalometry, limitations 222
cephalostat 71, 287, 289
chain of custody 270
chemical location of body 21–2
chemical pathology and toxicology 28–9
children
  age estimation, immature skeletons 56
  growth prediction 220–3
  indices of maturity 214–18
    bone age 214–16
    correlations 219
    dental age 216–17
    sexual age 217–18
  infant, criminal law 260–1
  missing children 203–4
  soft tissue thickness 182
  stillborn infant, and coroner's inquest 260
colour photography 133–4
communication, reporting and presentation of evidence
    245–8
communication skills 29
  forensic pathologist 29
computer assisted image reproduction 93–4
computer modelling 174, 187–99
  FACE computer-based system 171–2
  optical scanner 188
  recording of facial surface 187–9
  system layout 188
  see also three-dimensional models
coordinate systems, measurement of facial shape 170
coroner
  historical role 25–6
  inquests 260
corpse *see* remains
courtroom
  conversations outside 252
  entering/leaving 253
  environment 248
  presentation of evidence 248–9, 254–5
  see also evidence; witness box
cranial form
  base 206–7
  calvarium, settings for equipment 288
  growth, measurements 210
  orbital region 207
  radiography guides 287–90
  types 205
  see also skull
cranial index 205
cranial sutures *see* sutures
craniofacial anatomy 37–46
  age determination 55–9
  cranial base 42, 43
  cranial vault 42
  embryology and development 42–3
  explicit representations 174
  facial skeleton 42–3
  growth pattern 43–4

growth sites 44–6
importance of living face 3–4
individualizing factors 46
norma basalis (inferior) 41
norma frontalis 38–39
norma lateralis 40
norma occipitalis 40
norma verticalis (superior) 40–1
orbits 43–4, 102–3
ossification pattern 42
pathology 26–7
photographic superimposition 159–60
racial differences 40–1, 49–53
sex differences 39–40, 41, 55
see also anatomical landmarks; skull
craniofacial dissection 32–3, 95–104
  aims 96
  damaged face and head 96–7
  jaw removal 104
  neck upward 99–102
  procedures 97–9
  reconstruction 95–6
  scalp downwards 102–3
craniofacial superimposition *see* photographic
    superimposition
cranium, age estimation 56–8
crime
  compensation 262–3
  surveillance material video recording 14, 193–5
crime scene
  bloodstain pattern interpretation 19–20
  body location
    chemical 21–2
    physical 21–2
    visual 20–1
  exterior/interior photography 13–14
  initial assessment 11–12
  note-taking 14
  photogrammetry 22–3
  recording 13–16
  safety 18–19
  search techniques 15–16
  security and preservation 12–13
  sketches, plans and maps 14–15
  soils/botanical material 20
  specialized examination 19–24
  thermal imaging 23–4
  video recording 14
  zonal search 16
  see also evidential material; photography, of scene
criminal law 260–2
cytopathology 27

death
  clinical 85–6
  and contractual arrangements 259
  definition 258
  proof 263
decomposition 20, 86, 87, 90
dental age
  calcification 216
  calcification patterns/emergence dates 77–8

chronology of dental development 279–81
  deciduous teeth 279
  permanent teeth 280–1
index of maturity 216–17
dental identification 63–79
  age at death 75–9
  age changes 78–9
  comparative process 66–7
  crown form, Carabelli's trait 75
  general pattern agreement versus specific feature 73–5
  history 63–5
  incineration experiments 64
  life and death before birth 75–6
  maxillary incisors, shovelling 75
  necessity for expert opinion 65–6
  points of concordance 72
  post mortem radiography 71–3
  racial traits 75, 78
  Schour and Massler chart reliability 77
  teeth before birth 76–7
  third molars 77
dental records
  ante mortem chart (odontology) 68–9
  casts 64
  charting discrepancies, common 70
  charts compared with post mortem records 68–70
  Federation Dentaire Internationale (FDI) system 67,
      276–7
  fraud 70–1
  Haderup system 67
  inaccuracy and misinterpretation 69–70
  incompleteness 67–9
  Palmer-Zsigmondy notation 67, 277
  post mortem charts (odontology) 68–9
  radiography 64–5, 71–3
    bitewing radiographs 71–2, 74
    comparison of maxillae 74
    orthopantomograph 72
    panoramic 67–9
    points of concordance 72
    post mortem radiography 71–3
dentine, *levo-dextro* conversion of aspartic acid 79
dentition
  ageing and bone loss 226, 231
  anthropological notation 277–8
  charts, types 275–6
  development 210
  FDI notation 67, 276–7
  laboratory materials 283, 285
  radiography
    alignment 289, 290
    initial settings for equipment 288
    supplies 284–5
  teeth, occlusion 219
  Universal notation 277
dentures 178
dependants 258
desiccation 86
digital imaging, photography of scene 120
dinaric head form 219
DNA techniques 28
dolichocephaly 44, 219

dolichofacial growth pattern 220–1
dual-camera system, craniofacial photography 144–9

ear development 212
ears, superimposition techniques 160
embalming 87–88
   after autopsy 88
   forensic purposes 87
   public health considerations 87
   safety 87
epiphyses 214
   age estimation 56
ethnic differences 40–1, 49–53
euryprosopy (brachycephaly) 219, 221
evidence
   cross-examination 249–50
   examination-in-chief 248
   preparation 250–1
   re-examination 250
   reporting and presentation 245–55
evidential material
   chain of custody 270
   collection 16–18
   defined 10
   exchange principle 10–11
   packaging 17–18, 273
   priorities 16–18
   purpose of collection 10
   recovery of remains 267–71
   sampling and labelling 17
   scientific approach 11
   see also scene and evidence
examination-in-chief, witness box 248
exchange principle, evidential material 10–11
eyebrows, superimposition techniques 160
eyelids, reconstruction 183
eyes
   ageing changes 229–31
   photographic superimposition techniques 159
   superimposition techniques 159–60

face aligning system, craniofacial photography 146–7
FACE computer-based system 171–2
'faceprints' 193
facial anatomy *see* craniofacial anatomy
facial approximations 235–42
   assessment and comparisons of two renditions 238
   standard guidelines 236
facial growth
   height/depth 207–9
   upper/lower face 209
facial index 219
facial reconstruction 235
facial restoration 235
facial shape 165–76
   ageing in adulthood 225–31
     10 year periods 227–231
   biological age 214
   bone age 214–16
   bones, radiography, initial settings for equipment 288
   children 203–24
     changes in proportion 206, 214

   effects of make-up 215
   computer modelling 187–99
   creases 229
   defined 166
   gender differences 212–14
   height/width, upper and lower 207–9
   landmarks 170–1
   light line 189
   living face 3–4
   measurement 165–76
     2D and 3D point measurements 168–9
     3D surface scanning and digitizing 169
     coordinate systems 170
     image types and techniques 167–8
     reference points 171
   muscle groups 166–7
   properties 166–7
   reconstruction and approximation 177–85, 235–42
   registration 191–2
   representations and models 90–4
     3D models 173–4
     approximations 235–42
     images of face 171–3
     outlines 171
     point data 170–1
     replica fabrication 91–3
     techniques 235
   soft tissue thickness, various sources (*table*) 180
   types 219–20
   upper and lower height/width 207–9
   see also dentition; skull
facial skeleton 42–3
   see also craniofacial anatomy; mandible and maxilla
facial surface
   curvature, Gaussian and mean 192
   fundamental types 192
Federation Dentaire Internationale (FDI) system 67, 276–7
FELS method of scoring bone age 216
fetal skeleton
   age estimation 76
   teeth 76–7
fetus
   and coroner's inquest 260
   criminal law 260–1
film 107, 126–7, 142–3
film processing 117
fontanelles, closure 57
foramen magnum 41
forensic art approximations 235–42
   handling the response 242
   information to artist 240–1
   information to public 242
   laboratory materials 283–5
   successful identifications 240
forensic pathologist
   role 25–6
   training and skills 26–9
forensic report, sample document 293–6
foreseeability, and causation 261–2
formaldehyde 87
Forward Looking Infra-Red (FLIR) 24

Fourier shape analysis
  coefficients 171
  profile reconstruction 172–3
Frankfort horizontal 170, 181
  defined 38, 91
frontal sinuses 71, 206
funeral, time of 34–5

Gaussian and mean surface curvatures 192
glabella 39
glossary 297–8
gnathion 38, 208, 297
gonion 38, 208, 297
  bigonion diameter 208–9
Gouraud interpolation 189
Green River case, differing interpretations 239–40
Greulich and Pyle, *Skeletal Atlas* 216
grid search, crime scene 16
growth and maturation 204–23
  Scammon's curves 205

Haderup system, dental records 67
haematology 27
hair, ageing changes 230
hand-wrist radiographs 214
Haversian units (osteons)
  age estimation 59
  incineration, changes 64
health and safety
  autopsy 32
  mortuary 87
hepatitis B and C
  immunisation 19
  survival 18
historical aspects
  coroner 25–6
  dental identification 63–5
  photographic superimposition techniques 151–2
  preservation of remains 85–7
homelessness 6–7

identification 3–8, 257–65
  autopsy 25–36, 30–1
  difficulties 5, 66
  error 257–8
  legal context 7
  of living 263–4
  photographs and identity parades 263–4
  visual 4–6
  visual vs dental 66
identification number, photography of remains 131
immunology 28
impression material 179
infant *see* children
infra-red shutter 146
inquests 260
intercanthal distance 46, 207, 297
  photographic superimposition techniques 159–60
ischiopubic index, sex determination 55

juries 247

labelling, evidence collection 17
laboratory materials 283–5
landmarks *see* anatomical landmarks
laser scanning 169
lawyers, communication 246–7
legal skills 29
  forensic pathologist 29
lenses 106–7, 124, 126, 138, 145
leptoprosopy (dolichocephaly) 219, 221
light line, facial shape 189
light meters 125
lighting 107–8, 110–11, 124–5, 139–41, 146
  macrophotography 126
  multiple flash 119
  painting with light 118
  techniques 117–19, 127–8
lime 21–2
line search, crime scene 16
lips
  ageing changes 21, 227
  growth and development 212
  reconstruction 182–3
liquids
  embalming 88
  preservation 86
living, identification 263–4
long bones, age-related changes 59

malar tubercle 160
mandible and maxilla
  anatomy 38
  articulation repair 178
  bigonion diameter 208–9
  bone loss 226
  depth 209
  fetus 76
  infraorbital foramen 39
  mandibular symphysis closure 57
  maxilla depth 209
  pterygoid fovea 38
  radiography 74
    initial settings for equipment 288
    intra-oral film holder 290
    see also dental records
  remodelling 46
  removal in dissection 104
  sex differences 38–9, 55
maxillary sinuses 71
medical witness
  reporting and presentation of evidence 245–55
    communication 245–8
  see also evidence
medico-legal analysis 251–2
  guides and checklists 291–6
  medical records and notes 245–6
  sample forensic report 293–6
meningeal artery 40
mesocephaly 219
mesofacial growth pattern 220–1
metopic suture, closure 44, 57
microbiology 27–8
missing persons 203–4

missing persons (*cont.*)
  medical history 292
Moiré diffraction patterns 168–9
molecular biology 28
Mongoloid
  cranial traits 40, 41, 51
  dental traits 75
  orbit, and globe size 46
mortuary
  health and safety 87
  laboratory investigation 6–7
mortuary supplies 284
mouth, superimposition techniques 160

nasal bones 39
nasal bridge 46
nasal gutter 39
nasion 208, 298
natron 86
'natural consequence' 262
natural preservation 86
neck dissection 99–103
Negroid cranial traits 51
neuropathology 27
nose
  dissection 101
  nasolabial region 212
  reconstruction 183
  superimposition techniques 160
note-taking, crime scene and evidence 14
novus actus interveniens 262

occiput, age estimation 57
odontogram *see* dentition charts
orbits 43–4, 102–3
orthopantomograph (OPG) 72
ossification pattern and timescale 42, 56
  closure of sutures 44–5, 57
  thyroid cartilage 59
osteoarthritic changes 59
overall views (35mm lens) 113

packaging, evidence collection 17–18
palatal rugae 76
Palmer-Zsigmondy notation, dental records 67, 277
palpebral creases 229–30
palpebral fissure 183
parietal tuber 40
pelvis, sex determination 55
photogrammetry 22–3, 168
  crime scene 22–3
photographic superimposition techniques 151–64
  circum-maxillary 45
  comparison and determining identity 159–62
    ears 160
    eyebrows 160
    eyes 159–60
    mouth 160
    nose 160
    reliability 160–1
  history 151–2
  magnification and skull orientation 155–7

video 154–5, 171
photography
  accessories 125–6
  aperture and depth of field 141–2
  background 132
  camera and equipment *see* camera
  close-up equipment 113, 126
  colour 133–4
  crime scene and evidence 13–15
  cropping images 133
  depth of field 130–1, 141–2
  digital imaging 120
  dual-camera system 144–9
    face aligning system 146–7
    infra-red shutter release 146
    lens 145
    lighting 146
    subject photography 147–9
    support stand 144–5
  exposure 109–10, 128–30, 141
  film 107, 126–7, 142–3
    processing 117
  focus and depth of field 130–1
  identification 263–4
  lighting 107–8, 110–11, 124–5, 124–6, 126, 127–8, 139–41
    accessories 125–6
    macrophotography 126
    multiple flash 119
  of living person 137–49
    aperture and depth of field 141–2
    dual-camera system 144–9
    exposure controls 141
    film 142–3
    perspective and viewpoint distortion 139
    subject lighting 139–41
    subject positioning 143–4
  of remains 116–17, 123–35
    documentation 116
    identification number 131
    lighting techniques 124–8
    macrophotography 126, 134–5
    orientation photography 132–3
    perspective and viewpoint distortion 131–2, 139
    scale and identification number 131, 133
    see also camera
  of scene 105–21
    aerial photography 119–20
    background photography 132
    crime scene 13–14
    inadmissibility 111–12
    inside/outside 113–15
    lighting techniques 117–19, 127–8
    orientation photography 113
    overall views (35mm lens) 113
    policies and protocols 112–13
    textured pattern enhancement 117
physical/chemical location of body 21–2
plans and maps, crime scene and evidence 15
plaster of Paris 90
plastination, preservation 88
Polhemus 3D digitizer 169

post-autopsy procedures 35–6
post-cranial skeleton, sex determination 55
post-mortem *see* autopsy
powders, preservation 86
preservation
    arterial injection 86–7
    controlled drying 86
    embalming 87–8
    liquids 86
    natural 86
    plastination 88
    powders 86
    public health 87
    refrigeration and freezing 88
probate 259–60
pterion 40
pubic symphysis, age-related changes 58
pubis, precursor arc 55
public health, mortuary 32, 87
putrefaction 87, 90

race *see* anthropological assessment
racial differences 40–1, 49–53
radiography
    bitewing 72, 74
    dental records 64–5, 71–3
        panoramic 67–9
    guides 287–90
    initial settings for equipment 288
    intra-oral film holder 290
    maxillary anterior teeth 73
    periapical 73
    skull 31–2, 71
    supplies 284–5
    see also craniofacial anatomy
radius, ulna and fingers (RUS) scoring 216
reconstruction of putrefied tissues 90
records
    documentation of remains 116
    note-taking, crime scene and evidence 14
    see also dental records
recovery of remains 267–71
    surface remains 269
    see also burial sites
refrigeration and freezing 88
Reichert's cartilage 42
remains 85–94
    artificial preservation 86–9
    changes after death 85–6
    craniofacial dissection 32–3, 95–104
    duplication of remains 90–4
    natural preservation 86
    physical/chemical location 21–2
    property in dead body 259
    reconstruction of putrefied tissues 90
    restoration of appearance 89–90
    scene photography 116
    viewing conditions 89–90
    visual identification 4–6
    visual location 20–1
    see also autopsy; burial sites; identification
replication, acrylic resins 90–3

resins
    polymers, plastination 88
    replica fabrication 90–3
Ruxton case, photographic superimposition techniques 152

sacroiliac joint, auricular surface, age estimation 59
safety
    autopsy 32
    crime scene 18–19
    mortuary 87
sagittal suture
    early closure 44
    facial width 45
sampling, evidence collection 17
scale and identification number, photography 131, 133
scalp dissection 97–8, 102–3
scene and evidence, management 9–24
    appointment of coordinator 12
    evidence defined 10
    initial assessment 11–12
    initial examination 13
    material, chain of custody 270
    recording of crime scene 13–15
    safety 18–19
    security and scene preservation 12–13
    see also crime scene; evidential material; photography, of scene
sclerotomes 42
search techniques, crime scene and evidence 15–16
sella turcica 71
sex determination 39–41, 54–5
    cranium
        metrical characteristics 54–5
        morphological characteristics 54
    post-cranial skeleton 55
    skull 39–41, 54–5
sexual development stages 217–18
silicones, replication 90–3
skeletal age, indices of maturity 214–18
sketches, plans and maps, crime scene 14–15
skull
    computer assisted image reproduction 93–4
    duplication 178–81
    embryology and development 42–3
    facial reconstruction from skull 181–4, 198
        duplication of reconstruction 184–5
    growth and maturation 205–7, 211
    growth pattern 43–4
    growth sites 44–6
    malformation 44
    photographic superimposition techniques 151–64
    properties 166–7
    radiography 31–2, 71
        alignment 289, 290
        cephalostat 287, 289
        initial settings for equipment 288
    replica fabrication 91–3
        acrylic resin 90, 92–3
        comparison with original 92–3
        mould design and construction 91–2
        preparation 91

skull (*cont.*)
    sex differences 39–40, 41, 55
    see also cranial form
skull mounting and orientation device (SMOD) 156
soft tissues
    facial, children 182, 211–12
    gender differences 213–14
    photographic superimposition 159–60
    thickness, various locations 180
soils
    examination 20, 21–2
    preservation of remains 86
soils/botanical material, crime scene 20
somitomeres 42
spheno-ethmoidal angle 43
spheno-occipital synchondrosis
    basilar suture 41
    early closure 41, 45, 57–8
    growth 45
spiral search, crime scene 16
stereophotogrammetry 168
sternal rib, age-related changes 58
stomion 208
strip search, crime scene 16
styloid 42
superimposition *see* photographic superimposition
sutural bones 40
sutures 40, 41, 44–5
    basilar *see* spheno-occipital synchondrosis
    closure 41, 44, 45
        and ossification 44–5
        variability 57
    coronal 44
    craniofacial 45
    metopic 44, 57
    sagittal 44, 45

temporal bone 40, 42
thermal imaging 23–4
three-dimensional models 173–4
    facial reconstruction from skull 181–4
    see also computer modelling

three-dimensional surface digitizers 169
three-dimensional surface recordings
    data set visualization 189–90
    identification
        application to controlled entry 190–1
        registration method 191–2
    profile angle constancy 197
thyroid cartilage, ossification pattern and timescale 59
tort, creation and extinguishment 258
tortfeasor 258
toxicology 28–9
transference of evidence, exchange principle 10–11
trial
    attendance and dress 252–3
    see also courtroom; witness box

vault sutures *see* sutures
video identity assessment system (VIAS) 195
video recording
    Charge Coupled Device (CCD) 188
    crime scene 14
    with optical scanning 189–90
    superimposition techniques 154–5, 171
    surveillance material 14
        application to identification 193–5
        comparisons with databases 195–8

witness, reporting and presentation of evidence 245–55
witness box
    cross-examination 249–50
    dress and behaviour 253–5
    examination-in-chief 248
    presentation of evidence 248–9, 254–5
    re-examination 250
    taking the oath 253–4
wound
    description 33
    medical notes 292

zygomatic arch 39, 40, 100, 102
    anthropological traits 40–1
    bizygomatic diameter 208, 210